Testimonials

The Medicinal Forest Garden Handbook tells you everything you need to know to set up a resilient forest garden to provide food and medicine for body and soul. This book is eminently practical, addressing all the things you need to think about from the very first planning stages right through to harvesting and making your own medicinal preparations. Forty medicinal trees and shrubs are covered in detail, and there are recipes for making a range of medicines. I especially loved the inspiring examples of people who have put these ideas into practice in a wide variety of contexts.

Julie Bruton-Seal, artist, jeweller, photographer, herbalist and author

Anne has drawn on her vast experience to produce a beautifully practical guide to growing and using woody perennials for healing. Covering all aspects of plants care, harvest and use this book should become a standard for anyone growing these crops. For the growing number of agroforesters in the UK there is also great information on scaling up production to meet the demands of larger markets.

Ben Raskin, Head of Horticulture and Agroforestry at the Soil Association

This is an extremely comprehensive, multi-layered, informative book, as rich and diverse as a forest garden itself. Anne Stobart speaks from a place of authority and commitment, to bring us this wealth of detailed information and has created an invaluable guide for anyone interested in both forest gardening and medicinal trees and plants. Relevant for both small and large projects, it is a vital addition to any growers' bookshelf!

Glennie Kindred, author of *Walking with Trees* and *Letting in the Wild Edges*

Thanks to Anne Stobart, we have at last a book that explores the vast potential that forest gardens have for growing medicinal plants. Written by an expert in the field, meticulously researched and wide in scope, the book also touches on the many other health benefits of forest gardens.

Tomas Remiarz, permaculture practitioner and author of *Forest Gardening in Practice*

In the present climate of highlighted concern about climate change, this reference book shows what underused resources are in the world around us, and informs us in meticulously well researched fashion.

Colin Porter, ex-head Gardener RHS Rosemoor and chair of the Landscape Gardens Health Network

This book is a treasure trove of information. Anne (an experienced medical herbalist and grower of medicine), has deep insightful wisdoms that are beautifully articulated throughout the book. The book is in two main parts; Part 1 has detailed practical information on applications of tree medicine, designing, growing, harvesting and creating remedies and Part 2 provides a directory of 40 medicinal trees and shrubs.

Karen Lawton, one of the Seed SistAs from Sensory Solutions Herbal Evolution

As a nurseryman you learn something new every day, but after reading *The Medicinal Forest Garden Handbook* I discovered that we have a whole pharmacy in our back yard, with hundreds of medicines under hands' reach. The book is easy to read, clear, complete and furthermore, very practical.

Johan van den Berk, co-owner of Van den Berk Nurseries

Whether you want to grow a few medicinal trees or set up a larger-scale forest garden, you are in luck. Anne Stobart has distilled her personal experience and knowledge into the book that will guide your choices and set your course. Converting a former Sitka spruce forest into her own living forest garden has been a work of just under two decades. In the book she combines science with art and technique and explains why such a garden might be worthwhile on so many levels. She offers excellent descriptions of the plants she uses, harvesting techniques and ways to turn the harvest into medicinal preparations. It is all here: planting through to using, all set out in a clear style and a friendly encouraging, yet authoritative tone.

Barbara Segall, writer, herb gardener and author of several books, including *The Herb Garden Month by Month*

The Medicinal Forest Garden Handbook presents us with a unique and original exploration of environmental stewardship. The introductory chapters poignantly and in a visually stunning way, underscore the multigenerational value of medicinal forest gardens, while each botanical entry weaves the philosophical with the essential guidance needed for their creation.

Roy Upton, President of American Herbal Pharmacopoeia

The Medicinal Forest Garden Handbook is full of hope and inspiration. It lays out the methods for multi-layered forest farming and natural healing that will serve us long into the future. It offers gem after gem of practical insight into the healing wisdom of the herbal tradition – and how you can grow them and care for yourself, your loved ones and the world around, one tree at a time. All gleaned from Anne's experience as a Medical Herbalist and an expert in permaculture. It's both practical and visionary.

Sebastian Pole, Master Herbsmith and co-founder Pukka Herbs

Anne brings her experience as a practising medical herbalist to provide a thoroughly dependable and insightful resource. Her skill as a herbalist combined with her experience in permaculture and knowledge of the history of natural medicine means that Anne is an outstanding guide. This handbook is sure to establish itself as the key work in aiding the development of truly therapeutic forest gardens.

Peter Conway, Fellow of the National Institute of Medical Herbalists and the College of Practitioners of Phytotherapy and author of *The Consultation in Phytotherapy*

Based on her own experience of creating a forest garden of medicinal trees and shrubs from scratch, Stobart guides us expertly through all essentials, from planning and design, and practical horticulture, through to medicine making for both personal use and at a scale for marketing. Recipes for medicinal products and a directory of 40 detailed plant profiles are included, supported with a wealth of images, tables, sample projects, and research. The development of the garden as an educational experience for environmentally sustainable living is inspirational.

Vicki Pitman, clinical medical herbalist, and author of three books, including *Aromatherapy: A Practical Approach*

Not many people realize that the medicinal 'herbs' they use more than often were picked from a tree or a shrub. In this attractive and clearly written, well-referenced and effectively illustrated book, Anne Stobart clears this up thoroughly. Whilst doing so, she reveals a possible future with innovation in ecological farming. Our planet desperately needs these kinds of innovative lifestyle projects, where both agriculture and medicine convert into more sustainable human activities.

Tedje van Asseldonk, ethnobiologist and permaculture herb farmer www.mintal.eu, www.ethnobotany.nl

The Medicinal Forest Garden Handbook is exactly what it claims. Meticulously researched and resourced, it is a single volume guide to all aspects of medicinal plant growing, herb preparation and medicinal herb use. Plants come alive and at times you can almost sense the seeds ready to sprout! Anne Stobart's wealth of experience as herbalist, forest gardener and academic underpins this useful and beautifully illustrated book. Anyone into gardening, herb growing and herbal medicine will be keen to have it to hand.

Andrew Chevallier, past president of the National Institute of Medical Herbalists, and author of the *Encyclopedia of Herbal Medicine*

Anne Stobart has produced this beautiful practical guide to medicinal forest gardening full of interesting facts and useful advice for anyone interested in the medicinal properties of trees or wanting to expand their knowledge of forest gardens. An excellent resource for experts and amateurs alike, based on years of practical experience and containing a wealth of knowledge and insight.

Sally Westaway, Senior agroforestry researcher at the Organic Research Centre

Diversity is the key to a thriving forest garden, and Anne's inspirational book has unlocked a new layer of possibility and potential. We now have the knowledge and guidance to create our own perennial designs that not only heal our planet, but also ourselves.

Huw Richards, YouTuber, permaculturist and author of *Grow Food for Free*

The Medicinal Forest Garden Handbook

GROWING, HARVESTING AND USING
HEALING TREES AND SHRUBS IN A TEMPERATE CLIMATE

Anne Stobart

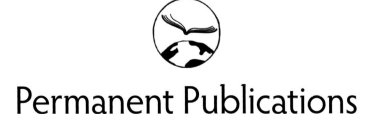

Permanent Publications

Published by
Permanent Publications
Hyden House Ltd
13 Clovelly Road
Portsmouth
PO4 8DL
United Kingdom
Tel: 01730 776 582
          international: +44 (0)1730
Email: enquiries@permaculture.co.uk
Web: www.permanentpublications.co.uk

Distributed in North America by
Chelsea Green Publishing Company, PO Box 428, White River Junction, VT 05001
www.chelseagreen.com

Photographs © Kay Piercy, unless stated otherwise in photograph acknowledgements on p.270

Designed by Two Plus George Limited, www.TwoPlusGeorge.co.uk

Printed in the UK by SRP Ltd, Bittern Road, Sowton Industrial Estate, Exeter EX2 7LW

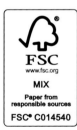

All paper from FSC certified mixed sources

The Forest Stewardship Council (FSC) is a non-profit international organisation established to promote the responsible management of the world's forests. Products carrying the FSC label are independently certified to assure consumers that they come from forests that are managed to meet the social, economic and ecological needs of present and future generations.

British Library Cataloguing-in-Publication Data
A catalogue record for this book is available from the British Library

ISBN 978 1 85623 332 3

Foreword

I love herbs, and I am especially passionate about medicinal trees and shrubs. This book is not only about how you can cultivate and harvest them, but it is also intended to provide you with the basis for creating your own medicinal planting design and herbal preparations. The medicinal forest garden provides a way to grow and harvest healing plants that draws on natural and sustainable processes to make efficient use of resources of light, space, soil and water. At a time when forests are regarded as key in combatting climate breakdown, what could be better than seizing the opportunity to promote health and biodiversity through planting more medicinal trees and shrubs!

The benefits of medicinal plants

As a consultant medical herbalist in the Western herbal medicine tradition, based in the UK, I have used many medicinal plants to help manage health and disease. I have also trained other professional herbal practitioners, developing systematic therapeutic approaches based on both tradition and scientific evidence. Carefully selected combinations of healing plants can be multifunctional in supporting good health, through addressing underlying health issues, providing relief of symptoms and preventing further problems. For myself, many of these healing plants are also an integral and enjoyable part of a pleasurable lifestyle, providing culinary and body care options and making wonderful gifts and artisan products. Not least, I have enjoyed growing many of these plants myself, providing an abundance of supplies for home and clinical practice.

Our medicinal forest garden

The tree-planting project I embarked on, with my partner in 2004, was the establishment of Holt Wood in Devon. Many important medicinal plants, although not native to the UK, can be readily grown in a temperate climate. So, I was enthusiastic about the possibility of developing cultivation and harvest of both native and introduced trees and shrubs. Our transformation of a redundant conifer plantation into a medicinal forest garden has provided an amazing opportunity to gain experience in growing many medicinal plants, from woody trees and shrubs to native wildflowers and other introduced herbs. However, most forest garden publications focus primarily on foods. So the idea for this book was born, to provide advice on growing and using medicinal plants in a forest garden context. This book is aimed at conveying our experience with medicinal trees and shrubs to a broad audience from home gardeners to foresters, from smallholders and permaculture designers to farmers.

Hopes for the future

Growing our own supplies of medicinal trees and shrubs could help to respond to the challenge of supplying an increasing demand for herbal remedies worldwide. There should be no need to continue relying on imports of many herbs, some of which are threatened in their native habitat or overly wild-harvested. Growers of all kinds can get involved in developing a more sustainable way with herbs, providing benefits for both domestic self-sufficiency and commercial market development. As I compiled examples for this book, I discovered that there are many growers and gardeners who are already cultivating and using medicinal plants in a host of different ways. Sadly, there is insufficient space to include details of everyone here. So, I hope there will be more opportunities for networking and spreading information about such initiatives. There are also many colleagues actively involved in education and health projects with herbal medicine. These include advisers on healthy lifestyles and nutrition, trainers of future herbal clinical practitioners, and forest school leaders inspiring the younger generation. Children can be amazed and enthused about the medicinal and many other possibilities that plants offer. As a 10-year-old said to a forest school leader, on hearing from her about the medicinal and other uses of a plant, "Wow, a plant can do all that!"

Contents

Note to readers

Warning

This book is not intended to replace professional advice from a qualified herbal or medical practitioner. Do not attempt to diagnose major health problems and treat yourself or others without professional advice, especially if you are pregnant or on prescribed medications.

This book is for Kay

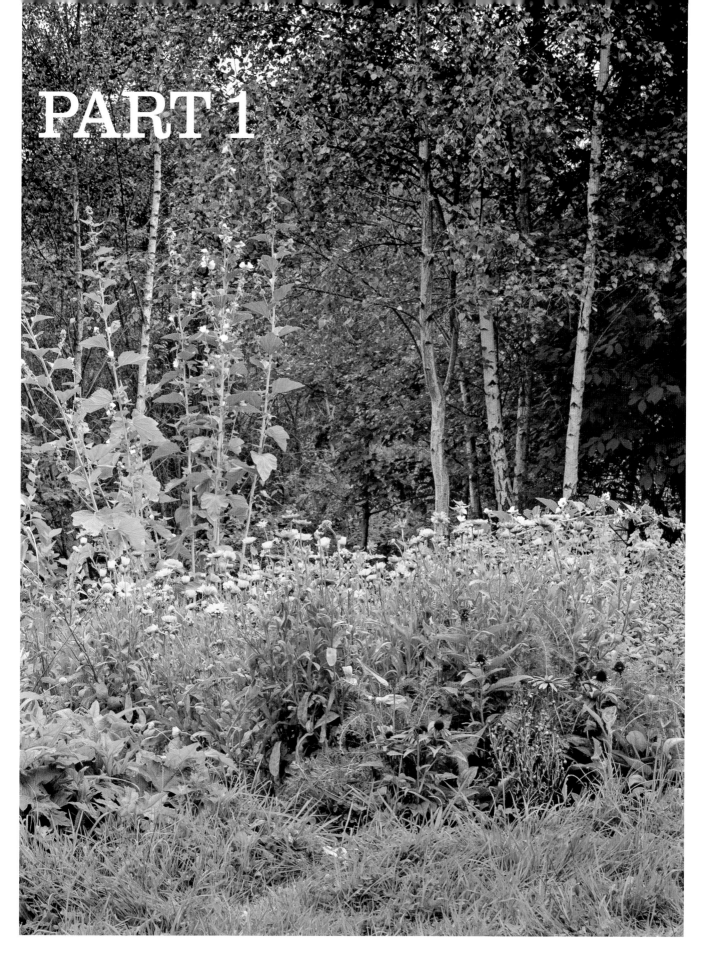

PART 1

Introduction

Why have a medicinal forest garden? In this introduction I explain the nature of a forest garden and explore the great potential of cultivating a medicinal forest garden. There is a compelling case for growing more medicinal plants sustainably, especially woody plants such as trees and shrubs. This case is supported from both economic and environmental perspectives. I provide an overview of increasing demands for medicinal plants worldwide and outline the threats to medicinal plant supplies due to habitat loss, climate change and overharvesting. At the end of this introduction, there is information about the structure of this book which may be helpful if you are deciding which parts of this book to read first.

The nature of forest gardens

The term 'forest garden' has been in use since the 1990s[1] although some writers have used other terms since, such as the 'woodland garden' and 'food forest'.[2] A forest garden is not just a collection of trees. Rather, it is the way in which these plants are brought together and managed that is characteristic of a forest garden. A forest garden can take many forms but is essentially 'a garden modelled on the structure of young natural woodland'.[3] To fully understand the nature of a forest garden, there are three key aspects to consider. First, the form of the forest garden draws on natural growth patterns, particularly in having multi-layered or 'stacked' plant species which are integrated in various ways.

Second, the forest garden is managed to a greater or lesser extent, particularly in terms of promoting soil health and diversity, and the management approach often draws on natural regenerative processes. Third, productivity in the forest garden is achieved in a sustainable way, primarily through ongoing supplies of foods that are harvested from a wide variety of plants.

The forest garden provides an environment that benefits soil organisms, perennial roots, fertility and availability of nutrients, and water management.[4] As leaves die off and accumulate as a mulch, and as roots die back, decomposition by micro-organisms provides nitrogen and other nutrients for the soil. Benefits from a forest garden style of cultivation include increased productivity, shade, improved soil management, pest and disease control, increased biodiversity and pollination, micro-climate modification, water management and carbon sequestration.[5] Many writers on forest gardens refer to a classical model of seven layers, from the upper canopy to the understorey and lower levels of shrubs, herbaceous plants, ground cover plants, roots and climbers. This level of categorisation can be much further subdivided, indeed 'the opportunities to fill every niche are endless'.[6] The forest garden has been described as 'a deliberately designed, high yielding, perennial plant system' for human sustenance.[7] A frequently used term is 'food forest', reflecting the primary focus on food crops such as leaves, fruit and nuts produced from a multi-layered woodland project.

What is a medicinal forest garden?

At Holt Wood, we started to use the phrase 'medicinal forest garden' because it so aptly describes the diversity and many layers of healing plants that have flourished since planting the medicinal woodland in 2005. My working definition has evolved for this book as:

> A medicinal forest garden is a natural or designed space including multi-layered plant species which is managed ethically and sustainably with potential for promoting health through a range of activities including harvest of medicinal plants.

This definition is deliberately broad in scope, in order to recognise that there can be many varied contexts for healing plants, from cottage gardens and parks to agroforestry and woodland. There is no 'one size fits all' medicinal forest garden! Medicinal plants, especially trees and shrubs, are often multifunctional and can co-exist within a forest garden having a wider range of purposes. Since health and diet are so closely intertwined, many food plants are recognised to have general health-promoting potential through their nutritional benefits (see The Forest Garden, p.4).

Resilience and forest gardening

A particular benefit claimed for forest gardening is increased resilience. The forest garden is likely to have greater biodiversity (range of species) and be designed with varied environments (range of light levels and soil characteristics), thus leading to greater resilience to climate extremes.[8] Biodiverse planting may also prove beneficial in combatting climate breakdown in large-scale tree planting. An example from China has shown that the 'richness' (i.e. greater range) of plantation species strongly increases productivity, and more complex plots increase biomass production and accumulate more carbon, nearly twice as much over an eight-year period compared to monocultures.[9] These results from research studies should encourage further multispecies forestry management strategies like forest gardening.

Threats to medicinal plant supplies

A significant threat is loss of habitat. Forests are particularly affected especially in tropical areas, and the range of threats includes increases in agriculture and settlements, fires and invasive plants, disturbances from war and mining.[10] In 2015, almost 4 billion hectares (30.6%) of the land area in the world was covered by forests. Of this total forested area, between 1990 and 2015, the areas of planted forest increased from 4% to 7%, but primary forest areas decreased, particularly tropical forested areas, and these are areas of irreplaceable biodiversity.[11] Actions to restore the planet's trees include the Reduced Emissions from Deforestation and Forest Degradation (REDD+) initiatives as part of global climate protection, originally proposed in 1997. These initiatives provide financial incentives to developing countries for reducing emissions related to conversion of forests to other uses.[12] REDD+ incorporates additional elements to focus on sustainable management and enhancement of forests, but full-scale implementation is yet to be achieved. The loss of habitat is a major source of concern in relation to medicinal plants. According to the State of the World's Plants 2017,[13] over a thousand important plant areas are under threat in Europe and the South Mediterranean, due to development and abandonment, agricultural intensification and inappropriate forest management. Tourism development is one of the most significant threats, due to disturbance and trampling or resort development with high impact in 136 locations.

Forests are also significantly affected by climate breakdown, not only by disruptive events of disturbances of heat, drought and storms but also by steady changes in the nature of climate.[14] In the Atlantic coastal zone of Europe, forest productivity may be increasing in some mountain areas as temperatures rise but decreasing in areas prone to drought stress. Insect and fungal population increases may cause substantial losses.[15] In the Continental zone of Europe, rising temperatures may mean greater productivity where sufficient water is available for trees to grow, but tree vitality will suffer in drier sites, especially where more wind, insect attacks and fungi are also likely. In the Mediterranean region,

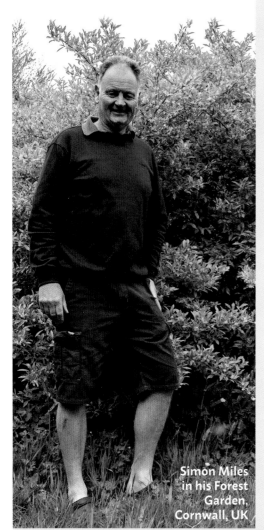

Simon Miles in his Forest Garden, Cornwall, UK

THE FOREST GARDEN – FOOD & MEDICINE TOGETHER

NAME: The Forest Garden

LOCATION: Near Falmouth, Cornwall, UK

ACTIVITY: Founder of The Forest Garden, Simon Miles is knowledgeable about herbal medicine, having trained as a Master Herbalist. He also has a background in horticulture. This well-established forest garden, of just over three acres, is near the coast in Cornwall, in south west England. The forest garden has been designed to efficiently produce tasty food, and supplies from medicinal and other useful plants. Many of the plants have both nutritional and medicinal effects, and are used by Simon in his clinical practice. The planting setup reflects the range of plants that grow best in a maritime climate where there is a salty wind, although there are less frequent frosts. Experience has shown which plants are most likely to succeed including the top fruit of selected Cornish apple, Asian pear, almond and other nut trees. Alongside these trees are many perennial bushes and herbs that can be used as companion plants to form multiple layers in a low maintenance design. Edible landscape design advice is available on perennial plants to suit particular requirements, and is supported by education through courses, as well as supplies of some hard-to-find plants.

KEY POINT: Herbal medicine and food can work well together in forest gardening layers.

INFO: www.theforestgarden.co.uk

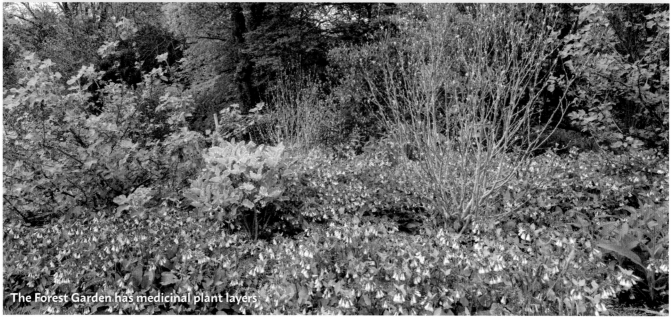

The Forest Garden has medicinal plant layers

increasing carbon dioxide levels will enhance photosynthesis, perhaps increasing growth by 30-50% for young broadleaved trees.[16] Overall, the distribution of tree species is likely to alter as trees become vulnerable to the changes.

While habitat loss and climate breakdown are the most significant threats to medicinal plants, the possibility of overharvesting remains a concern. It has been estimated that over 28,000 plants have medicinal uses worldwide.[17] According to Traffic International,[18] between 60-90% of medicinal plants are collected from the wild, particularly in forests, and conservation status is unknown for at least 93% of these species. Some 1280 medicinal plants are listed in the Convention on International Trade in Endangered Species of Wild Fauna and Flora (CITES). The CITES Secretariat has recognised that the greatest use of non-timber forest products is related to medicinal trade, and much of this trade is carried out through online networks that are particularly hard to trace.[19] Efforts to regulate use of medicinal non-timber forest products through certification are made more complex due to the wide range of herbal products, their seasonality, different end uses and insecure harvesting rights.[20] Alternatives to wild-harvested plants may be possible through cultivation for sustainable supplies, especially significant where these plants are 'destructively harvested for their bark, roots or the whole plant'.[21] Cultivation can include simulation of natural woodland environments, such as in developments supported in the US by United Plant Savers. This may be a way forward to protect some endangered species (see United Plant Savers Botanical Sanctuary, p.6). An advantage of cultivating plants in conditions similar to the wild is the sustainable harvest, and controls can be applied to ensure organic or other suitable standards are maintained.[22]

Potential for cultivating medicinal plants including trees and shrubs

The growing of medicinal plants on a small scale has considerable potential for increasing the supply of medicinal and aromatic plants in response to rising demand. Small woodlands can have a key role to play. In 2004, a survey published by Plantlife in the UK made recommendations that included support for cultivation through partnerships with small-scale growers.[23] A recent European study suggests a role for agroforestry or agriculture with trees:

> With dwindling supplies from natural sources and increasing global demand, the MAPs [medicinal and aromatic plants] will need to be cultivated to ensure their regular supply as well as conservation. Since many of the MAPs are grown under forest cover and are shade tolerant, agroforestry offers a convenient strategy for promoting their cultivation and conservation.[24]

The possibilities of further commercially exploiting by-products of forestry have been well established in the US context.[25] There are numerous possible connections between markets for non-timber forest products in areas such as floristry and cosmetics as well as health care.

In the US, the potential for valuable medicinal crops has benefitted from advice and support to farmers and woodland owners. Since 2004, Jeanine Davis and colleagues at North Carolina State University, US, have been working with local farmers to produce medicinal herbs for commerce. Funds were made available to farmers, so that they learned to grow, harvest, clean, dry and market a range of herbs including ginseng (*Panax quinquefolius*) and goldenseal (*Hydrastis canadensis*).[26] These crops can be profitable but farmers were unfamiliar with them and needed more support, from practical information through to research and shared-use facilities for processing. In the UK, surveys have previously identified a buoyant market for medicinal herbs but a lack of home production for a variety of reasons.[27] The potential problems of low prices for raw materials and high labour costs of harvesting could be counteracted by identification of more efficient cultivation methods,

CONSERVING NATURAL HABITATS WITH MEDICINAL PLANTS IN THE US

NAME: United Plant Savers Botanical Sanctuary

LOCATION: Center for Medicinal Plant Conservation, Ohio, US

ACTIVITY: Founded in 1994, United Plant Savers exists to promote medicinal plant conservation in the US. In Ohio, the Goldenseal Botanical Sanctuary provides a haven for plant lovers and all interested in the conservation of medicinal plants. Based on a 379 acre plot of land, previously degraded by mining activities, much of the site has been carefully planted and a new visitor centre has been opened. Visitors can follow marked medicine trails in the restored woodland, seeing medicinal trees and other healing plants. The Sanctuary also hosts demonstrations of shade cultivation and examples of prairie plants such as *Echinacea* species. An internship programme runs each year which provides an opportunity for visitors to become involved in the maintenance and development of the sanctuary. United Plant Savers advises on sustainable cultivation methods, and also maintains a list of 'at-risk' plants including woodland plants such as ginseng and goldenseal.

KEY POINT: Restoration of natural habitats provides real opportunities to learn about the conservation of medicinal plants in the US.

INFO: www.unitedplantsavers.org

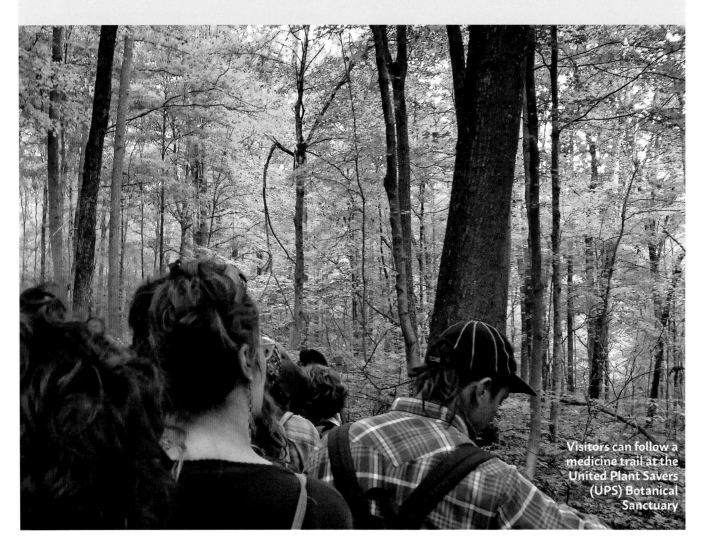

Visitors can follow a medicine trail at the United Plant Savers (UPS) Botanical Sanctuary

co-operative processing and organic premiums, with ways of combining cultivation with other activities to provide an economic return.

Agroforestry and permaculture

Changing agricultural practices have brought rising interest in the potential of agroforestry. Part of the renaissance of such new approaches has been due to the success of permaculture design principles in creating productive sites, by drawing on examples from nature, and moving away from monocrop styles of growing. There is also an important ethical basis inherent in seeking to achieve more sustainable ways of growing and living. This can be seen in the three ethical principles associated with permaculture developments: they should be good for the planet (earth care), good for people (people care), and ensure that surplus produce is fairly used (fair shares). The transformational approach of permaculture is well adapted to fostering resilience as well as flexibility in response to change.[28]

Quality control and medicinal plants

An advantage of cultivation over wild-harvesting is the potential for producing top quality herb products. There have been concerns regarding the quality and provenance of herb supplies and products that are sold over the counter. In the UK, a study of St John's wort (*Hypericum perforatum*) products, which used high performance thin layer chromatography alongside spectroscopy, found that over one-third (36%) of the products were adulterated.[29] As in previous studies on ginkgo products, the commercial products of the highest quality were those with European traditional herbal registration licences rather than unlicensed products.[30] In North America, a study based on DNA barcodes, including elder, ginkgo and walnut, found that only two out of 12 suppliers had products without plant substitution, use of fillers or contamination.[31] If the costs of testing for purity could be reduced then such DNA testing could be used more widely to provide authentication of herbal products both in cultivation and wild-harvesting.[32]

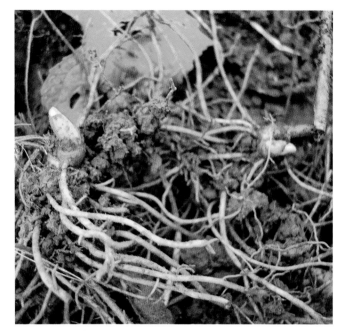

Goldenseal (*Hydrastis canadensis*) plant from sustainable cultivation in woodland

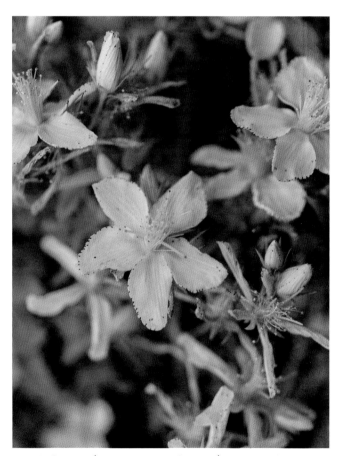

St John's wort (*Hypericum perforatum*) is sold over the counter as an antidepressant

Demand for medicinal plants worldwide

Although medicinal plants are used worldwide, just 12 countries make up 80% of world trade by value in medicinal plants, and the US, Germany and Hong Kong are the most important trade centres.[33] The main exporters of medicinal plants are China, exporting over 1.3 billion kg in 2013, as well as India, Canada, Germany and the US. Most of the source countries, where herbs are harvested, export botanicals after little processing, dried and packed into large containers. The main importers by value are Hong Kong, China, the US, Germany and Japan.[34] However, detailed statistics are not easy to come by for trade in the world herbal market, mainly because import and export data are poorly defined.[35] A few plant species are specifically recorded in the data, such as liquorice and ginseng, but most of the remaining plants are categorised together as 'medicinal and aromatic' plants.

Even though the statistics may not be itemised in terms of individual medicinal plants, growth of interest in traditional and complementary medicine worldwide has become increasingly well documented in both industrialised and developing countries.[36] In Europe, demand for herbal medicinal products has been rising:

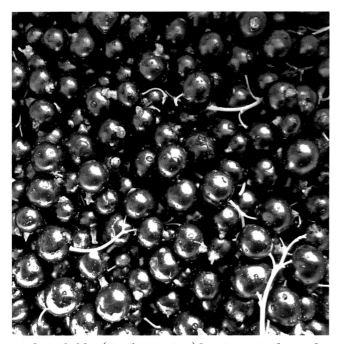

Medicinal elder (*Sambucus nigra*) berries are in demand

statistics published in March 2017[37] showed that retail sales in Germany in 2015 had increased 5.9% from the previous year, reaching 1.6 billion Euros. The top three categories of herbal remedies were products for coughs, respiratory tract diseases, and colds and flu, and altogether these three product categories accounted for over half of sales.[38] Sales of some herbal supplements continue to be popular in the US, whether through supermarkets, health-food stores or mail order online. For example, supermarket sales of extracts of elderberry (*Sambucus nigra*) increased by 34.7% from 2016 to 2017.[39]

Demand for traceability and sustainability

Apart from over-the-counter herbal remedies for common complaints, medicinal and aromatic plants also feature strongly in personal care products. The global organic personal care market was estimated at US$10.16 billion in 2015, and rising consumer awareness is expected to drive further growth in sales of organic products.[40] Growth potential in the market is evident for skin care, hair care, oral care and, particularly, anti-ageing products. Ironically, new innovations such as forest-derived health-related products and services, may contribute to growing the market in Western countries but may be damaging for the survival of some plants in the wild.[41] Wild-harvesting is the main way in which these medicinal and other plants for health supplements and cosmetics worldwide are sourced for trade. This wild-harvesting trade can provide an important source of income for poor or disadvantaged people in rural communities, particularly women who rely on forest products.[42] However, since demand for medicinal plants is likely to continue to rise, this will increase pressure on wild-harvested sources.[43] Amongst consumers there is greater interest in provenance of ingredients in products,[44] and growing numbers of people making as well as using natural remedies.[45] This interest in sustainability is encouraging the natural products industry to improve the traceability of botanical supplies, making the supply chain more transparent.[46] Progress is being made in reporting on sustainability by forward-looking herbal businesses such as Pukka Herbs and Weleda.[47]

About this book

This book is in two main parts. Part 1 consists of seven chapters that deal with general principles and advice, from designing with medicinal trees to harvest and use, with many practical examples. Chapter 1 provides a backdrop of how herbal medicines work, especially trees and their phytochemistry. At the end of Chapter 1 there is a quick access listing of the 40 trees and shrubs detailed in Part 2 (see pp.23-24). If you want to design a medicinal forest garden then go straight to Chapter 2. If you are keen to focus on practical aspects of establishing and maintaining a medicinal forest garden then jump to Chapter 3. Propagation and sourcing of plants is covered in Chapter 4. For details of best practices in harvesting and making herbal preparations then see Chapters 5 and 6. Finally, Chapter 7 provides some suggestions regarding scaling up to a higher level of growing, including commercial possibilities. Part 2 provides a concise A to Z listing by Latin name of individual profiles of 40 trees and shrubs suitable for a temperate climate. Each profile entry provides details of the species relevant to successful cultivation, as well as advice on parts for harvesting, possible indications for use, and relevant research examples and other key information.

Sources used

Throughout this book there are reference sources, provided in the endnotes, and there is a selected bibliography. The Plant List hosted by Kew Gardens provides up-to-date accepted scientific plant names.[48] Online sources such as the Plants for a Future database[49] and North American horticultural information sites have provided much cultivation information. For clinical and scientific studies, keyword searches in PubMed have identified additional examples of published research in a range of disciplines from forestry to medicine and phytochemistry.[50] This book focuses on the northern temperate climate for growing medicinal plants. The temperate zones have distinct summer and winter seasons, and native temperate forests are diverse, including conifers and deciduous trees. I have included several trees and shrubs which are almost hardy in these temperate areas if given some protection. These semi-hardy medicinal plants may have increasing potential for cultivation in a warming climate. I have excluded species that are more suitable for boreal, southern or tropical climates. All measurements are given in metric and there is a conversion table for metric and imperial measurements in Appendix 1. A glossary is provided in Appendix 2. Towards the end of the book are further useful appendices on herbaceous medicinal plants (Appendix 3), climate zones (Appendix 4 and 5) and links to organisations and other resources (Appendix 6).

CHAPTER 1

The Medicinal Uses of Trees and Shrubs

This chapter underpins the important role of medicinal trees and shrubs in the wider context of herbal medicine. Many of these woody healing plants are in use today as part of traditional systems around the world. This chapter provides an overview of research into traditions of use of herbal medicines, particularly trees and shrubs, as well as the practices of herbal medicine today. The study of individual plant constituents has increased our understanding of the actual and potential uses of plants in health and disease. You may already have come to know plants around you through cultivation or spending time out with nature, and will readily recognise aromas, colours and tastes that reflect some of a plant's constituents. Here, the medicinal actions of key herbal constituents are briefly outlined with indications of medicinal plant uses, with examples in preventative health, antibiotics, cancer and ageing treatments. There is considerable evidence for the wider health benefits of trees in the environment, contributing to both mental and physical health. Finally, I look at how some of the actions of plant constituents may be useful in aid for common ailments. The chapter ends with a quick access listing providing a guide to 40 trees and shrubs which are described in much more detail in Part 2 of this book.

Medicinal plants and traditional uses

An incredible range of medicinal plants can be found in many different contexts. From gardens of all kinds: cottage, botanic, hospice and parks, to agricultural, forestry and wilder environments: fields, marshes, moors, mountains and woods, there are plants at every level from ground to overstorey that have traditional uses for health. Many of these plants are trees and shrubs. For the purpose of this book, a tree is generally a plant with a woody stem having branches at some distance from the ground whereas a shrub has multiple stems arising from the ground and is smaller than a tree.[1] Many of these healing plants can now be identified as containing key constituents which often explain not only some of their traditionally observed actions, but also indicate further possibilities for use.[2]

Some examples of past use of tree preparations for medicinal purposes can give an idea of the range of complaints that were treated. Externally, alder (*Alnus glutinosa*) bark was used as a decoction for bathing swellings and was traditionally used for sore throat and ague. Few folklore records are reported of the use of this tree, although the ripe cones were drunk in tea for gout on the Somerset-Dorset border, and the leaves were crushed and laid on burns in Norfolk.[3] Another tree, elder (*Sambucus nigra*), provided leaves that when bruised could be rubbed on the skin or worn in a hat to repel flies, and they were traditionally used to make a 'green ointment' used for piles, tumours and swellings. A longstanding remedy was oak (*Quercus robur* or *petraea*). According to Richard Elkes in 1651, the advice given to an old soldier was to boil oak bark for stomach upsets:

> Carrie in your Knap-sacke a piece of steele to
> heat red hot, and quench it in your beer, water,
> or milke, and as you travel gather the leaves and

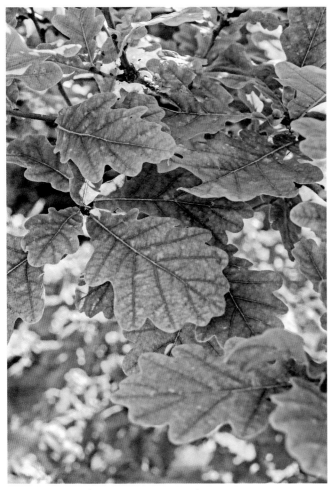

Quercus robur (and related species) has astringent tannin-rich bark

barke of the Oake, and the leaves of the black-Thorn, a bagge of Salt and Oatmeale, that if the Flux should take you, you might helpe your selfe.[4]

Oak bark does have some antiseptic effect. These remedies could have been effective although we now know that the particular type of tannin found in oak bark means that it should not be used internally for long periods.

Of course, the use of plants for healing purposes is nothing new, since the medical uses of plants have been explored in many traditions throughout the world for centuries. Ethnobotany is the systematic study of traditional knowledge and customs of people and their relationships with plants. Started as a discipline in the later nineteenth century, ethnobotany began by collecting data about plant uses, particularly in countries of northern and southern Americas, Asia[5] and Africa.[6] Later studies were carried out in Europe,[7] and in the twenty-first century the focus has turned towards reaping ideas for pharmaceutical drug discovery rather than recording traditional practices.[8] Ethnobotanical studies provide us with examples of the kinds of preparations used by indigenous peoples, but some of these preparation methods may have fallen out of use. For example, the use of fire on tree parts such as bark, leaves, flowers and cones, is not often seen for medicinal purposes: the Inuktitut of Canada once burned and inhaled the smoke of alder (*Alnus viridis*) to treat rheumatism and as an insecticide against mosquitoes, the Antrim of Ireland inhaled the smoke and smouldering twigs of ash (*Fraxinus excelsior*) as a worm treatment, and in the Ubage Valley of France, elder (*Sambucus nigra*) flowers were used to provide smoke for fumigating eye problems.[9]

New plant introductions

There are also many examples of introduced plants, including shrubs and trees, that have medicinal value. In the past, knowledge about plants for medicinal use travelled widely across continents and many plants, including trees, were transported to new areas as exotic introductions.[10] For example, plants brought to the UK from Europe and Asia, some attributed to the Romans, included sweet chestnut, walnut and mulberry.[11] By the end of the sixteenth century,[12] there were over 100 foreign trees and shrubs in cultivation in the UK, including some North American introductions such as arbor vitae (*Thuja occidentalis*). Many more introductions were made in the seventeenth century, when botanic gardens were being established in the UK including Oxford (1621), Chelsea Physic Garden (1674) and Edinburgh (1680). In the nineteenth and twentieth centuries, more plants were collected from China, Japan, South America and the Himalayas.[13] Many introduced plants, once claimed to provide medicinal actions, nowadays are more highly regarded for their ornamental value.

Herbal medicine today – practitioners and remedies

Worldwide, there are numerous traditional systems of healthcare still in existence, and the World Health Organization (WHO) has recognised the importance of such provision, whether known as traditional medicine or complementary medicine. Four development objectives for traditional medicine have been identified by the WHO:

- to develop policy to integrate traditional medicine,
- to promote the knowledge base supporting safety, efficacy and quality,
- to increase availability and affordability,
- to promote rational therapeutic use of traditional medicine.

In 2013, the progress in achieving these objectives was reviewed, and the WHO sought more action from member states.[14] Despite these efforts, recognition of traditional medicine practitioners continues to vary considerably throughout the world. While traditional Chinese medicine and Ayurvedic practitioners are well integrated and supported to some extent within national medical systems, there are many barriers to traditional practices in other countries of Europe and North America. In these Western contexts where evidence-based medicine holds sway, the use of traditional or complementary medicine approaches is largely denigrated even where there is research evidence for positive outcomes. Clinical complementary medicine practitioners have formed professional bodies and sought to provide self-regulation based on training, standards and ethical guidelines.[15] Practitioners of herbal medicine are trained to use holistic approaches to treatment alongside knowledge of orthodox clinical approaches and the pharmacological actions of plants. Rather than providing over-the-counter remedies and symptomatic treatment, the clinical herbal practitioner takes a detailed case history and aims to identify underlying issues that may be treated with combinations of medicinal herbs and diet.

The use of herbal remedies is dependent on knowledge about plants, which is usually formulated in herbal monographs providing details of constituents, actions, preparations and indications alongside research and traditional uses. There is a process for recognition in the European Union of herbal remedies with evidence of longstanding traditional use, and monographs are compiled. In the US, Europe and UK there have been extensive efforts to establish accurate and detailed monographs to help improve standards of supplies of herbs. Safety and efficacy issues, rightly, have come to the fore and handbooks with pharmacopoeia standards help to clarify any possibilities of adverse effects or other considerations.[16] However, where herbal monographs are based solely on 'evidence-based' studies, they do not always benefit from associated historical information such as traditional experience with safe forms of use and dosage.

Synergy and the approach of herbal medicine

Many research studies into the actions of medicinal plants continue to try to isolate single active constituents. But some researchers have pointed out the advantages of plant combinations and whole plant extracts.[17] Containing many constituents, the whole plant extract shows synergy with enhancements of activity enabled by different constituents. Synergistic effects can make whole plant extracts more effective, for example by enabling greater absorption. Some lipophilic plant constituents readily dissolve in fats or oils and are able to cross cell walls to produce antimicrobial effects. Other constituents, such as flavonoids, are able to inhibit DNA synthesis or energy metabolism in microbial cells and further undermine the spread of disease.[18] A study on treatments for dry eye found that natural extracts of bilberry fruit were more effective than purified anthocyanins: the plant constituents were acting together synergistically for greater effect.[19] However, research into herbal medicines continues to suffer from lack of support. Reviews may point towards efficacy but call for more studies, and lack of funding prevents further detailed investigation unless a commercial prospect is seen.

Using plants in health and disease

Preventative health care and plants

Plants may be considered not only for treating disease but are also key contributors to many aspects of preventative health. The benefits of plant-rich diets are widely recognised. For example, berry fruits are often considered as 'superfoods' due to their high content of vitamins, fibre and phenolic compounds. The bright colours of many berries, from blackberries and raspberries (*Rubus* species) to bilberries (*Vaccinium* species) and chokeberries (*Aronia melanocarpa*), blackcurrants (*Ribes nigrum*) and elderberries (*Sambucus nigra*) are due to anthocyanins. Studies show that the leaves of these plants are also rich in these phenolic constituents, and these by-products could be used rather than wasted when berries are harvested.[20] Not only can individual plants contribute to health but also the diverse range of plant species helps to promote health. The existence of forests has been shown to contribute to child health overall, through beneficial effects on children's diets. When forest access and children's diet were reviewed in 27 developing countries, the greatest dietary diversity was found for households living within 3km of a forested area with 40% tree cover. This diversity was significant in providing micronutrients such as vitamin A and iron, showing that forest conservation can have a direct impact on health and mortality.[21]

Plants that fight bacteria

Many of the trees and shrubs mentioned in this book have powerful antibacterial effects. Coniferous trees such as the Douglas fir (*Pseudotsuga menziesii*), Scots pine (*Pinus sylvestris*) and juniper (*Juniperus communis*) all contain antiseptic essential oils. Other aromatic trees include eucalyptus (*Eucalyptus* species), sweet bay (*Laurus nobilis*) and sweet gum (*Liquidambar styraciflua*). A number of woody shrubs considered as ornamentals are also useful in this respect, having antiseptic properties, such as forsythia (*Forsythia suspensa*) and myrtle (*Myrtus communis*). Some bacterial challenges to human health have outstripped the resources available and threaten catastrophe, such as the spread of methicillin-resistant *Staphylococcus aureus* (MRSA), which appears to defy modern antibiotics. It is possible that new treatments may be found from natural sources, such as the use of isoflavonoids from plants as antimicrobials.[22] Other studies of extracts of common plants, such as nettle (*Urtica dioica*) and rosemary (*Rosmarinus officinalis*), also show high antibacterial potential.[23]

Using plants to beat cancer

Cancer accounted for 8.8m deaths globally in 2015.[24] Natural products have attracted attention as possible aides to cancer treatment, either in direct use or as leads for further drug development. Extracts from the yew (*Taxus* species) are used in a range of cancers. Paclitaxel (known in commerce as taxol) was originally extracted from the bark of the Pacific yew (*Taxus brevifolia*) though it can now be made from precursors in the needles of yew family members such as common yew (*T. baccata*). This drug targets β tubulin to prevent

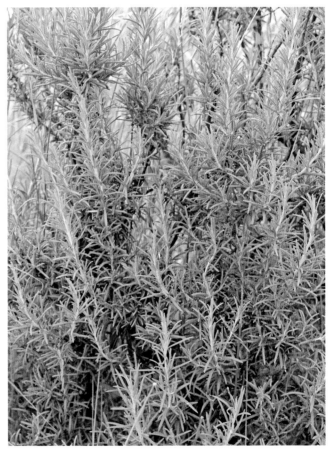

Rosemary (*Rosmarinus officinalis*) **contains antibacterial essential oils**

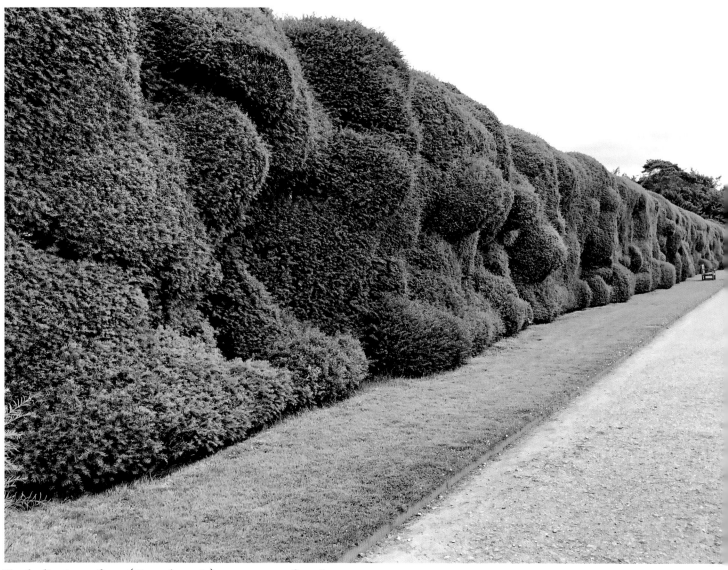

Fresh clippings of yew (*Taxus baccata*) are a source of taxol

proper mitotic spindle assembly, so causing the death of replicating cancer cells. Various formulations have been developed to direct the paclitaxel in the body to a tumour location, and further synthetic derivatives such as docetaxel and cabazitaxel have now been developed for clinical use.[25] A range of other plant constituents are being investigated for possible use in cancer treatments. One example is betulinic acid, a triterpene which can be obtained from birch (*Betula pendula*) bark. Betulinic acid appears to be cytotoxic in a wide range of cancer types; the mechanism of action includes causing mitochondrial collapse in cells and other effects

including limiting the blood supply and speed of metastasis. Synergistic effects with other anticancer drugs have also been found. Betulinic acid is slightly soluble in water, and research is under way to find methods of use or derivatives which are readily available to the body.[26] Another example, berberine, has also been suggested to have considerable potential in cancer treatments. Berberine is found in plants such as barberry (*Berberis vulgaris*) and Oregon grape root (*Berberis aquifolium*). It has been shown that berberine exhibits preferential selectivity for human pancreatic cancer cells compared to other cells.[27]

Ageing, anti-oxidants and healing plants

Anti-oxidant and anti-inflammatory effects are widespread in plant extracts, and can contribute to slowing the effects of the ageing process. In particular, research is being carried out to develop ways to use plants to treat some of the diseases associated with neurological ageing. For example, Alzheimer's disease is known to involve abnormal clumping together of Tau proteins in a way that disrupts the neurons in the brain. These proteins collect together to form paired helical filaments which are a hallmark of Alzheimer's disease. One study looked at 200,000 compounds to see if any would stop or alter this aggregation. Using various tests the study showed that several types of plant anthraquinones were able to inhibit the formation of the paired helical filaments and these included emodin, daunorubicin and adriamycin.[28] Emodin is a widely found constituent in plants as diverse as alder (*Alnus glutinosa*), alder buckthorn (*Frangula alnus*) and rhubarb (*Rheum officinale*).[29]

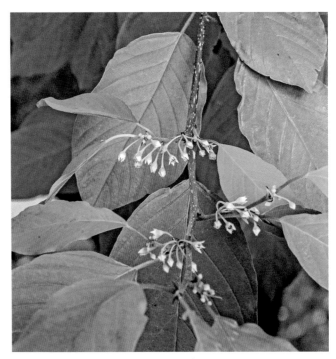

Alder buckthorn (*Frangula alnus*) contains anthraquinones such as emodin

Trees and health in the environment
Green infrastructure

Wider ecosystems and human health are related in many ways, and biodiversity, in forests and elsewhere, remains crucial for the health of a large proportion of the world population.[30] Trees are a significant component of the 'green infrastructure' of parks, gardens, forests, farmland and open spaces, 'an interconnected network of green space that conserves natural ecosystem values and functions and provides associated benefits to human populations'.[31] Ecosystem services have been identified in four categories to which trees contribute:

- provisioning (food, medicine and water),
- regulating (climate, flood control, soil fertility, pollination, disease modulation),
- cultural (recreation, spiritual and mental health)
- supporting (soil formation, nutrient and water cycling).

Trees are good for the urban environment too. This was recognised by John Evelyn in earlier times, writing about trees in 1661. He wrote of how 'a mass of sweet smelling trees, bushes and plants would be planted to surround and vivify London'.[32] Today, we understand better the mechanisms of health improvement in urban areas through trees which include shading in heat, reduction of ultraviolet radiation, reduction of wind speed, reduction of air pollution, encouraging physical activity in green space, and reduction of stress and noise levels.[33]

The benefits of trees in urban areas

In the urban context of Toronto, people living in neighbourhoods with a higher density of street trees reported significantly fewer cardio-metabolic conditions (hypertension, high blood sugar, obesity, high cholesterol, heart disease, stroke and diabetes).[34] In real terms, after adjusting for income and other factors, this study showed that 10 more trees in a city block equated to being seven years younger, and the equivalent of $10,000 per annum extra income. Overall, urban trees provide more benefits than cost in planting and maintenance, yet the need for these trees is not readily understood.

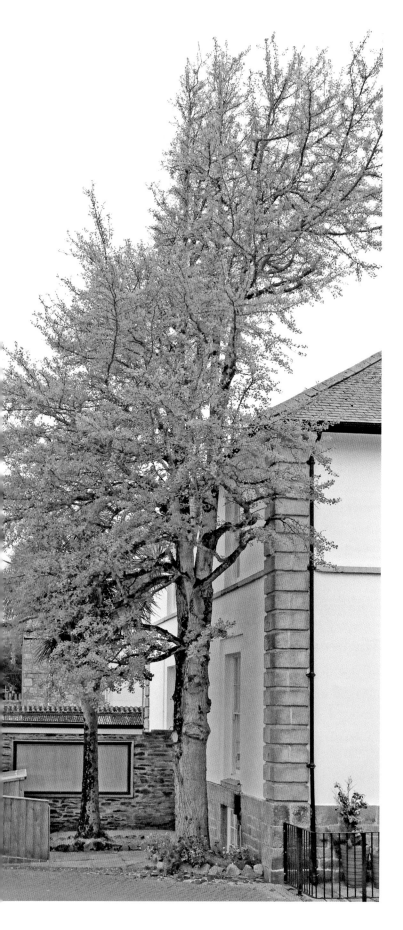

Forest bathing

A forest environment can provide measurable benefits for individual health – ranging from speedier physical recovery from illness to improvement of mental health, reductions of stress and mortality to improving outcomes in pregnancy.[35] Shinrin-yoku or 'experiencing the forest atmosphere' has become popular for its therapeutic effect: physical changes have been identified, such as an improved immune system arising from forest visits.[36] Forest bathing or walking in woods research studies have shown recognisable health benefits for depression and hypertension.[37] A randomised controlled trial with women aged over 60 years old in Korea showed that just one hour of walking around a forested area improved arterial stiffness and pulmonary function.[38] A review of 20 trials found that both diastolic and systolic blood pressure in the forest environment were significantly lower than in a non-forest environment, particularly in older people.[39] Further reviews are needed to confirm the positive effects of forest therapy in circulatory conditions, inflammation, stress, anxiety and depression.[40] In addition to supporting physical health, trees in formal arrangements can provide cathedral-like spaces for reflection and restoration of mental health.

Trees and spiritual regeneration

Whilst we know that trees can contribute to physical and mental health, there is also an unescapable aspect of spirituality in the ways that we relate to them and nature. In some cultures, there are inbuilt connections to the land which provide an ongoing link with nature over generations. A great example of the living link with trees and forests can be seen in the 'hytte' of Norwegian culture. On page 18 you can see an example of this in practice.

LEFT: Ginkgo (*Ginkgo biloba*) can tolerate urban pollution

RIGHT: Sweet gum trees form a living cathedral in Porto, Portugal

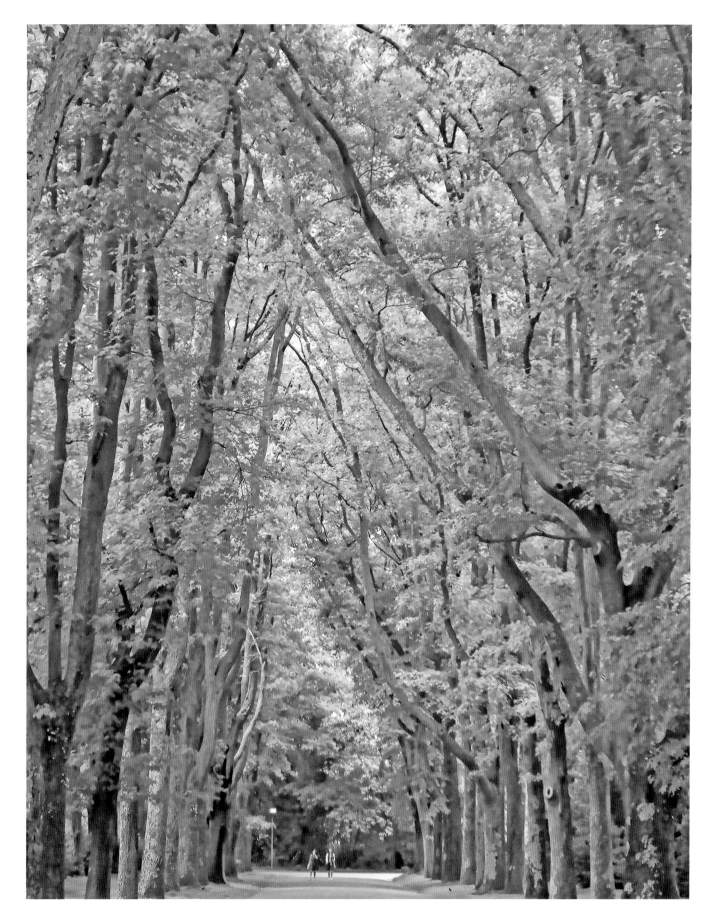

FOREST BATHING AND DEEP RELAXATION IN NORWAY

NAME: Karen With is a hardworking educator and celebrant based in south west England. She is half-Norwegian, and has access to a small cabin or 'hytte' in a wooded river valley, 20km from Oslo.

LOCATION: Kjaglidalen, Norway, about 30km from Oslo

ACTIVITY: Karen says "Wider health benefits from trees include immersion/forest bathing. Central to Norwegian lives is the 'hytte', either by the sea, in the mountains or in the forest. My whole life has involved temporarily living immersed in nature. Seeing the natural world through these cultural lenses has enabled me to tune in and rejuvenate. Through reconnecting with self and forming intimate relationship with certain trees, the layers fall away and deep relaxation occurs. Living a more simple life off-grid is regenerating and soul-enriching and such a tonic! A deeper connection occurs and the benefits of foraging and managing fuel for heating connects me to the cycle of life. What a gift such places/times are in our fragmented world, spending time in forest retreat offers wellbeing as well as a refreshing sense of renewal, whilst relating to the trees."

KEY POINT: Trees are an integral part of cultural engagement with nature, contributing to rejuvenation, reconnection and renewal.

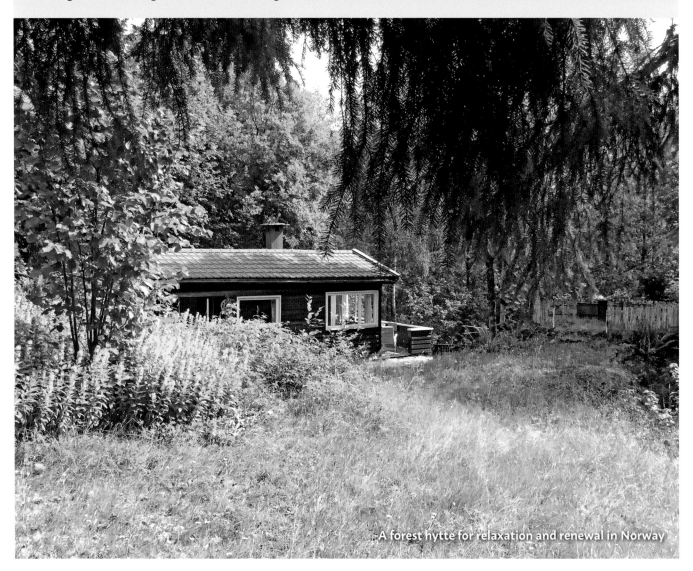

A forest hytte for relaxation and renewal in Norway

Phytochemistry and plant constituents

Phytochemistry refers to the study of chemical constituents of plants, and often there are hundreds of chemicals involved in just one plant. Many key active constituents of medicinal plants are secondary metabolites, not essential to plant life but useful in defence, protecting from predators and environmental damage.[41] The three main groups of secondary metabolites are phenols, terpenoids and alkaloids, and examples are shown in the table below.[42] Many plant constituents can be fitted into more than one of the categories shown. Other significant groups of plant constituents include saponins, which produce a soap-like foam when shaken with water, and polysaccharides or sugar-like complexes that can be found as gums, mucilages and resins.

Phenols

Phenolic plant constituents contain aromatic hydrocarbon rings, such as the polyphenolic molecules known as tannins which are astringent and drying in their actions. One of the earliest and most well-known phenolic plant constituents to be chemically identified is salicin, a phenolic glycoside found in the leaves and bark of willow (*Salix* species) trees.[43] Willow bark has long been used to relieve fever, having anti-inflammatory and painkilling effects, a predecessor to commercial aspirin, acetylsalicylic acid, developed in the twentieth century as less irritating to the stomach.[44] A Cochrane systematic review assessed the effectiveness of herbal medicines for low back pain, including white willow (*Salix alba*) bark and found evidence of improvement.[45] Phenolic compounds can have other effects including anti-oxidant activity as well as antibacterial effects. A survey of phytoextracts of

Examples of secondary metabolites in medicinal plants

Plant examples	Key constituents	Actions and possible effects
Oak (*Quercus robur*) Agrimony (*Agrimonia eupatoria*) Avens (*Geum urbanum*)	Polyphenolic tannins	External astringent drying effect to aid the healing of spots and wounds Internal soothing of sore throats
St John's wort (*Hypericum perforatum*) Bilberry (*Vaccinium* species) Blackberry (*Rubus fruticosus*) Hawthorn (*Crataegus monogyna*)	Phenolic flavones and flavonoids e.g. quercitin, genistein, myricetin Also anthocyanins, widely found blue, purple or red pigments in fruits	Have anti-inflammatory effects and strengthen the circulatory system, helping to repair connective tissue and blood vessels
Alder buckthorn (*Frangula alnus*) Curled dock (*Rumex crispus*)	Anthraquinones	Laxative due to stimulation of intestinal muscle
Birch (*Betula pendula*) Pine (*Pinus sylvestris*) Snow gum (*Eucalyptus pauciflora*) Black peppermint (*Mentha* x *piperita vulgaris*)	Monoterpenes e.g. geraniol, limonene, menthol, camphor characteristic of aromatic volatile essential oils	Antiseptic and support the immune system Some terpenes are calming for digestion
Mugwort (*Artemisia vulgaris*) Myrtle (*Myrtus communis*)	Sesquiterpenes e.g. farnesol, artemisinin	Antimicrobial effects Can affect the nervous system
Barberry (*Berberis vulgaris*) Oregon grape root (*Berberis aquifolium*) Bittersweet (*Solanum dulcamara*)	Alkaloids e.g. ephedrine, berberine	Affect the nervous system, may be stimulant or depressant depending on plant
Marsh mallow (*Althaea officinalis*)	Mucilages, polysaccharides	Soothe and reduce inflammation
Liquorice (*Glycyrrhiza glabra*)	Saponins or soap-like substances	Can reduce inflammation and are somewhat emetic and used as expectorants

relevance in skin care, with emphasis on phenolic acids and flavonoids, found that many could be derived from tree barks including sweet chestnut (*Castanea sativa*), sea buckthorn (*Elaeagnus rhamnoides*), mulberry (*Morus alba*) and pomegranate (*Punica granatum*).[46] Extracts from a range of tree barks were evaluated for their radical-scavenging activity, and showed antibacterial effects on gram-positive *Staphylococcus* species, as well as other benefits to the skin.[47] Not only are new constituents constantly being identified, but also new uses have been proposed for parts of trees previously considered as waste, such as the knots in timber discarded in processing in forestry. A new polyphenolic lignan and stilbenoid mixture extracted from the knots of Scots pine (*Pinus sylvestris*) has shown promise for use in prostate cancer.[48]

Terpenes

Terpenes are unsaturated hydrocarbons and are widespread in plants, giving rise to terpenoids (also known as isoprenoids) in plant extracts, including the chemicals producing the aroma of essential oils. We are familiar with many of these essential oils in aromatic herbs such as mints, as well as sweet-smelling citrus and pine trees. Terpenes occur in various subclasses such as monoterpenes, sesquiterpenes and diterpenes, and have important anti-inflammatory, anti-oxidant, antiviral and antibacterial properties. Artemisin is a sesquiterpene lactone used in malaria treatment, and it was originally derived from sweet wormwood (*Artemisia annua*) in the daisy family (Asteraceae). Terpenes can form the basis for steroid hormones, and some triterpenes are created by plants for defence against insects. These triterpenoid chemicals can mimic the hormones used by insect plant-eaters, and this disrupts moulting processes, so that their metabolism is seriously affected.[49]

Alkaloids

Alkaloids are best known as the nitrogen-containing plant constituents that affect the nervous system, including some important opiate drugs in the poppy or Papaveraceae family, and other active chemicals such as caffeine from coffee (*Caffea arabica*). Used with care,

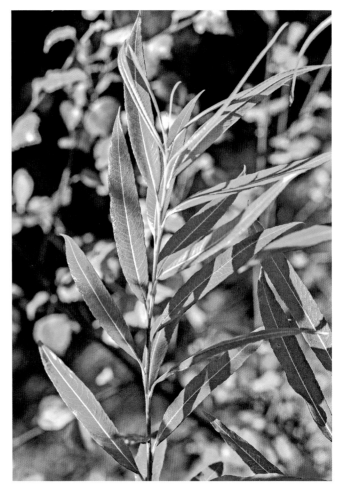

White willow (*Salix alba*) leaves and bark are rich in phenols with anti-inflammatory actions

the alkaloids can have positive effects, and efforts to extract alkaloids from forestry residues are of continuing commercial interest.[50] Taxol, or paclitaxel, is an alkaloid derived from yew trees, or *Taxus* species. Some significant plant-based alkaloids are reported in the *State of the World's Plants 2017*, including an extract of the alkaloid galantamine from snowdrops (*Galanthus* species) and daffodils (*Narcissus* species), which is used in treating Alzheimer's disease.[51] Berberine, also mentioned earlier, is an alkaloid found in many plants including the barberry and the ornamental Oregon grape (*Berberis* species), readily recognised by its bright yellow colour. The effects of this alkaloid include lowering of blood cholesterol and glucose, making it of interest in a range of metabolic disorders.[52]

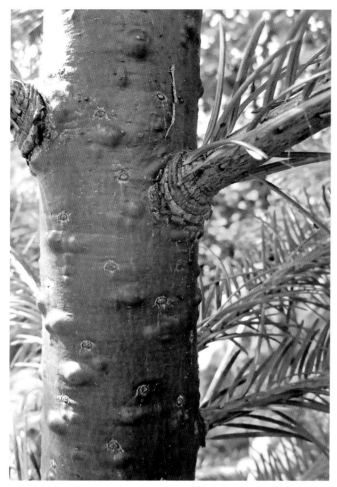

Douglas fir (*Pseudotsuga menziesii*) bark essential oils contain terpenes

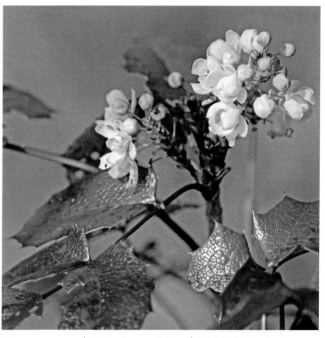

Oregon grape (*Berberis aquifolium*) is rich in berberine, an alkaloid

Phytochemistry in action

Using plants in common ailments

Many plant constituents have desirable actions in providing immediate aid for common ailments (see table on following page). Knowledge of the phytochemistry of plants may be helpful in explaining the actions of individual plants, but is not essential for using them. If treatment of acute conditions is given then it must always be followed through, for example by keeping the person warm, accompanying them home, checking on how they are over the following 24 hours, and referring to a qualified clinical practitioner if symptoms do not resolve. Acute treatment provides short-term relief and encourages healing: it does not take the place of a full consultation with a medical practitioner or professional medical herbalist who will take a detailed case history in which medical history, medications, systems, diet etc. are considered. Immediate aid for minor complaints with herbal remedies may involve herbs offering anodyne pain relief. Further action may be anti-inflammatory providing reduction of swelling, redness and heat or antispasmodic to relax muscles and reduce tension. Other helpful actions would be to soothe irritation (demulcent or emollient) and also to provide some antiseptic or antimicrobial effect. As a general rule when dealing with cuts, bites, bruises, first make sure the area is clean. However, it is important to know your plants! Always seek advice from a qualified clinical practitioner if symptoms persist! Some conditions should always be

Herbal actions and some common ailments

Herbal action	Example of plant
Astringent – an action of plants that are rich in tannins which reduce secretions. The effect of the tannins is styptic, ideal for stopping blood flow.	Bramble (*Rubus fruticosus*) has both leaves and roots with astringent effects, used in folklore for many skin disorders from spots, sores to burns and boils. Yarrow (*Achillea millefolium*) is an example of a vulnerary herb that promotes wound repair. The effect of stopping a nosebleed was traditionally achieved by rolling up and inserting a leaf into the nose.
Anti-inflammatory – many plants contain compounds which have an anti-inflammatory action.	Meadowsweet (*Filipendula ulmaria*) contains natural aspirin-like chemicals in the flowering tops and can be used in a tea to reduce pain. Willow species (*Salix alba, S. diaphnoides*) contain substantial tannin and salicin in the bark and this can be used fresh or dried.
Antiseptic – an antiseptic action is especially found in plants containing aromatic oils or volatile ingredients.	Pine (*Pinus* species) and larch (*Pinus larix*) are sources of resin exuding from the bark, and this can be distilled to produce a powerful antiseptic essential oil. Wild garlic (*Allium ursinum*) contains pungent, volatile ingredients rich in sulphur, and the juice of the plant can be diluted with water and applied direct.
Antispasmodic – the antispasmodic action provides a reduction of pain and tension and can be a result of constituents such as alkaloids which relax muscles.	Cherry (*Prunus* species) bark has some antispasmodic effect for the relief of dry coughs. Cramp bark (*Viburnum opulus*) contains the bitter glucoside viburnine as well as valerianic acid and can be taken in a decoction for all kinds of cramps and spasms.

referred for medical help, and these include trauma, severe bleeding, breathing difficulties, very high temperature (especially in children), eye problems and severe allergic response.

Medicinal plants to grow and use today

There are thousands of plants which have medicinal uses, far too many to list here. The many traditional uses of medicinal plants, including trees and shrubs, are being revealed through research evidence, though much more remains to be done in terms of clinical studies. Medicinal trees and shrubs provide a win-win outcome, since not only can they supply complex and efficacious remedies but they also help to improve the environment. In the table on pp.23-24, you can see a quick access list of the 40 trees and shrubs which are fully detailed in the Part 2 Directory in this book. These trees and shrubs have been selected to provide a sample for possible inclusion in a medicinal forest garden. Listed alphabetically by common name, each plant is also identified by its Latin species name. The parts used with sample preparations and indications are given. Cultivation details are also provided for each plant including likely maximum height, climate zone, and soil and light preferences. If you turn to Appendix 3 you can see a further alphabetical list of 50 herbaceous plants summarising cultivation details and therapeutic uses, that may be grown and used alongside medicinal trees and shrubs.

Quick access listing of 40 trees and shrubs in Part 2 Directory

Common name	Latin name	Parts used	Sample indications	Sample preparations	Potential height (m)	USDA climate zone	Soil preference	Sun and shade needs	Page no. in this book
Alder buckthorn	*Frangula alnus*	Bark, berries	Constipation	Powder, tincture	5	3	Moist acid soil	Sun or light shade	p.161
Arbor vitae	*Thuja occidentalis*	Leafy twigs	Colds and flu, warts	Infusion, tincture	15	3	Moist well-drained soil	Sun or light shade	p.216
Ash	*Fraxinus excelsior*	Bark, leaves, seeds	Arthritis, viral infections	Infusion, poultice, powder	30	4	Most moist soils	Sun	p.163
Bilberry	*Vaccinium myrtillus*	Leaves, fruit	Poor circulation, cystitis, high blood fats	Infusion, tincture	0.5	3	Well-drained acidic soil	Light shade	p.221
Bird cherry	*Prunus padus*	Bark, fruit stalks, resin	Dry cough, cystitis	Decoction, syrup, tincture	16	3	Most moist soils	Sun or light shade	p.195
Black chokeberry	*Aronia melanocarpa*	Fruit, leaf	Respiratory infections	Fruit leather, infusion, syrup	2	5a	Most soils	Sun or light shade	p.126
Blackcurrant	*Ribes nigrum*	Leaves, fruit	Sore throat, colds, flu, cystitis, stress	Gargle, glycerite, infusion, tincture	1.8	4	Moist acid soil	Sun or light shade	p.201
Black mulberry	*Morus nigra*	Leaves, fruit	Lowering blood sugars, colds, sore throat	Infusion, tincture, gargle	10	5	Moist well-drained soil	Sun or light shade	p.187
Broom	*Cytisus scoparius*	Flowering shoots	Hypotension, fluid retention, arthritis	Infusion, tincture, decoction	2	5	Dry acid soil	Sun or light shade	p.144
Chaste tree	*Vitex agnus-castus*	Leaves, fruit	Premenstrual tension, menopause	Infusion, inhalation, tincture	3	8a	Dry or well-drained soils	Sun	p.227
Cramp bark	*Viburnum opulus*	Bark	Painful periods, threatened miscarriage, poor circulation	Powder, tincture	3	3	Most moist soils	Sun or light shade	p.224
Dog rose	*Rosa canina*	Leaves, flowers, fruit	Infections, cardiovascular and degenerative diseases	Decoction, infusion, syrup	3.5	3	Most well-drained soils	Sun	p.203
Douglas fir	*Pseudotsuga menziesii*	Leaves, bark, resin	Coughs, colds, sore throats	Hydrosol, inhalation, infusion	60	5a	Moist well-drained acid soil	Sun	p.198
Elder	*Sambucus nigra*	Flowers, fruit	Colds and flu	Infusion, syrup, tincture, vinegar	6	5	Most moist soils	Sun or light shade	p.213
Fig	*Ficus carica*	Fruit, leaves, latex	High cholesterol, skin diseases	Infusion	6	8	Most soils	Sun	p.155
Forsythia	*Forsythia suspensa*	Flowers, fruits, leaves	Sore throats and colds, urinary infection	Infusion, decoction, syrup	3	5	Most soils	Sun or light shade	p.158
Fringe tree	*Chionanthus virginicus*	Root and stem bark	Liver and gallbladder disorders	Tincture	5	5a	Rich moist soil	Sun or light shade	p.139
Ginkgo	*Ginkgo biloba*	Leaves, seeds	Poor circulation, anxiety, dementia	Infusion, powder, tincture	30	5a	Most soils	Sun	p.167
Hawthorn	*Crataegus monogyna*	Flowers, leaves, fruits	Hypertension and anxiety	Infusion, tincture	10	4	Any moist soil	Sun or light shade	p.141
Horse chestnut	*Aesculus hippocastanum*	Seed, bark, leaf	Venous congestion, haemorrhoids, varicose veins	Venous congestion, haemorrhoids, varicose veins	30	4	Most soils	Sun or light shade	p.124
Juniper	*Juniperus communis*	Leaves, fruit	Cystitis, insect repellent	Infusion, tincture, lotion	9	4	Well-drained soil, slightly alkaline	Sun or light shade	p.175

Quick access listing continued

Common name	Latin name	Parts used	Sample indications	Sample preparations	Potential height (m)	USDA climate zone	Soil preference	Sun and shade needs	Page no. in this book
Lily magnolia	*Magnolia liliiflora*	Flowers, bark	Sinusitis	Decoction, infusion	4	7	Slightly acidic moist well-drained soil	Sun or light shade	p.183
Myrtle	*Myrtus communis*	Leaves, fruit	Dyspepsia, cystitis, bronchitis, skin complaints	Hydrosol, infusion, tincture, gargle	4.5	8	Dry or well-drained soil	Sun	p.189
Oregon grape	*Berberis aquifolium*	Bark, roots	Skin disorders	Decoction, tincture	3	5	Most well-drained soils	Shade	p.129
Prickly ash	*Zanthoxylum americanum*	Leaves, bark, fruit	Leg cramps, rheumatism	Powder, tincture	4	4	Moist well-drained soil especially alkaline soils	Sun or light shade	p.230
Raspberry	*Rubus idaeus*	Leaves, fruit	Painful periods, sore throat, childbirth	Gargle, infusion, tincture, vinegar	1.5	4	Moist acidic well-drained soil	Sun or light shade	p.208
Red root	*Ceanothus americanus*	Bark, leaves, root	Catarrh, sore throat and swollen glands	Infusion, tincture	1	5	Poor dry soils	Sun or light shade	p.137
Rosemary	*Rosmarinus officinalis*	Leaves, flowers	Digestion, anxiety, memory	Hydrosol, infusion, tincture	2	6	Most soils including alkaline soils	Sun	p.206
Scots pine	*Pinus sylvestris*	Leaves, bark, resin	Sinusitis, bronchitis, rheumatism	Infusion, inhalation, tincture	35	2	Light acidic soil	Sun or light shade	p.193
Sea buckthorn	*Elaeagnus rhamnoides*	Fruit, leaves	Immune support	Infusion, juice, vinegar	6	3	Most soils	Sun	p.147
Siberian ginseng	*Eleutherococcus senticosus*	Bark, leaves, rhizomes	Exhaustion and stress	Infusion, powder, tincture	3	3	Rich, moist well-drained soil	Sun or light shade	p.149
Silver birch	*Betula pendula*	Bark, buds, leaves	Skin, rheumatism and urinary complaints	Infusion, glycerite, tincture	25	2	Poor acid soils	Sun	p.131
Small-leaved lime	*Tilia cordata*	Flowers, leaves	Anxiety, insomnia, hypertension	Infusion, tincture	30	3	Moist well-drained alkaline soils	Sun or light shade	p.219
Snow gum	*Eucalyptus pauciflora*	Bark, leaves	Coughs and colds	Hydrosol, infusion	12	8	Poor well-drained soil	Sun	p.152
Sweet bay	*Laurus nobilis*	Leaves, fruit	Indigestion, colds	Hydrosol, infusion, lotion	10	7	Most well-drained soils	Sun or light shade	p.178
Sweet chestnut	*Castanea sativa*	Leaves and seeds	Coughs and colds	Infusion	30	5	Poor acid and well-drained soils	Sun	p.135
Sweet gum	*Liquidambar styraciflua*	Leaves, bark	Catarrh, coughs, colds	Infusion, lotion, syrup	30	5	Well-drained acidic soil	Sun or light shade	p.180
Violet willow	*Salix daphnoides*	Leaves, bark	Back and joint pain, headache, insomnia	Infusion, powder, gargle	6	5	Moist neutral to acid soil	Sun	p.210
Walnut	*Juglans regia*	Bark, fruit, leaves	Constipation, eczema, dandruff, athlete's foot	Infusion, tincture	30	5	Well-drained soil	Sun	p.172
Witch hazel	*Hamamelis virginiana*	Leafy twigs, bark	Skin wounds and bites, acne, eczema, sprains	Decoction, distillation	5	5	Moist acid soil	Sun or light shade	p.169

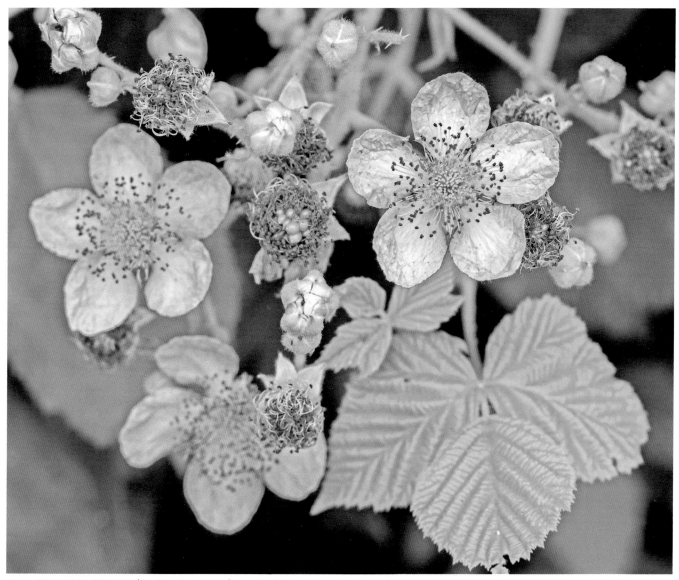

Bramble or blackberry (*Rubus fruticosus*) is a highly astringent remedy

Conclusion

Understanding of the principal components of medicinal plants helps us to see how traditional uses may have been well justified, and can also provide the basis for extending to further possible uses. The potential discovery of commercially viable new drugs may be a driver for ongoing research. However, there is much to be gained from a holistic perspective appreciating the actions and synergy of constituents in whole plant extracts, and using them in an integrated way with other health-promoting elements of diet and lifestyle.

Learning about the medicinal actions of a plant from an expert herbal practitioner is a starting point for possible use. A good way to learn more about the traditional and modern uses of plants is to go on a local walk with a medical herbalist (see page 26). These walks allow you to learn about identification features which place each plant in a particular family or genus. Plants in the same family often have similar chemical compositions, so that familiarity with the uses of one plant can give clues as to the uses of a close relation. For further information there are courses available, from use of herbs for common ailments to professional practitioner training.[53]

HERBAL MEDICINE IN ALEXANDRA PARK FOOD FOREST

LOCATION: Glasgow, Scotland

ACTIVITY: Learning about medicinal plants is an activity offered at the Alexandra Park Food Forest. Based in the heart of a major city, the Glasgow food forest was planted as part of the Helping Britain Blossom project (now the Orchard Project). As Clem Sandison (shown here) explains, a free training course was the starting point for making the initial design, bringing together local residents to learn about growing fruit and help plant an orchard for the community. Various fruiting trees and shrubs have been planted in a forest garden design, which includes a wildflower meadow and beds with herbs. The trees and shrubs are establishing well in mulched areas on an open sloping site surrounded by a public park. Some further courses are offered including a popular course introducing medicinal plants, which is run by local medical herbalist Catriona Gibson. Catriona has completed a substantial training programme in botanical therapeutics with clinical training and is a registered medical herbalist with the National Institute of Medical Herbalists. She also has much expertise in foraging and can show people how to make seasonal food and medicine preparations.

KEY POINT: Many benefits can be obtained from collaboration between forest gardens and herbal medicine practitioners to encourage interest in both edible and medicinal plants.

INFO: www.facebook.com/AllyParkFoodForest

CONTACT: www.catrionagibson.co.uk/services

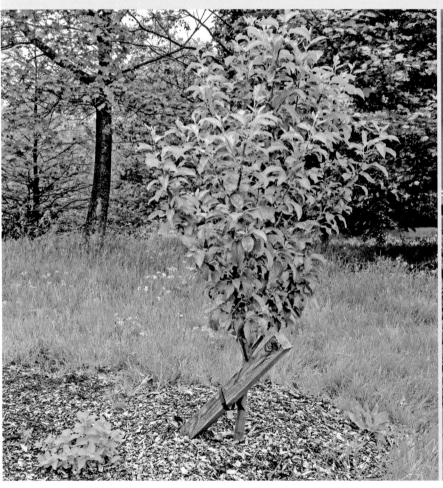

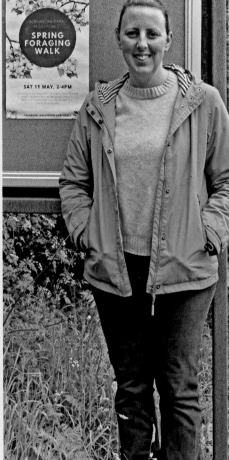

CHAPTER 2

Designing

Medicinal plants, including trees and shrubs, can be part of a planting project from a small cottage garden to a large woodland. In this chapter I aim to identify key considerations and processes involved in designing a medicinal forest garden, whether small or large. As I explain, thinking about purpose is a good starting point, followed by observation of the space available and existing resources. A design plan brings together purpose and resources. To help the design process, permaculture principles are described which help to maximise resource use and sustainability. Suggestions about choosing suitable medicinal trees, shrubs and other plants are addressed here, providing guidance on native and introduced medicinal species and their site preferences. As a brief guide to this process of planning, an assessment toolkit checklist (see on right) describes the main elements in this design process.

Identifying purpose

The starting point for any kind of planning or design involves gathering details about your overall purpose and aims. A good design is important for a forest garden since it will likely live for a long time and, although change is possible, making changes can be increasingly costly in terms of energy and other resources. Surprisingly perhaps, there may be quite a number of differing reasons for wanting to establish a medicinal forest garden. The following questions can assist in teasing out these reasons and identifying aims which can be reflected in the design.[1]

Assessment toolkit checklist

Stage of design	Elements
(a) Identifying purpose	- overall aim and objectives - ethical stance and regenerative aims - key products wanted and target audience - skills desired and any other benefits
(b) Observation and survey of site and resources	- produce base map with boundaries and topography - identify soil nature, existing species, vegetation and wildlife - list resources available on site including water and water management - factors to consider such as canopy shade, other limitations - history (including organic or other accreditation) and climate - existing skills and budget
(c) Analysis with choices and opportunities	- plan with identified zones and key features - suggested plant lists with analysis of possible uses - if commercial then retail and wholesale possibilities - costings, operations and indication of sources - design summary – overall plan, issues, possibilities
(d) Advice on implementation	- timescale - ongoing monitoring and evaluation

A. Are you keen to learn to recognise and cultivate a wide range of medicinal plants including trees and shrubs? Are you wanting to grow herbs for interest in their historical and traditional uses? Identification and accuracy will be paramount for you if recreating planting designs with significant historical plants. This might lead to a garden intended for training in botanical identification, enabling teaching and learning about herbal medicine, or perhaps a hospital or hospice garden intended to provide an environment that can promote wellbeing and health. Such a garden may not involve much harvesting but can provide a focus for learning to identify a wide range of plants and providing information about their medicinal properties amongst students, patients, visitors and the community at large.

B. Do you want to grow a selection of herbs to use for personal or family health complaints? Are you interested in harvesting medicinal plants, including trees and shrubs, and processing them to store or make your own remedies? You may desire to have greater self-sufficiency in herbal medicines for general health, common conditions and first aid. You may need sufficient quantities for hand-harvesting for a family. These medicinal plants might be integrated with other supplies in a forest garden providing fruit, nuts, firewood etc. This garden could provide small-scale harvesting of a range of plants for teas, tinctures, syrups and other preparations. Such a garden may be shared by the family, friends and volunteers so that there could be a number of users keen on gaining practical skills in growing and harvesting and making herbal preparations.

C. Are you keen to grow certain medicinal herbs, including trees and shrubs, for wider sharing, for use in a clinical practice or commercial reasons? Are you interested in making herbal products for sale? You may want to grow and harvest selected medicinal plants in substantial quantities. You may need access to specialised equipment for processing the crop, including ground preparation, weed management, dryers, cutters and grinders. The products could be dried or fresh herbs, or processed to have added value, such as powder for capsules, cut herbs for tea bags, specialist preparations such as cordials and

spirits. There could be associated activity in the project from nursery plant production to running a market stall or farm shop. The range of medicinal plant species harvested may be limited, but larger harvests will need extra help and good storage. Such a project may involve additional staff and/or trained volunteers to implement consistent quality standards for growing and production.

The above three aims are not exclusive. You might not fit clearly into any of the groups, but it will help in planning if you can identify the ways you want to use medicinal plants. Having clarified your purpose, this will be a good point at which you can identify the level of human resources already available to put into the forest garden, whether contributions of experience, labour, equipment or finance. There may be individuals involved who have positive skills to offer, for example, with experience of organic gardening approaches or making herbal medicines. Establishment and ongoing maintenance will include some labour input so a rough estimate is needed of how much help is available and how often it can be provided. Existing equipment and buildings can be identified, from hand and power tools to greenhouses and sheds. The financial input that is potentially available should be identified, whether capital spending for purchase of land, funds for purchase of plants and fencing, insurance and repairs. Once your purpose and aims are clearer, many of these human resources will begin to fit into place, or if not available will need to be sought out!

Observation and survey

Having identified purpose and aims, the permaculture design process continues with close observation of an intended site. This will assist drawing up a base map indicating boundaries and key points or areas, to which other features can be added. A survey of the site enables a record to be made of the situation or physical form (slope, features) and climate (region and microclimate), water sources, soil, existing vegetation and other ecological characteristics. These kinds of details will need to be considered when looking for a suitable site for a new project. The base map can be drawn to scale and show movement of winds, path of the sun, contours and water movement, boundaries and key features, vegetation, human, wildlife and other elements. As you record your observations you may also have ideas about how different parts of the site might be adapted or used. It is worth recording these additional ideas at this stage, so that they may be considered in finalising a design plan.[2]

Climate

Overall the 'situation' of a planting site refers to the amount of light and warmth, usually determined by the orientation and slope of the site. A site needs to be assessed in terms of the path of the sun through the seasons, as well as general climate. Local climate can be variable. Frost is less likely in coastal areas. On slopes cold air tends to move downwards, but frost pockets may occur at the bottom. Some shelter from wind may be provided by existing trees or other features such as buildings. General climate levels for a region regarding tempe-ature variation are useful, particularly to indicate likelihood of the lowest winter temperatures. This kind of information is readily indicated by zones, and Appendix 4 and 5 provide maps of climate zones for Europe and the US respectively.

Water

Existing streams, ponds and other sources of water including piped supplies are important to identify. The underlying geology and the contours of a site will contribute to the way in which water moves around, so that some areas may accumulate moisture while others are freely drained. Certain herbs, trees and shrubs positively prefer moisture while others cannot tolerate wet soil and poor drainage. Thus steep and stony areas may not suit agriculture but may be well drained and ideal for certain medicinal trees and shrubs.[3] For example, both ginkgo (*Ginkgo biloba*) and walnut (*Juglans regia*) are suitable for sloping sites.[4] For trees there is another consideration: the deeper soil condition. Some soils are 'panned' at some level, having a hard and impenetrable layer which impedes drainage and water. This can prevent deeper roots and limit tree growth beyond a certain point.

If trees are to be grown to full potential then the soil may need to be broken up at a greater depth.

Soil

A guide to the nature of the soil is to observe existing vegetation, for example, dock (*Rumex*) species are characteristic of poorly drained sites; nettle (*Urtica dioica*) grows especially well in rich soil. Previous use of a site can affect the nature of the soil, and observation of existing vegetation may be indicative of this. A distinction is often made between so-called 'ancient' woodland (existing since before 1600) and more recent woodland, and the older the woodland the more likely it will have accumulated a greater range of native species.[5] Some areas may have been cleared of trees yet retain characteristics of previous woodland such as local names or indicator plants. Wild Garlic (*Allium ursinum*) and cramp bark (*Viburnum opulus*) are two of the indicator species which point to woodland of 'ancient' standing.[6] If you have an existing woodland then you may be able to identify the range of plants occurring with one of the particular woodland communities included in a national vegetation classification system.[7] There may be plants of medicinal value already in place.[8]

Medicinal plants differ greatly in their soil preferences, some being very tolerant and others not. A simple soil texture test indicator is to manually feel the soil.[9] A sandy soil will not readily form into a ball and breaks up easily, feeling quite gritty. A clay soil will readily form a ball, feeling sticky, and does not readily break up. A loamy soil is a mixture of sand and clay. Testing the soil for fertility indicators (such as nitrogen content) and acidity can be done professionally, or alternatively you can obtain a test kit at garden centres. Many herbs will grow fairly well even in poor soils, but can vary in their requirement for acidity or alkalinity.[10] Most trees and shrubs can access nutrients when the acidity indicator (pH) is in the range 5.5-7.0. Some shrubs such as bilberries (*Vaccinium myrtillus*) prefer a very acidic soil, less than pH 5.5. The tables on p.30 and p.31 give indications of medicinal plants with preferences for acidic and alkaline soils, respectively.

Choosing a new site

You may be in a position to choose your site for a new medicinal forest garden. From the point of view of medicinal plant growing, my experience is that a site with a variety of different growing environments is best. This enables a wider range of different plant species to be included. So, for example, if you wish to include plants that need full sunlight as well as plants that prefer shade, you will need both open ground and some tree cover. Likewise, if you wish to grow moisture-loving plants then a pond or stream within or on the boundary of a site is helpful. For plants that like dry and stony soil, a free-draining slope is ideal. These environments can be created to some extent by planting trees to create shade and digging out water courses to provide drainage and water-filled areas. You may also be able to create smaller pockets of ideal conditions for particular plants, such as sheltered areas for those that are less hardy, more alkaline areas through additions of calcium and so on.

Other considerations

If you are buying or renting a site, then it is important to check a number of things:

1. Are all rights to the land available, as fishing and hunting rights may have been sold separately? There may be public rights of way across the land to consider.

2. Check neighbouring activities, as a nearby road or a farm using fertilisers and pesticides may not be ideal.

Medicinal plant suggestions for acidic soil (below pH=6.5)

Layer	Common name	Latin name	Example of use
Tree	Ash	*Fraxinus excelsior*	Leaves can be used as a laxative
	Sweet bay	*Laurus nobilis*	Leaf infusion to boost appetite and as antibacterial
	Fringe tree	*Chionanthus virginicus*	Bark used in digestive, liver and gallbladder complaints
	Elder	*Sambucus nigra*	Flower infusion and berry syrup for colds and flu
Shrub	Witch hazel	*Hamamelis virginiana*	Distilled water is astringent and anti-inflammatory, used as a skin tonic and for insect bites
Bush	Bilberry	*Vaccinium myrtillus*	Leaf infusion antiseptic and diuretic
	Blackberry	*Rubus fruticosus*	Infusion of leaves astringent for gargle and mouthwash
Herb	Elecampane	*Inula helenium*	Root antiseptic and expectorant in syrup for respiratory complaints
	Lemon balm	*Melissa officinalis*	Herb infusion carminative for digestion and nerves
	Angelica	*Angelica archangelica*	Seeds and root antispasmodic for digestive and urinary complaints
	Burdock	*Arctium lappa*	Decoction of roots used in detoxification
	Marigold	*Calendula officinalis*	Infused oil or ointment for burns, wounds, athlete's foot
	Nettle	*Urtica dioica*	Leaf infusion for arthritis and cystitis
Climber	Cleavers	*Galium aparine*	Herb infusion as a diuretic and lymphatic cleanser
	Hops	*Humulus lupulus*	Bitter herb infusion for digestion and insomnia
Ground layer	Strawberry	*Fragaria vesca*	Leaf infusion is astringent and toning

3. Is the site accessible for all people who may be involved? Examine roads and tracks to ensure you have vehicular access and parking when needed.

4. Enquire as to geological and water surveys, tree preservation orders, protected species, to clarify if any restrictions apply to the land.

5. Consider facilities in place such as shelter and toilets for people on site. Clarify if additional insurance for public liability is required for visitors and volunteers.

6. Check for protective measures such as deer fencing – if not in place then this may need to be budgeted for.

If you are clearing existing woodland in order to replant, be aware that there may be restrictions on the amount of timber which can be cut without a licence.[11] If you want to set up buildings or structures for processing and storage then there may be some planning controls to consider. In the UK, there is a category of 'permitted development' allowed in relation to 'reasonably necessary' activities for forestry operations, such as a tool store or access route.[12] However, forestry is not a clearly defined activity so some types of growing and processing may be considered as agricultural, and subject to different planning regulations. The important point here is to contact the local planning authority for further advice. See the case study on transforming a redundant conifer plantation (Holt Wood, p.32).

Medicinal plant suggestions for neutral and alkaline soil (above pH=7)

Layer	Common name	Latin name	Possible uses
Tree	Hawthorn	Crataegus monogyna	Flowers and fruits used for moderating blood pressure and as a heart tonic
	Ginkgo	Ginkgo biloba	Leaf infusion for circulation
	Sweet bay	Laurus nobilis	Leaves infused in oil as insect repellent, as an inhalation in respiratory disorders
	Bird cherry	Prunus padus	Bark decoction in syrup for persistent cough, or resin for inhalation
	Arbor vitae	Thuja occidentalis	Leafy twig tea or inhalation for respiratory complaints
	Cramp bark	Viburnum opulus	Bark in powder or tincture used as antispasmodic for period pains
Shrub	Barberry	Berberis vulgaris	Stem and root bark tincture as gallbladder tonic and antibiotic
	Juniper	Juniperus communis	Berries in infusion for cystitis, and leaf essential oil as insect deterrent
	New Jersey tea	Ceanothus americanus	Roots and bark used in respiratory complaints
	Weeping forsythia	Forsythia suspensa	Flowers and fruit are antiseptic, and used in respiratory complaints
Herb	Oregano	Origanum vulgare	Herb is antiseptic, sedative and expectorant
	Borage	Borago officinalis	Leaf infusion for fevers and respiratory complaints, seed oil for skin
	St John's wort	Hypericum perforatum	Infusion in oil or water of flowers for wounds, ulcers and skin problems
	Sage	Salvia officinalis	Leaf infusion as gargle for sore mouth or throat
	Goldenrod	Solidago virgaurea	Flowering tops infusion for urinary infections
	Mullein	Verbascum thapsus	Flowers infused in oil are used as ear drops
Climber	Honeysuckle	Lonicera periclymenum	Flowers in syrup are expectorant for respiratory complaints
Ground layer	Lady's mantle	Alchemilla vulgaris	Leaf infusion is astringent and used in diarrhoea and heavy periods
	Yarrow	Achillea millefolium	Herb infusion used in colds and flu
	Self-heal	Prunella vulgaris	Herb used in poultice for skin complaints and as an astringent in sore throat or diarrhoea

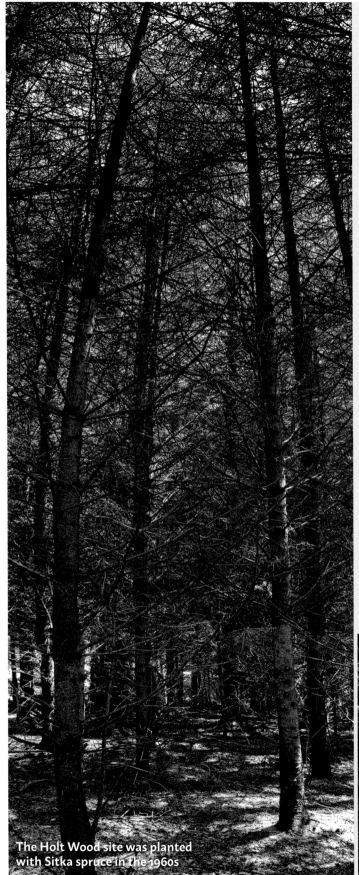

The Holt Wood site was planted with Sitka spruce in the 1960s

TRANSFORMING A CONIFER PLANTATION WITH MEDICINAL TREES

NAME: Holt Wood Herbs

LOCATION: Devon, UK

ACTIVITY: The Holt Wood Herbs project was started to provide herbal supplies for a medical herbalist practitioner and to develop a range of expertise in cultivating and harvesting medicinal trees and shrubs. Purchased in 2004, the original site of 2.5 acres was a plantation of Sitka spruce, estimated at 35-40 years of age. A management plan was prepared for felling and replanting with a mixture of introduced and native tree species. A new design based on permaculture principles was developed to incorporate a wide range of medicinal plants from upper storey to ground level. A licence was agreed with the Forestry Commission for felling the conifers, and a grant obtained towards the costs of planting trees. Since 2005, Holt Wood has developed as a flourishing medicinal forest garden with trees, shrubs and other plants, offering courses to help others.

KEY POINT: A redundant conifer plantation can be transformed by design with medicinal trees and shrubs.

INFO: www.holtwoodherbs.com

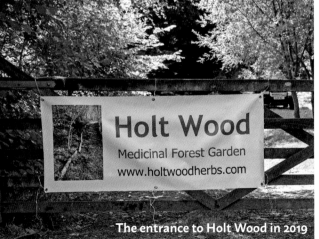

Holt Wood
Medicinal Forest Garden
www.holtwoodherbs.com

The entrance to Holt Wood in 2019

Analysis and design with permaculture principles

Producing a design plan brings together the main purpose and aims with analysis of existing resources and site, to embody the actual reality of a project. The plan can demonstrate energy efficient approaches, recycling opportunities, nutrient and water conservation, benefits of biodiversity, key features and care for the soil, and other 'whole system' ways of thinking. Many of the elements will be multifunctional. Within the plan there can be an indication of zones to show expected levels of activity or intervention. Generally, zones 0-5 are placed in relation to human habitation, the nearest being zone 0 and the furthest being zone 5. The most intense activity takes place in zone 0. The list in the table on the right draws on zones and typical activities at Holt Wood.

Other design features

Ideally, the design plan can provide plenty of edges offering opportunities for multiple layers of planting. Levels of light are so important as sources of energy for plants. Many medicinal plants will do best in sunlight or light shade, and so it is important to create spaces in the medicinal forest garden design that will remain open. One way to do this is to think in terms of open beds or areas, and another is to include wide paths or rides between woodland areas that help to improve access to various parts of the site. Water is a precious resource, and the design plan should indicate how water will be used and conserved. 'The goal is to use water as many times as possible before it reaches the sink',[13] that is, before the water is lost from the landscape. Use of ponds and swales, or ditches that lie along a contour, will help to catch water and slow it down as it drains away down a slope. The swale is designed so that it is level and water collects and then slowly soaks into the ground. In the case of Elder Farm, medicinal trees are part of the design of water management, planted along contours as swales (Elder Farm, p.34).

Energy and resource efficiency zones at Holt Wood

Zones of activity at Holt Wood	Activities
Zone 0	Centre of activities – accommodation, first aid, eating area, compost loo. This is a high maintenance, high use area.
Zone 1	Annual herbs, herbs that are often harvested for tea or flowers such as marigolds, mints, St John's wort, tool store, herb dryer, washing and processing area and other high use activities, compost bin, log store.
Zone 2	Vegetables, perennial herbs, greenhouse or polytunnel, water storage, items involving regular harvest and/or watering over a period, nursery crops, growing on cuttings, frequent use area.
Zone 3	Fruiting bushes, rides and meadow area needing repeat clearing/cutting, understorey and hedge plants involving repeat visits and picking in season such as rose, blackberry, birch, lime, additional water storage, for access at certain times of year.
Zone 4	Forestry, main crops from coppice or pollard which are annually pruned/harvested such as coppiced cramp bark, pollarded willow and witch hazel, camping, field shelters, occasional use.
Zone 5	Wild zone, where nature is in charge and little or no intervention needed apart from making paths for access, limited use and access.

MEDICINAL TREES AND WATER MANAGEMENT

NAME: Elder Farm

LOCATION: Elder Farm is an off-grid medicinal herb farm established on the Ecological Land Co-operative's first site in South West England.

ACTIVITY: Helen Kearney, medical herbalist and husband Stuart have goals of reconnecting people with sustainable growing methods and with the amazing healing power of plants. Their 5.5 acre herb farm is based on permaculture principles, and has successfully gained organic accreditation. The site slopes, and is wet in winter and dry in summer. Medicinal trees have been planted along contour lines in order to create 'tree swales', such as elder (*Sambucus nigra*) and witch hazel (*Hamamelis virginiana*), and have been mulched to help their establishment. The trees will provide medicinal supplies and help to manage water, by slowing run-off and spreading water horizontally to reduce soil erosion. Leaf fall will add organic matter to the soil, and further useful plants such as meadowsweet (*Filipendula ulmaria*) can be interplanted. Elder Farm has developed as a successful business based on a variety of activities, including wholesale herbs and herbal preparations for sale, and herbal training programmes.

KEY POINT: By design, trees can have multiple functions, for example being used to help manage water run-off as well as to provide medicinal supplies.

INFO: www.elderfarm.co.uk

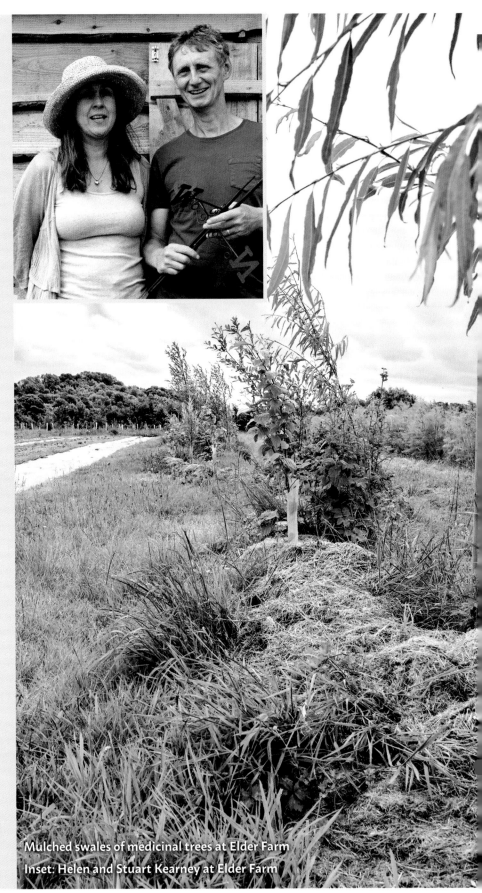

Mulched swales of medicinal trees at Elder Farm
Inset: Helen and Stuart Kearney at Elder Farm

Multifunctional elements

Building relationships between elements of the plan is fundamental to permaculture design. Ideally, every element can have many functions, and is placed in a way that supports others. Medicinal plants too can have a number of functions.[14] Many are also food plants for humans. For example, raspberry (*Rubus idaeus*) provides a medicinal tea from leaves, and also food from fruits. Many medicinal plant species can contribute as food plants for insects and animals, adding to biodiversity and wildlife; alder buckthorn (*Frangula alnus*) supplies a laxative bark, and is also a food plant for the yellow brimstone (*Gonepteryx rhamni*) butterfly.

There are a number of ways in which medicinal plants can contribute to soil improvement in addition to their natural leaf fall adding to the soil layer:

- Coppiced willow (*Salix* species) and other coppiced shrubs provide waste from unused smaller stems, which is an ideal source for making chipped mulch.

- Comfrey (*Symphytum officinale*) and other deep-rooting plants access soil nutrients and supply them to the soil through subsequent leaf fall.

- Broom (*Cytisus scoparius*) and other members of the pea family (Leguminaceae) add nitrogen to the soil through nitrogen-fixing bacteria in nodules on their roots. A study of walnut trees found that they benefitted from planting with companion trees, specifically when grown with nitrogen-fixing autumn olive (*Elaeagnus umbellata*); they showed greater height and nitrogen levels, fewer multiple stems and finer branches.[15]

Medicinal plants can benefit from mixed plantings in other ways, such as from other plants contributing ground cover, while others can encourage beneficial insects. Weed management is a function of many lower-growing medicinal plants. For example, strawberry (*Fragaria vesca*) provides ground cover as well as medicinal tea from leaves and edible fruits (more ground cover plants are suggested in the following section). Some herbs with flowering tops can contribute benefits of attracting insect predators, such as wild carrot (*Daucus carota*). Aromatic medicinal plants can also help deter insect pests. Within agroforestry, an unexpected beneficial interaction between species has recently been identified: lemon balm (*Melissa officinalis*) has a higher essential oil content when planted in alleys between cherry trees grown for timber.[16] It is likely that the delay to flowering in lemon balm which arises due to the extra shade of the trees is a contributory factor to increasing essential oil in the leaves.

Plant selection and sustainability

Choice of plants to produce planting lists should take into consideration what we already know about climate breakdown effects. The key changes expected, apart from an overall increase in temperature, are extreme weather events including heat waves and drought, intense rainfall and flooding, increasing wind, storm and fire frequency.[17] In relation to European agroforestry, it has been recommended that additional 'adaptive capacity'[18] is needed to increase resistance and resilience. Greater variety in tree species and more structural diversity using trees of different ages and sizes are recommended. Introducing trees with provenances from more southerly distributions may also be beneficial. Such measures can help to maintain the general health of trees to resist weather disturbance and disease. A diverse planting such as that of a medicinal forest garden is likely to have the most resilience in the face of environmental change.

The medicinal forest garden is designed to accommodate a variety of plants in layers from the ground to the overstorey. As we saw above, key considerations are the situation, climate and the nature of the soil, from acid to alkaline, and whether soil has good drainage or often remains waterlogged. We also have to think about how plants can be managed in the longer term and those plants which may need particular care. It is a good idea to locate trees and shrubs in a design sketch before planning other planting. In a forest-like environment, shade is largely determined by the height of trees and the extent of tree canopy. In the early stages of establishment of a medicinal forest garden, it may be hard to imagine that shade will ever be a problem.

As trees establish they will soon begin to limit the light reaching the understorey and ground level. The extent of shade can vary with the species of tree, for example lime trees (*Tilia* species) with fairly large leaves, produce more shade than smaller leaved trees such as birch trees (*Betula* species).[19] However, many herbs will tolerate a light or dappled shade such as that found along a woodland edge, and it makes sense to include plenty of edges, whether straight or curved, where more light-demanding plants will be comfortable.

Layers

Choosing plants for the medicinal forest garden involves considering the niches available at various levels of light availability. For example, there may be an overstorey of taller trees, such as birch (*Betula pendula*), oak (*Quercus* species) and limeflower (*Tilia cordata*), and an understorey of smaller trees and large shrubs, such as hawthorn (*Crataegus monogyna*), Siberian ginseng (*Eleutherococcus senticosus*) and prickly ash bark (*Zanthoxylum americanum*). Then there is a layer of smaller shrubs and taller perennial herbs, such as wormwood (*Artemisia absinthum*) and mullein (*Verbascum thapsus*). Some of these herbs can provide effective ground cover in shadier areas, such as greater celandine (*Chelidonum majus*). Layers of lower growing herbs and surface-spreading plants can fill in the gaps, providing further ground cover, such as lady's mantle (*Alchemilla vulgaris*), lungwort (*Pulmonaria officinalis*), self-heal (*Prunella vulgaris*) and yarrow (*Achillea millefolium*).

Extra layers

In amongst the other layers of plants is a climber layer; these are plants which can grow over structures of trees and shrubs, such as honeysuckle (*Lonicera periclymenum*), hops (*Humulus lupulus*), passionflower (*Passiflora incarnata*) and woody nightshade (*Solanum nigra*).

There is another layer which is not always considered. This is a 'surface' layer of plants, including lichens, mosses and fungi, usually attached to other plants or may be found on features such as dead wood or stones. There is insufficient space here to cover these kinds of plants in much detail, so just a few examples will be mentioned. Lichens are symbiotic partnerships of fungi and algae or bacteria, and many are slow-growing and good indicators of levels of pollution.[20] *Usnea* species are lichens found worldwide growing on host trees, which have antibacterial properties, with many traditional uses including poultices for skin infections and burns, and teas for respiratory complaints. There is antioxidant potential of polyphenols shown in a review of more than 75 different lichens,[21] while other actions include antiviral, antibiotic and antitumour.[22] Mosses have also long been used in wound dressing, having benefits in stopping blood flow and reducing inflammation and infection.[23]

It is worth considering whether a design can incorporate fungi. Pharmacological uses of mushrooms are now much better understood.[24] Mushrooms provide a source of polysaccharides, particularly beta-glucans and polysaccharide-protein complexes with anticancer and immunostimulating properties. The fruiting bodies also contain triterpenes, lactones, alkaloids and other compounds.[25] Some fungi require inoculation of suitable logs (such as shitake, *Lentinus edodes*) but there are also those that will probably arrive of their own accord, such as turkeytail (*Trametes versicolor*). If you are keen to include mushrooms then you should plan for some areas of dead wood and log piles in relatively shaded parts of the site.

Plant guilds for health

The above sections focus on multiple functions in the forest garden design, and suggest combinations of plants that may work well together. In permaculture design, there is an emphasis on integrating plants together in guilds. A plant guild provides a focus on a selection of plants which will comfortably grow and complement each other, maximising space and resources, and often benefiting from each other's contribution.[26] Many herb gardens reflect the idea of guilds in bringing together selections of herbs that can grow well together, although these combinations may be limited to one or two herbaceous plant layers. Within a design for the medicinal forest garden, we can be more adventurous in

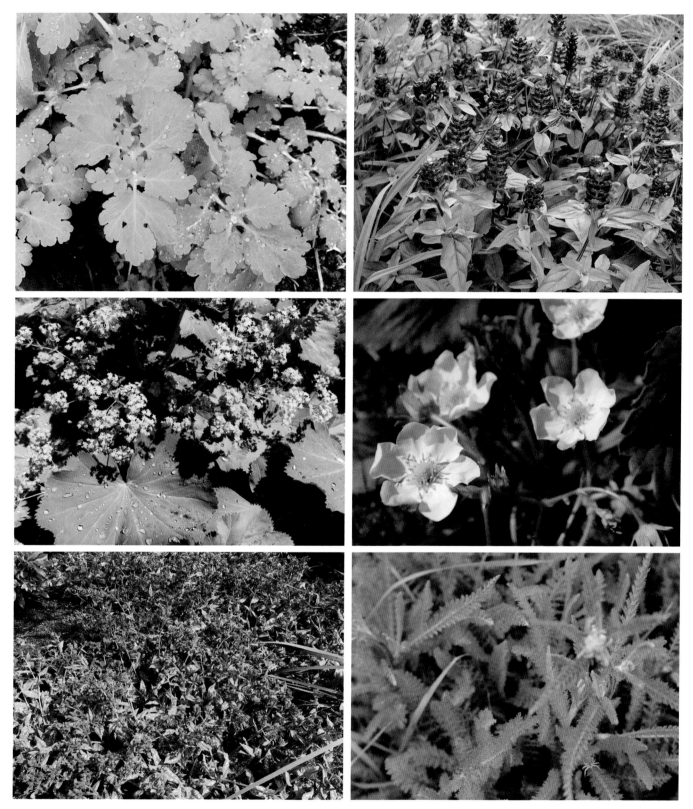

Ground cover plants include (left to right, from top) greater celandine (*Chelidonum majus*), selfheal (*Prunella vulgaris*), lady's mantle (*Alchemillla vulgaris*), strawberry (*Fragaria species*), lungwort (*Pulmonaria officinalis*) and yarrow (*Achillea millefolium*)

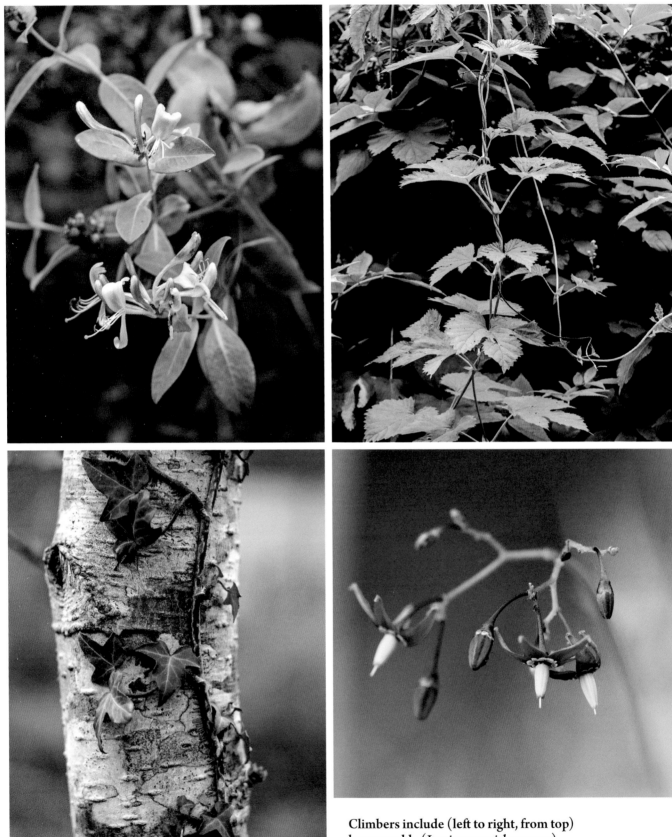

Climbers include (left to right, from top)
honeysuckle (*Lonicera periclymenum*),
hops (*Humulus lupulus*), ivy (*Hedera helix*) and
woody nightshade (*Solanum nigra*)

choosing healing plants of many layers. A starting point for designing a medicinal plant guild may be a focus on particular health issues or complaints. For example, we could focus on a guild of medicinal plants suitable for use in women's health conditions. This guild would include a tree layer of cramp bark for period pains and chasteberry for hormonal regulation. A shrub layer would include raspberry for a uterine tonic. A herb layer could consist of nettles for supporting iron levels and yarrow for cystitis. A climber might be the hop, an oestrogenic plant promoting digestion and sleep. Some further suggestions for other key health issues suited to guild creation are given in the table on the following page.

Longer-term management and coppicing

Planning for maintenance of the medicinal forest garden depends considerably on how plants are going to be used. If you have a particular interest in cutting herbs for making medicinal teas then little further maintenance may be needed. But, at some point, you have to consider how the medicinal forest garden is going to age. As the canopy of trees and larger shrubs closes over (this can happen within 10-15 years), the remaining plants may suffer and disappear, less flowering and fruiting will take place, and conditions become difficult for maintaining a diverse planting. It is good to have some idea of the longer-term size and shape of plants, as well as stronger growing plants which may come to dominate and shade or crowd out others. If plants are to be regularly coppiced then selection of species and varieties can be somewhat freer. Trees that coppice freely (that is they will produce shoots when cut to the ground) include many broadleaf species such as ash (*Fraxinus excelsior*), oak (*Quercus robur*), lime (*Tilia* species), alder (*Alnus glutinosa*), willow (*Salix* species) and sweet chestnut (*Castanea sativa*). Generally conifers will not coppice or prune readily although there are some exceptions, mainly juniper (*Juniperus communis*) and yew (*Taxus baccata*). However, 'stump culture' can be practised with some conifers – this is the practice of cutting down to a stump with some lower branches retained, then

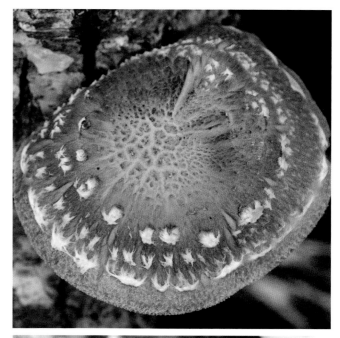

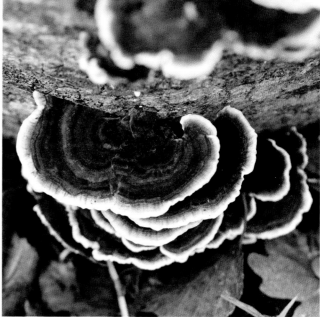

Mushrooms: baby shitake (*Lentinus edodes*) mushrooms on oak logs (top); turkey tail (*Trametes versicolor*) mushrooms on ash logs (bottom)

Medicinal plant guild suggestions

Health focus	Plants	Uses	Notes
Women's health conditions	Cramp bark Chasteberry Raspberry Yarrow Lady's mantle	Painful periods Hormonal regulation Uterine tonic Cystitis Toning for heavy periods	Coppicing will help to maintain bark and leaf production and provide light for lower plants.
Arthritis and rheumatism	Willow Ash Cramp bark Nettle	Anti-inflammatory Anti-inflammatory Antispasmodic Diuretic	These plants like rich, moist conditions, and growth might be controlled with coppicing.
Coughs and colds	Sweet gum Bird cherry Eucalyptus Magnolia Elderflower Forsythia	Colds and coughs Dry cough Colds and coughs Sinusitis Colds and flu Sore throat	These are mostly trees and shrubs that could form a hedge for flowers and leaves.
Anxiety and stress	Limeflower Siberian ginseng Passionflower Valerian Hops	Restlessness Stress Anxiety Sleeplessness Anxiety	These are woodland plants, ideal for a shady glade.
Circulation and heart support	Ginkgo Hawthorn Prickly ash Nettle Yarrow	Promotes circulation Lowers blood pressure Promotes circulation Diuretic and iron support Lowers blood pressure	Some prickly plants here could make a hedge or barrier.
Digestion and elimination	Alder buckthorn Sweet bay Wormwood Lemon balm	Bitter and laxative Digestive support Bitter Digestive support	All are plants that can do well in light shade.

allowing these to grow on, one to form a new leader.[27] North American trees that coppice freely include western balsam poplar (*Populus trichocarpa*) and sweet gum (*Liquidambar styraciflua*). Many of the less hardy trees and shrubs also coppice vigorously, including eucalyptus (*Eucalyptus* species). Aspen (*Populus tremula*) produces suckers freely but does not coppice well, and wild cherry (*Prunus avium*) produces suckers if the parent tree is damaged or felled.[28]

If left alone, newly planted trees or freshly cut coppice remain 'open' in the first 3-4 years. After 5-8 years the canopy closes and shade eliminates much of the lower levels of foliage.[29] Coppiced areas in a design are ideal for creating light conditions on a regular basis but care should be taken that they will be large enough. Generally it is considered that an area of at least 1,000m² (or one-quarter of an acre) should be coppiced at a time. The reason for this is that trees and shrubs surrounding a newly coppiced section of ground will rapidly lean and grow into the lighter area, and soon close up the tree canopy. This problem may also affect paths and rides, and so it is worth considering wider access routes through the wooded areas. In smaller sites, slow-growing or smaller varieties of trees should be selected unless regular pruning or coppicing and pollarding is carried out (see Medicinal Cottage Garden, opposite).

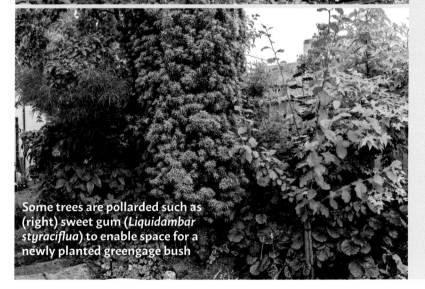

DESIGNING A MEDICINAL FOREST GARDEN FOR A SMALL SPACE

NAME: Medicinal cottage garden in Devon

LOCATION: A small Devon garden, measuring barely 7m by 10m, associated with a cottage originally built in the sixteenth century.

ACTIVITY: This cottage garden was taken over in 1990 by a medical herbalist, and was a bare grassy lawn sloping down towards the house. The soil was heavy and calcium-rich due to decades of chucking out broken pots and other household waste. Now the garden has been terraced and planted with multiple layers of medicinal herbs, arranged according to plant preferences, in addition to culinary herbs for the kitchen. A stone wall and small greenhouse provide shelter for less hardy plants. Warmth-loving Mediterranean herbs like sage and lavender are placed by the sunny wall, while moisture-loving herbs are situated around a small pond. A range of trees and shrubs have been added over the years, kept to manageable size by pruning, including alder buckthorn (*Frangula alnus*), barberry (*Berberis* spp.), fig (*Ficus carica*), fringe tree (*Chionanthus virginicus*), ginkgo (*Ginkgo biloba*) and mulberry (*Morus nigra*). Frequent pruning has the advantage of providing small harvests for medicinal purposes and plenty of young woody growth is available for propagation of medicinal trees and shrubs.

KEY POINT: Limited space is not such a drawback if medicinal plants can be grown in multiple layers, ideal for small harvests and also to provide propagation material from specimen plants.

'This small garden includes (left) alder buckthorn (*Frangula alnus*) and (right) herbs such as lady's mantle (*Alchemilla vulgaris*) and wormwood (*Artemisia absinthum*)

Some trees are pollarded such as (right) sweet gum (*Liquidambar styraciflua*) to enable space for a newly planted greengage bush

Designing with special care plants

Some plants have reputations as being dangerous, and special care is needed if they may be found growing in the area, or are to be included in the medicinal forest garden. Physically, certain plants are especially thorny or irritating and harvests require careful handling, so that protection is needed with stout gloves, such as prickly ash (*Zanthoxylum americanum*). Some plants look good enough to eat, for example red berries of the guelder rose (*Viburnum opulus*), but are so bitter they're practically inedible. The berries of potato (*Solanaceae*) family members such as deadly nightshade (*Atropa belladonna*) are toxic and can seriously affect the nervous system. Certain parts of a plant may be toxic while other parts are actually edible, such as the poisonous seeds of yew (*Taxus baccata*) in their edible red fleshy coating. Harder to distinguish though, and extremely toxic, are some alkaloid-containing plants of the carrot (Apiaceae) family, for example wild angelica (*Angelica sylvestris*) may be confused with hemlock (*Conium maculatum*) which contains toxic alkaloids.

While a dangerous reputation may be deserved in a few cases, and such plants are best avoided, most plants are safe if correctly identified, treated with respect and used in appropriate quantities. Ideally, a practical way forward is to carry out a risk assessment as to whether any plants may be mistaken, eaten, handled or used inappropriately. The risk assessment should also consider people who may be unfamiliar with these plants and associated risks and how they can avoid them, such as children or visitors. The risk of harm can be significantly reduced by ensuring clear advice is given to enable accurate plant identification, making people aware of possible dangers. In some cases these special care plants can be included as teaching aids to assist learning about the risks.

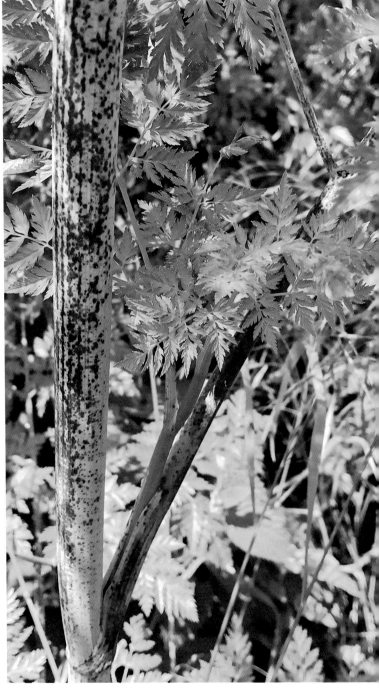

Poisonous hemlock (*Conium maculatum*) has purple blotches on the stem

Introduced medicinal plant species

A forest garden based solely on native species would be very limited in the range of crops produced.[30] Native plants can provide a range of medicinal uses but then we would have a much-reduced repertoire of herbal remedies. With regard to introduced medicinal plants in the UK, there are a number of considerations that I think are relevant, including past and present use, environmental benefits and future climate change. Firstly, there are many plants well established in the herbal dispensary which have been imported and widely used in Europe for many years, from Oriental herbs and spices to barks and roots from the Americas and herbs from the tropics. Thus, we already have a well-established tradition of use of introduced medicinal remedies. Second, a large proportion of Asian and North American plants that thrive in a temperate climate have been shown, often as ornamentals, to succeed in UK and European conditions. If we can grow these ourselves then we may help to offset the environmental costs of transporting these plants from other countries. Third, as climate changes and habitats are destroyed, we must consider greater use of cultivated plants in place of plants which are over-harvested or struggling in their native habitats. In order to maintain a range of medicinal actions for treating all kinds of complaints, we may need to further develop substitutes for threatened plants, whether native or introduced. For these reasons, overall, I think that it is acceptable to benefit from selected desirable introduced trees, shrubs and other medicinal plants, provided that they are well managed.

Invasive plants

Understanding the spread of plants worldwide is fundamental to appreciating the role of invasive plants in responding to imbalances in the environment. A plant that is medicinal in one region may be invasive in another, yet may have potential benefits in controlling pollution or restoring landscape.[31] However, some introduced plant species are a problem due to uncontrolled and opportunistic spreading by seed or root. I recommend avoidance, unless a specialist control and management plan can be formulated. This is because any medicinal benefit is likely to be outweighed by environmental disadvantages which may be very difficult to control or reverse. The key to the control of invasive species is early recognition and intervention. The advice of the UK Department for Environment, Food and Rural Affairs (DEFRA) is for land managers to have a strategy.[32] Only a minority of non-native species are environmentally harmful. Prevention and early intervention are much more successful and cost-effective than later control or eradication – thus it is important to have effective early warning systems. However, if a plant can be managed effectively, then it may be appropriate to use. For example, buddleia (*Buddleja asiatica*) from Asia is considered invasive in the UK and Australia – yet it could provide medicinal benefits since the leaves give an essential oil on distillation containing monoterpenes and sesquiterpenes with antibacterial action against pathogens such as *Shigella boydii*.[33] In the Part 2 Directory listings I have indicated where plants are regarded as potentially invasive, so that this can be taken into account when choosing plants.

Planting numbers and spacing

After deciding on which trees, shrubs and other plants are desired, then the next step is to determine the number of particular trees and shrubs needed. For example, several elder trees may be sufficient to produce enough harvest of elderflowers for making cordial or dried tea for a household. In contrast, several hundred elder trees might be required for commercial planting and harvest. Having approximate numbers of plants will allow a costing. A sketch design using the base map and cut-out pieces of card to represent key features, trees and shrubs is a good way to play around with a design to see what can be fitted in. Areas for smaller plants, climbers and ground cover can also be designated on the base map. Spacing of plants will be a key element of any plan, and more space is often needed between plants than you might think. A wider spacing of trees and shrubs means fewer plants and lower cost, and also less thinning, but can lead to slower growth rates at early stages due to lack of mutual protection.[34] In plantations, trees are usually spaced very close together at 1.5-2.5m, so that a density of 2m × 2m gives 2500 plants per hectare. This kind of spacing may be appropriate if canopy cover is desired at an early stage, and thinning is planned. Where trees are intended to be grown as standards, a wide spacing of 1m × 10m gives 100 plants per hectare, and this would be suitable for specimen trees allowed to grow to their full size. A common mistake when planting new trees and shrubs is to plant them too close together, as even smaller trees may need to be spaced at least 3-5m apart, depending on the likely crown size at maturity. A sketch of the proposed planting can help to identify realistic spacing. Closer spacing can be considered if you are going to regularly coppice medicinal trees and shrubs, for example cramp bark (*Viburnum opulus*) can be as close as 1m, and this approach fits well with use of bark from 2-3 year old trees.

Changes in design and practice

Although a design plan may appear to have considered all aspects of a proposed project, it is unlikely that everything will turn out perfectly. Most permaculture designs build in a monitoring and review process to evaluate progress towards the original aims. As you go about the medicinal forest garden, you will notice things that need attention. In terms of care of the environment, there may be plants that could do with more light and less competition, moist areas that could be transformed with the addition of more suitable plants, structures that need repair, and other enhancements to consider. In terms of care of people, there may become apparent a need for a restful seat or somewhere to relax, improved access with wider paths, tree branches that should be taken down for safety, additional training needs and so on.

In terms of productivity and ethical sharing, there may be new developments that could be added to the design in order to boost harvests or reach new audiences. You may find too that your aims have shifted as you realise the further possibilities ahead, so that longer-term changes are needed. Ideally the design plan should start out with a view over 10 years, and be reviewed at least every five years.

If you are not already committed to monitoring and recording progress in relation to your design plan, then you should start right now. You can keep notes in a diary format (we do this at Holt Wood using an A4 diary, each double page spread ruled up into five columns so that we can easily compare five years at a time). Alternatively, you can set up folders with separate sections for

(a) inputs (such as hours of labour, plants brought in, tools, manure and straw and other soil additives),

(b) observations (animals, insects, wild flowers, weather, first flowering, rainfall),

(c) operations (hours spent on site, repairs made, activities, visitors and volunteers),

(d) outputs (species harvested, weight of produce, number of items etc.).

You can also add photographic and video evidence to the records. The sooner you start keeping records, the sooner you will find that these written notes quickly build into a fascinating record of your journey with a medicinal forest garden. These records can be used to support future planning, and are essential if you wish to move further towards accreditation and commercial production (more on this in Chapter 7).

CHAPTER 3
Establishing and Maintaining

In this chapter you will find advice on establishing medicinal trees, shrubs and other plants, from initial planting to ongoing sustainable management. Suggestions are given which may be applicable in both small and larger scale planting, based on organic management approaches. Good site preparation is an important starting point for success, followed by planned planting and protection. Improvement and maintenance of soil condition are emphasised here, including use of a range of mulches. The practices of coppicing and pollarding in both small and large plantings are described for ongoing management and sustainable harvests. Finally, there is some consideration of how to monitor ongoing progress and change. In this chapter I also include risk assessment and health and safety aspects, with suggestions about tools needed.

Establishing and maintaining a medicinal forest garden is likely to require more intervention than maintaining a natural woodland. One of the aims of forest gardening is to mimic nature and produce a relatively steady state with considerable self-maintenance. However, without intervention, new woodland is likely to continue evolving into a full canopy, and no garden is likely to continue to be fully productive without some management. Rather than seeing natural regeneration alone as providing for continuing supplies, the medicinal forest gardener has to take an active management approach to ensure future supplies. Initially, this involves the establishment of a range of native or introduced plant species, promoting a multi-layered and biodiverse habitat. For ongoing medicinal plant harvests, there will be more interventions which promote the shape or form of plants required,

such as coppicing and pollarding. These are processes which adjust the layers in a less than natural way, yet they can prolong life and result in sustainable harvests.

Site preparation and planting season

A forest garden is likely to have a number of layers, from low ground plants up to shrubs and trees of various sizes. If you are starting with a 'clear' site such as a field then the larger elements, the trees and some shrubs, will be the ones to be established initially (later in this section there are suggestions for adding plants to existing woodland). To implement the design plan, you need to consider the environmental conditions (planting season, site conditions, irrigation needs), additional resources (site preparation, soil mulches, adequate protection), as well as personnel (those doing the planting and the tools and training that they will need). The best time for planting trees and shrubs is in the winter dormant period. The timing of the planting season for bare-root tree seedlings is partly determined by moisture requirements for root growth which continues in autumn for up to two weeks after shoot growth finishes, and restarts earlier than spring shoot growth. Late autumn to winter planting allows for a period of root growth before bud break. So late October to late November is the earliest time, though evergreens from warmer climates prefer to grow into a warming soil so spring planting is somewhat better for them, that is February to March. Other herbaceous plants may be added in spring or after the last frosts depending on hardiness. All plantings can suffer in a dry spring as the roots need to penetrate and establish in the surrounding soil, and increasing water demand from the foliage causes stress. Container-grown stock can be planted throughout the year, so long as moisture needs can be met, and it is important to keep the root system as intact as possible when removed from the container. Irrigate directly after planting and for some weeks afterwards, keeping soil weed-free and mulched.[1]

Clearing the site

Site preparation is needed to help ensure good establishment. Clearfelling, that is the removal of some or all of the existing trees, may be needed on some sites such as old conifer plantations. Clearance of such sites is likely to need professional forestry contractors unless you are prepared to undergo training in the safe use of chainsaws. Forestry contractors can also advise on the

sale of timber or process it for later use on site. Care is needed to avoid too much soil compaction from the use of vehicles to remove logs; alternatively horse-drawn extraction of logs may be possible. Remaining brushwood should be stacked for removal or burned in several different sites to avoid damaging the soil (the wood ash can be stored under cover for later use as a mulch to supplement nutrition of fruiting trees and shrubs). An alternative use of logs and brushwood can be considered in constructing hugelkultur raised beds.[2] If the site is waterlogged, unless trees are to be planted which will appreciate damp conditions, then drainage channels will be needed. Scrub can be cleared using a tractor-mounted flail mower or a brush cutter. Where machines are not used, screefing is the removal of top surface vegetation with a spade or mattock, so removing competing plants.[3] Your design plan should provide locations for planting and this can be used to mark out the ground. In some areas, a deer fence (at least 2m high) will be needed around the planting area to ensure that plants can establish well, otherwise, plants may need individual protection from predators (see the section

LEFT TO RIGHT
Site clearance in a conifer plantation
After tree felling a site is marked out for planting
Deer fencing is likely to be needed in some areas

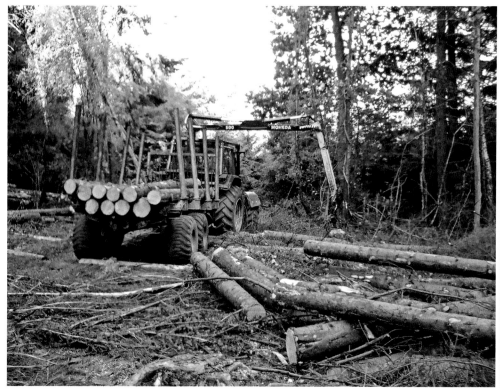
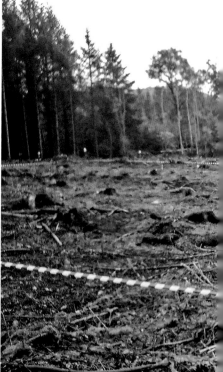

on establishing plants below). The boundaries of specific areas can be identified with string or tape stretched between posts, and posts are more readily seen with removable markers such as plastic bottles (which can then be recycled). Rows or lines can be further identified with posts or canes. Markers for individual tree and shrub locations may be used such as bamboo canes, and these may also serve as support for tree guards. Sand or pebbles can be used to outline smaller areas of planting where soil has been cleared.

Existing woodland

Planting into an existing woodland area needs some extra consideration in preparing the site. Since there are relatively few plants that grow well in full shade, it is likely that some trees or other plants will have to be cleared to make sufficient space available. In the planned context of a forest garden it is intended that plants will co-exist on an ongoing basis, often taking up niches at different levels. The main issues are access to light and the level of competition from other plants for water and nutrients. For greatest success, prepare the ground to

ensure the least competition for water and nutrients, and thin or cut back higher layers of vegetation to ensure the best possible light levels. Provide a mulch to hold back additional growth of nearby plants. Monitor to ensure that other plants do not become dominant. Repeated cutting is likely to be needed to allow new plants to become established.

Safe working practices

Whether you are doing everything yourself with family and friends, or involving paid workers and volunteers in your activities, it is essential to provide safety advice and take precautions to avoid potential injuries. Completing a risk assessment in advance which relates to the activity and location will help to identify possible problems and how they may be dealt with (see example on p.49). Ideally, advise everyone in advance of suitable clothing to wear on the day. Check the site before starting for obvious hazards and ensure tools are in good condition. Start the day with a welcome and advise on procedure if an accident or emergency arises, where to meet, location of first aid and telephone. Check that everyone

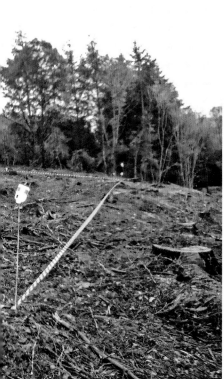
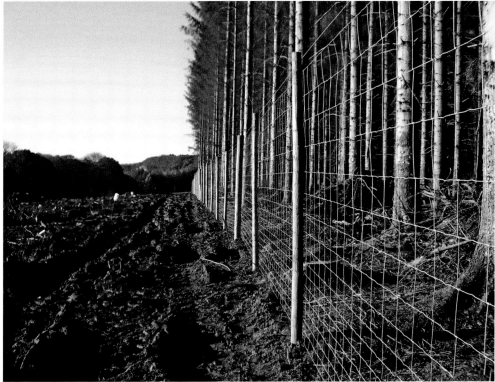

is wearing suitable shoes/boots and any other necessary protection such as long sleeves, hats and gloves. Access to toilet and rest facilities must also be considered and, if possible, provide hand washing facilities or hand sterilising gel. Provide clear instructions on tasks and make sure that equipment and procedures are explained. It may not have been formalised but there should be someone clearly responsible for overseeing planting, a person who can demonstrate and explain purpose and techniques, involve helpers in decision-making, and be contacted if there is a problem or questions about the work. The benefits of planning ahead include more effective planting, confidence and enjoyment for all, with possibilities of learning new skills.[4]

Establishing plants

Success in establishment of planting involves recognition of the following three main factors: choice of suitable species with well-grown plants with good root-to-shoot ratios; handling conditions including keeping the root ball moist with good planting technique; and good aftercare.[5] Success in planting out young trees requires us to take care to protect the roots. John Evelyn wrote of this in 1670, referring back to ancient Greek advice:

> [Take] great caution in planting to preserve the Roots, and especially the Earth, adhering to the smallest Fibers, which should by no means be shaken off, as most of our Gardners do to trim and quicken them ... not at all considering, that those tender Hairs are the very mouths and Vehicles which suck in the nutriment, and transfuse into all the parts of the Tree.[6]

John Evelyn was right in his emphasis on 'tender' roots, since tree roots can dry out within minutes of exposure and need to be covered and in the shade at all times. Plants should be wrapped in a moist cloth or in strong plastic bags to avoid damage and loss of moisture, and they should not be uncovered until the planting position is ready. It may be necessary to 'divide and wrap' bare-root plants into smaller groups before taking them to different parts of a planting site. If planting has to be delayed then bare-root trees and shrubs can be heeled in temporarily, laying them down with their roots in a shallow pit covered with soil to protect from frost or further moisture loss. Where many plants are to be put in high-density schemes, notch or 'nick' planting can be used, and this is especially suitable for bare-root seedlings. For this, a slit is cut into the ground with a spade, tree roots are inserted and the stem is held vertically while soil is firmed. Larger planting pits can be used for larger trees or shrubs in pots. Final planting should ensure that soil is level and does not encroach on the stem. After planting, mulching to conserve moisture and reduce growth of other plants around the newly planted tree is beneficial. At Holt Wood we use cardboard with organic mulch or clippings, although plastic mulch mats are available.

Young plants need to be protected from grazing animals and rodents. For protection from basal damage by voles and rabbits, tree guards of plastic spirals are available in 45cm and 60cm lengths, or larger stock guards can be used to prevent cattle or deer munching higher up the plant. Apart from fencing and plastic guards you can use prickly shrub clippings and branches, such as hawthorn or juniper, placed around the base of the plant and its growing tips. Seedlings are not usually supported with stakes as wind movement helps to trigger root growth to increase anchorage and encourage growth of the main stem. If a stake is to be used for very windy sites, then it should be about one-third of the tree height, and is usually secured upright on the windward side of the tree. Any tree tie must be removed after successful establishment and no later than two seasons after planting, otherwise it can girdle and kill the growing tree.[7]

Mycorrhizas and trees

A mycorrhiza is a symbiotic association between a fungus and a plant. The plant provides sugars for the fungus and the fungus supplies water and nutrients to the plant via the roots. Resilience in the health of trees and shrubs depends considerably on the ability to take up nutrients and water, so mycorrhizas are considered beneficial. Mycorrhizal fungi benefit from no-dig or shallow cultivation, mulching and cover crops.[8] Several

Sample risk assessment for a forest garden activity

Risk Assessment Form			
Contact name			
Organisation name, address, telephone			
Email			
Description of activity *Clearing and marking out locations and planting out seedlings in forest garden project*			
Type of hazard	Persons at risk	Controls to minimise risk	Further actions
1. Weather extremes of rain or cold	*Workers and volunteers*	*Advise participants of suitable clothing in advance* *Area under cover, either shed or tent for duration of events*	*Make spare clothing, hats and gloves available* *Contact details provided in case of need for cancellation*
2. Tripping hazard from uneven ground and roots/stumps	*Workers and volunteers*	*Warning to all visitors in pre-visit advice of uneven ground and need to wear walking shoes/boots*	*Preview paths and remove stumps where possible – otherwise mark with highly visible sticks*
3. Fire hazards from bonfires and flammable material	*Workers and volunteers*	*Fires only permitted in specific areas – brazier used for heating food and bonfires kept to a minimum*	*No smoking in area close to cars, fuel or portable gas supply* *Fire paddles available*
4. Use of hand tools such as spades, secateurs and tree saws a source of possible damage	*Workers and volunteers*	*Health and safety advice given to ensure cutting away from body* *Tools checked over prior to each use*	*Hand tools well maintained and sharpened for each event*
5. Petrol powered equipment including brushcutters has potential for accidents	*Workers and volunteers*	*Only staff with suitable experience and training to use power equipment* *Signs provided when tree-felling*	*Plan to ensure machinery not in use in area of planting*
Risk assessment completed by (name in print)	Signature		
Date of risk assessment			

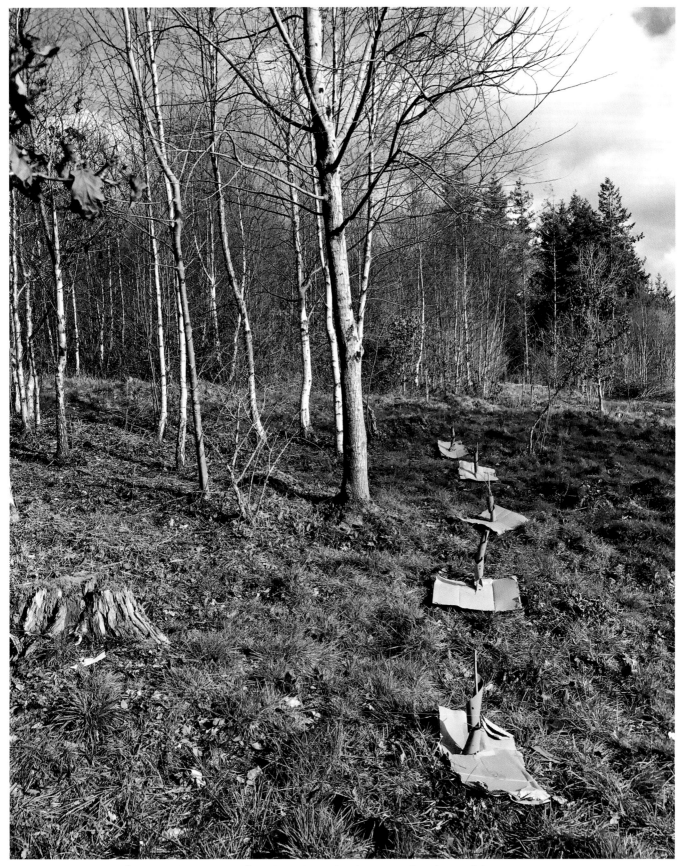

Planting witch hazel (*Hamamelis virginiana*) with cardboard to be covered with a mulch

types of mycorrhizal fungi have been identified, ectomycorrhizas (found in around 10% of plant families, mostly woody plants, for example surrounding the roots in pine, birch, oak and willow species) and arbuscular mycorrhizas (found in around 90% of plant families). Hedgerows are significant reservoirs of mycorrhizal and other beneficial organisms.[9]

Knowledge of exactly what the effects of mycorrhizas are on plants is limited, especially as most research so far has focused on intensively grown commercial crops such as tomatoes, or valuable tropical tree crops such as coffee.[10] Soil mycorrhizas can increase the nutritional value of food crops, including content of secondary metabolites of anti-oxidants such as phenolics,[11] although an increased uptake of pollutants is also possible.[12] So, it is likely that mycorrhizas can help to promote medicinal constituents in plants, especially where soils are poor or consist of heavy clay. In the context of the medicinal forest garden, mycorrhizal fungi can be encouraged through the use of inoculation of young plants. Inoculation of tree seedlings with mycorrhizal fungi may be carried out when repotting the seedlings, and can lead to faster and more effective establishment of plants. Seedlings are dipped in a solution, or granules are sprinkled into planting holes. In addition, good soil management with little disturbance and plenty of mulching is likely to encourage mycorrhizal fungi. Mulching with chipped woody material can also promote the growth of the mycorrhizal fungi to benefit trees and shrubs.

Ongoing maintenance and management

A forest garden planting of medicinal trees and shrubs does need ongoing interventions to maintain health and diversity. Without intervention, the natural processes in the formation of forests will ensure that certain species come to dominate, canopy gaps will be filled and much ground flora will disappear. Long-term observation of Lady Park Wood in the Wye Valley, a coppiced wood left undisturbed since 1944, shows a loss of diversity in flora and fauna, alongside the growth of some dangerously unstable timber trees.[13] Without active management,

the regeneration and health of many plants will be undermined. A positive approach can improve the soil, control pests and weeds, and maintain tree health.

Tools

A range of hand tools are useful in the forest garden context, particularly for pruning and coppicing, such as loppers, secateurs and tree saws. Use of a scythe may be very suitable for keeping paths and rides clear. In general, tools should be appropriate to the job in hand and must be kept sharp. It is best to have a regular schedule for cleaning and sharpening tools. Cleaning of tools is worthwhile to avoid the risk of transfering disease when working on plants. Brush off soil from forks and spades, and use a scouring pad and washing-up liquid soap. Blades can be wiped with a disinfectant or methylated spirit. It is best to keep sharp tools in containers or covered in bags. At Holt Wood we make covers for pruning tools and saws out of the legs of old jeans and these can be readily washed.

Power tools can make a considerable saving in labour especially for larger or repetitive jobs. Our early days at Holt Wood seemed to focus substantially on use of strimmers and brushcutters to enable young trees and shrubs to establish. Until recently, these mostly ran on petrol-based fuels, a potential source of pollution not particularly desirable in the medicinal forest garden. Improvements in design and reduced costs mean that cordless power tools using heavy duty rechargeable batteries can be considered. The cordless chainsaw is effective for use on cutting branches and thinning smaller trees, and a biologically degradable chainsaw oil is available. Use of power tools to cut branches or stems of trees for bark requires personnel who have suitable training and clothing as well as serviced and properly maintained power tools. The table on p.53 gives suggestions for safe working practices when cutting or coppicing trees and shrubs.

Soil improvement and ground cover

Soil in a natural forest receives inputs of nitrogen from various sources – bird and animal droppings, nitrogen-fixing bacteria in the soil, nitrogen-fixing

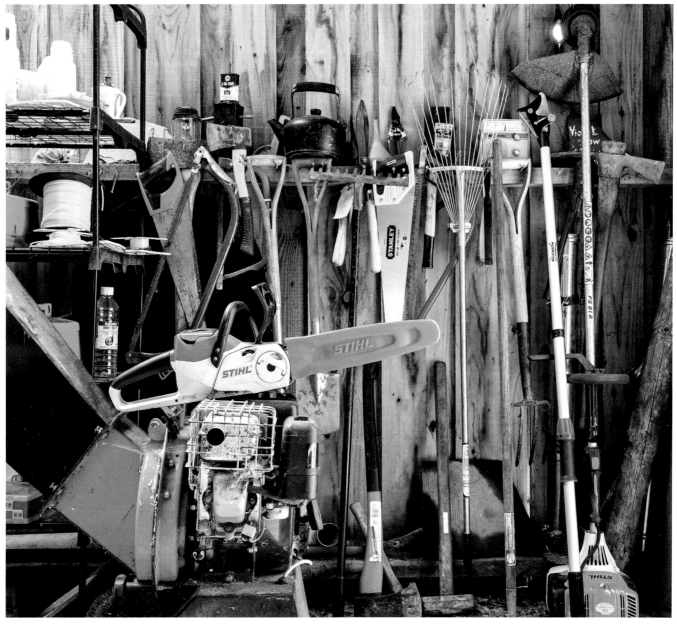

A selection of useful tools includes secateurs, tree saw, chainsaw and brushcutter

plants, and atmospheric deposits – other nutrients such as minerals are drawn from the soil aided by fungi. Additional nitrogen is not usually needed for young seedlings, indeed the application of fertilisers such as nitrates may suppress mycorrhizal development. Nitrogen-fixing trees and shrubs include bayberry (*Myrica* species) and autumn olive (*Elaeagnus* species) as well as members of the pea family (Fabaceae). In moist soils, alder (*Alnus* species) can be used to promote nitrogen. In a forest garden harvested for fruit, more nutrients may be needed to support plants and replace nutrients lost in harvests. However, most medicinal trees and shrubs, apart from those producing fruits such as hawthorn and elder, need little by way of additional nutrients. If extra fertility is needed, then it can be added as mulches around plants drawing from material grown in the forest garden such as chopped comfrey leaves, and wood ash from bonfires.[14]

Safe working in the medicinal forest garden when coppicing

Safety issue	Safety advice
Safety	• Do not stand near a tree likely to fall, or near anyone using a sharp hand tool or a power tool • Always walk forwards and look out for partially hidden stumps which are easy to fall over • If you cannot lift something comfortably (bending legs at the knee) then get help • Have a well-equipped first aid kit with dressings, bandages, adhesive tape, scissors, clean water and ensure the first aid kit is visible and accessible • Ensure that one person has first aid training which is up to date • Keep equipment and clothes out of the working area and away from fires, and be aware of wind direction which can change easily
Tools	• Ensure edge tools are sharpened every session • Show new helpers how to use a tool correctly • Dogs and children must be continually supervised if present • Never cut towards your body with an edge tool as it can bounce • Never cut above your head • When trees are felled, ensure that 180 degrees area in front is clear of people before final cut • Clear up as you work
Clothing	• Boots and gloves are usually essential, and trousers should be worn and tucked into socks • Above the waist wear clothes that allow movement but not a loose or dangling scarf or anything which can snag • Chainsaw operators must wear approved protective clothing including safety helmet, visor, ear muffs, steel capped boots, padded gloves and padded trousers • Have warm clothes to put on when you take a break

Adapted from Tabor R, Mummery C and Homewood N. (1997) *A Guide to the Techniques of Coppice Management*, Felixstowe Ferry, Suffolk: Woodland Craft Supplies, pp.4-6.

Ongoing weed suppression is helped by mulching to provide ground cover. Mulches can be organic, sheet or mineral.[15] Organic mulches include farmyard manure, leaf mould, straw, chopped prunings, bark chips, and all of these help to suppress weed seedlings, increase soil temperature and moisture, and add nutrition or fungal matter, improving soil in the longer term. Decomposition of the organic mulch depends on the kind of material and our experience at Holt Wood is that finer and damper materials decompose quickly and will not effectively suppress perennials unless placed on top of a sheet mulch. Sheet mulches include cardboard shreds, felt, fibre sheets and woven polyethylene, and these can provide some weed-suppressant capability although they can 'puddle' on top if moisture does not readily drain through. The woven fibre kinds of mulch mat material cost more but do let moisture through. Recycled cardboard costs little or nothing and decomposes more slowly if laid down in double or triple layers. Mineral mulches of coarse sand or grit can help suppress annuals and improve drainage but do not add to nutrition and can be readily re-infested by undesirable weeds. Some minerals can reduce levels of acidity, such as limestone chips. Application of surface soil treatments such as biochar is likely to be beneficial.[16] Biochar is a form of charcoal, a fine-grained residue from incomplete combustion which has a high surface area. It is extremely porous and provides for retention of water and water-soluble nutrients. It provides a habitat for the development of many beneficial soil organisms, and plant roots are more frequently found in soil areas treated with biochar.[17]

Maintaining tree health

Without regular management, the more vigorous trees and shrubs will outgrow the others, suppressing growth and reducing diversity. Light reaching the understorey and herb layer will be reduced. There are likely to be benefits in pruning to maintain health and good harvests. As with orchard fruit trees, much of pruning is focused on taking out diseased or dead branches, and enabling a good airflow around the tree or shrub. If flowers and fruits are wanted, it is important to know what sort of cycle of pruning is best. For hedgerow species such as

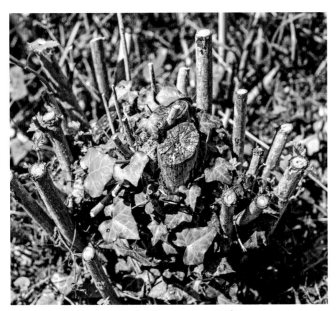

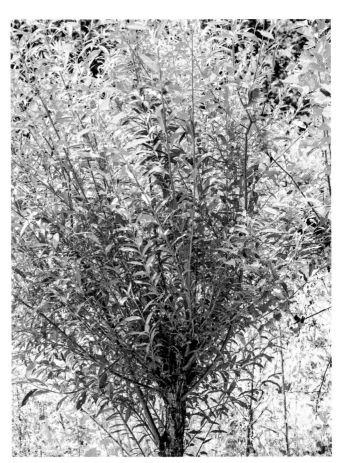

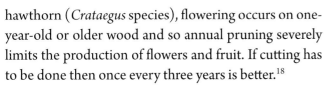
Coppiced cramp bark (*Viburnum opulus*)

Pollarded white willow (*Salix alba*)

hawthorn (*Crataegus* species), flowering occurs on one-year-old or older wood and so annual pruning severely limits the production of flowers and fruit. If cutting has to be done then once every three years is better.[18]

In the medicinal forest garden, coppicing suits some trees and shrubs well, as it keeps size down and produces supplies of young bark, for example cramp bark (*Viburnum opulus*). Coppicing is an ancient technique of cutting back established trees and shrubs to the ground in winter to produce new growth on the cut stumps.[19] In the UK, the technique was used in the past for the production of many types of wood for charcoal making, fuel, furniture, tools and many other items.[20] The coppicing technique was also used to produce considerable quantities of bark for tanning purposes. This kind of management began to decline as coke fuels were increasingly used in the eighteenth century, with further decline in the nineteenth and twentieth

centuries as coppice products were needed less, tanning increasingly used chemicals other than bark, and priorities were changed for land use. Many coppiced woodlands were abandoned or replaced.

A form of coppicing at a higher level in the tree is known as pollarding, generally done at a height of 1-2m or above. Pollarding is an ancient practice too, involving the lopping of branches back to a tree stem at variable heights, sometimes in hedgerows and also in pastures. The previously extensive use of pollarding produced animal fodder for later use, but was gradually reduced with enclosure and agricultural changes. Pollarded trees were once extremely common, although not always recorded on maps, and few massive and ancient pollards remain today. Within Europe, there are many longstanding traditions of coppicing and pollarding, and some are in continuing use in forest management.[21] The use of pollarding is particularly suitable for a number of

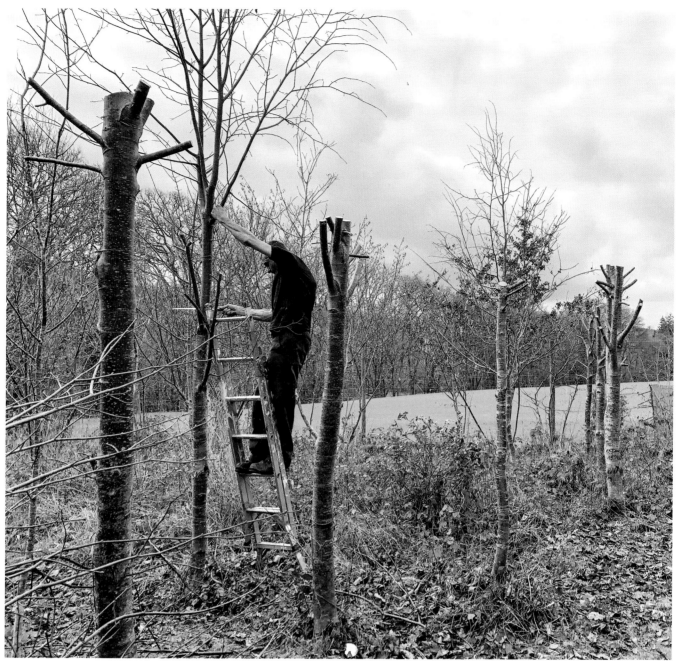

Pollarding lime (*Tilia × europea*)

medicinal trees such as willow (*Salix alba*) and lime (*Tilia × europea*). However, at Holt Wood we have found that some trees are so vigorous in responding to pollarding that they need careful subsequent management to 'thin' or reduce the number of sprouting shoots, especially white willow (*Salix alba*) and hawthorn (*Crataegus monogyna*). Pollarding at above shoulder height will require use of steps or ladders, and extra care is needed in the use of sharp/power tools to remove branches.

Tree damage and pests

Damage to trees can occur from deliberate activities of coppicing and pruning or from weather disruption and pests, and always needs to be checked.[22] Superficial wounds are repaired by the tree itself through production of a new layer of bark. The general practice is to allow wounds to heal naturally or carry out minor trimming to leave an organic, free-draining shape and the smallest possible wound size. A garlic extract can provide an antifungal wash if appropriate.[23] Typically, a large head of garlic cloves can be peeled and crushed and placed in 500ml of hot water to stand overnight. The following day the mixture can be strained and the remaining liquid diluted up to 10 times for application as a spray or wash.

Pest control does not need to involve killing all known pests. Indeed in the forest garden mimicking nature, there is more emphasis on sustainable pest management which occurs naturally through encouraging predators. The level of damage may be acceptable if sufficient harvests and plant health can be maintained. Squirrels may be a problem as they can ringbark young stems of trees. Field voles may be a problem in areas of mulch, as their tunnelling exposes roots. A varied environment can help to encourage natural predators of these creatures, providing cover for animals such as foxes and birds of prey.

Tree health

Tree health is much supported by good soil and good management, but a barrage of new diseases are being found. In the past, according to recent research, most trees were felled when comparatively young, so it was unusual for trees to survive more than 50 years. There was also considerably more pollarding in the past so that trees of a substantial age were repeatedly producing new growth. Management practices have changed to encourage the biodiversity of insects and animals, usually resulting in a considerable accumulation of dead wood. Nowadays the dead wood is welcome in supporting biodiversity but it can also provide a host for tree pathogens. In the past this material would probably have been collected as fuel, and trees in poor health were usually felled and cleared. The biggest threat to trees at present appears to be from climate breakdown and from spreading diseases, such as fungal infections in water, which are difficult to control. There has been an increase in epidemic disease with a succession of invasive bacteria, insects and fungi, due in part to international trade: Dutch elm disease (*Ophiostoma ulmi*) was disseminated by the elm bark beetle; horse chestnuts suffered bleeding canker; chestnut leaf miner (*Cameraria*

ohridella) followed with destructive larvae; and chalara fungus (*Hymenoscyphus fraxineus*) caused ash crown dieback.[24] Ultimately the health of trees requires significant changes in management practices and the Tree Charter identifies important steps that need to be taken (see table below).

Tree Charter proposals for tree health

1   Bring all woods into management. Managed woods are more resilient to the threats of pests, disease and climate change than neglected woods.

2   Provide clear, good practice guidelines on planting and management. Informed decisions about species choice can ensure the best chance of newly planted trees thriving to create, replenish or buffer woodland habitats.

3   Ensure diversity of trees across the landscape. Woodland habitats dominated by one species of tree are vulnerable, because the impact of a pest or disease that affects that species could decimate the landscape.

4   Let woods breathe. A crowded wood leads to weaker trees more vulnerable to threats.

5   Actively manage orchards for the future. Orchards need active management to endure.

6   Act fast on pests and invasive species. Woods can be irreparably damaged when populations of destructive animals and plants get out of control.

7   Invest in research to find solutions to tree diseases. Knowledge is our greatest tool in protecting the woods and trees of the future.

8   Ensure an early warning system for tree disease and pests. We need to monitor for threats closely to ensure problems are identified before they get out of control.

9   Maintain a disease-free supply chain for trees and timber. Preventing the spread of disease is better than treatment.

Adapted from https://treecharter.uk/pdf/Charter-for-Trees2CWoods-and-People.pdf

Monitoring
the medicinal forest garden

In chapter 2, I concluded with a recommendation to start monitoring and evaluating progress. Keeping an ongoing record of inputs, observations, operations and outputs can not only help to evaluate how things are going in a project but also provide important data for research on a wider scale. However, it is unlikely that any two medicinal forest gardens will be the same, and this means that research to identify useful information and good practices presents some challenges. Each project will vary according to purpose, species composition, environment of soil and temperature etc., labour contributed, and end products produced. Ideally we need to look at more examples, compare experiences of growing techniques and different species and compile records of harvesting outcomes and productivity. Gathering these kinds of details could provide the basis for audits to inform others of practical experience and good practice. A further way to develop research would be to focus on the three main ethical principles of permaculture design and measure the contribution of medicinal forest gardens. This could be done by evaluating:

(a) environmental benefits (growth rates, forest services, increased biodiversity, range of species, resilience and sustainability);

(b) benefits to people (involvement of the community, volunteers, educational opportunities, measures of health and self-help);

(c) sharing and reinvestment opportunities (impact on local economy, markets and small businesses).

CHAPTER 4
Propagation and Provenance

Locating sources for medicinal trees and shrubs can be a real challenge. Seed may be readily available for many annual and perennial healing herbs but not so easily found for native or woody species. Most garden centres sell plant varieties that are optimised for colourful appearance or particular traits of shape or size, rather than original species with medicinal traits. So an early issue may be how do you get your plants? Chapter 4 is aimed at providing suggestions to help with medicinal plant propagation and sourcing. The main forms of propagation are briefly covered, from seed to cuttings and other methods such as layering and root division. Finding some desired plant species may require tree nursery supplies and so there is advice on this kind of provision. The provenance, or place of origin, of trees and shrubs is something to consider too, as we seek to adapt in the light of climate breakdown. The more you can do to maintain your own seed supplies the better, for self use or sharing, and this chapter includes a section on seed saving and storing.

Growing your own plants is very rewarding. Not too much equipment is required to get started. You need clean pots and trays, a thermometer, clear plastic bags and ties, a sharp knife or secateurs, a small watering can with rose, plant labels and a permanent marker. Much can be done on a windowsill. If you wish to extend the possibilities, then access to a greenhouse or polytunnel provides an ideal location for sowing trays or growing on more plants in a protected environment.

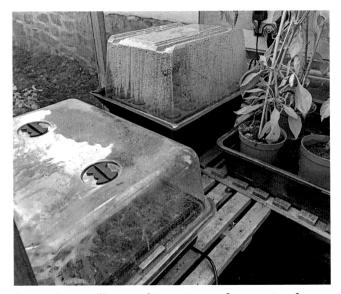

A greenhouse allows earlier sowing and protection for young plants from cuttings

Growing from seed

Growing from seed remains the most cost-effective way of producing many medicinal plants. It is an ideal approach if large numbers of shrubs or trees are to be grown, or if the plant you want is not available to buy. See the table on the following page for examples of medicinal plants suitable for propagation by seed and suggested times of sowing (though many seeds will germinate outside these times).

Seed that is dispersed by plants in early summer can germinate quickly in warm and moist conditions. If not sown immediately when ripe, some tree seeds also need a further warm period for the seed embryo to form properly. Further pre-treatments before sowing may be required for success in the sowing of many plants,

Propagation of medicinal plants by seed

Latin name	Common name	Treatment	Indoor sowing	Outdoor sowing
Achillea millefolium	Yarrow		Apr-May	
Alchemilla xanthochlora	Lady's mantle			Apr-May
Althaea officinalis	Mallow			Oct-Nov
Berberis vulgaris	Barberry	Stratify 6-8 weeks cold		Oct-Nov
Betula pendula	Birch	Stratification needed Needs light so surface sow		Oct
Borago officinalis	Borage			Apr-May
Calendula officinalis	Marigold		Mar-May	
Filipendula ulmaria	Meadowsweet		Feb-Mar	
Ginkgo biloba	Ginkgo			Sept-Oct
Hypericum perforatum	St John's wort	Needs light, so surface sow		Mar-April
Inula helenium	Elecampane		Mar-Apr	
Lavandula angustifolia	Lavender		Feb-Apr	
Nepeta cataria	Catmint		Feb-Apr	
Passiflora incarnata	Maypop	Needs pre-soaking	Jan	
Plantago major	Plantain			Mar-Apr
Rheum palmatum	Wild rhubarb		Feb-Mar	
Scutellaria laterifolia	Skullcap			Mar-Apr
Stachys betonica	Wood betony		Mar-Apr	
Tanacetum parthenium	Feverfew		Mar-Apr	
Vaccinium myrtillus	Bilberry	May need stratification	Oct-Nov	
Verbascum thapsus	Mullein	Needs light	Feb-Apr	
Verbena officinalis	Vervain		Feb-May	
Viola tricolor	Heartsease		Jan-May	

whether fresh or stored. Use of stratification, placing seeds in cold temperatures, is needed to trigger breakdown of the growth-inhibiting hormones in many seeds.[1] If not sown in the autumn period, many tree seeds (*Betula, Juniperus, Liquidambar, Prunus, Viburnum* species) require cold stratification at near freezing temperature, in cold and moist conditions before they will produce a radicle and shoot.[2] For stratification of small amounts of seed, place in a 50/50 mix of moist compost and grit or sand and keep in a ziplock polythene bag with a label in the refrigerator. Larger quantities of seed requiring stratification are best sown in pots outside in a cold frame. Additionally some seed coats (*Rhamnus* species and legumes of the Fabaceae family) are hard and impermeable to water.[3] These seeds need to be scarified or abraded in order to germinate. This can be done by nicking the seed coat or rubbing with sandpaper to expose a little of the paler endosperm within. There is some variation between plants in the requirement for these special treatments and so it is advisable to check the individual tree and shrub descriptions in the Directory in Part 2.

Seed sowing

Most growers use plastic seed trays or pots as they are available in many sizes and are reusable if cleaned and washed. Seed compost can be placed in the container and firmed, then moistened and allowed to drain. Further compost can be added so that the container is filled within 2cm of the top. Fine seeds can be sown directly onto this medium, with a little sand sprinkled over, whereas other seeds are sown to a depth of two or three times their diameter. Some seeds need light to germinate and do not need covering. A layer of grit of 2-3mm can be used to cover the medium. The pots or trays can be placed on a windowsill indoors or in a cold frame, or unheated greenhouse. A clear cover helps to retain moisture and additional warmth may be needed for some species. As the seedlings germinate and become large enough to handle (by the leaves and not the stem) the young seedlings can be transplanted to a wider spacing or individual pots. Some seeds germinate unevenly, so that a proportion emerge in the first spring and then others in the following spring. It is a good idea to label seed trays and pots clearly so they can be left for two complete springs. If left outdoors you may need to cover tray or pots with mesh to protect from mice.

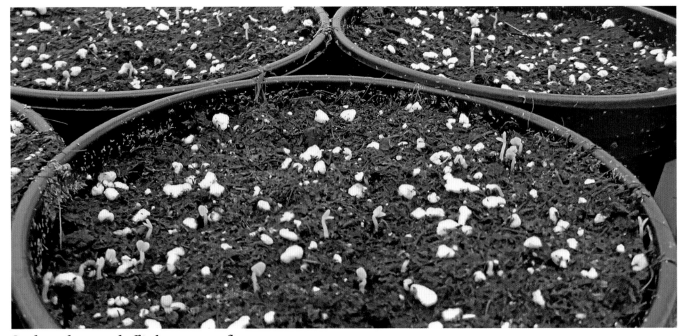

Seeds can be started off in large pots or flat trays

Composts for seed sowing may be purchased, and offer a sterile growing medium giving a moisture-retaining but free-draining medium that is needed for seeds to germinate. You can also mix your own version of seed compost. Mixtures of moisture-retaining material (peat alternatives, bark, compost, vermiculite) with drainage material (coarse sand) are suggested in different proportions by various authors.[4] At Holt Wood, we have found a mix of equal parts of peat-free potting compost and sand works well for stratifying or starting off seeds. As alternatives to peat and vermiculite, some authors recommend coir (coconut fibre) or leaf mould for up to 50% of the constituents of seed-sowing compost.

Some elements of a seed compost can be created from existing resources grown on site. Leaf mould, or composted leaves, provides an alternative to peat. It is made by collecting fallen leaves (not evergreen leaves) in autumn and placing in layers in a bin or in black polythene sacks with a few small holes. Add some water if the leaves are very dry, and leave them to break down slowly over 1-2 years. The process can be sped up to one year if some grass mowings are incorporated. This dark brown crumbly leaf mould can be sieved to make a compost or used as a mulch. At Holt Wood we are experimenting with use of bracken fern (*Pteridinium aquilinum*) to make compost since it is prolific and needs to be controlled in its spread. Bracken can be harvested up to June for compost making but should not be cut later as it produces spores in July. We have also found that bracken needs to be wilted on the ground for a few days before gathering up into bags, otherwise it turns into a wet mess. Bark is another alternative to consider; it can be chipped and aged. Both bracken and bark can be added to the compost heap and allowed to decompose before use.[5] However, it should be noted that these kinds of material are likely to produce a somewhat more acidic compost than that available commercially.

Growing on

Growing on refers to the process of transplanting a seedling so that it has sufficient warmth, light and nutrition to continue growing and form a well-grown plant suitable for planting out. Once seeds have germinated

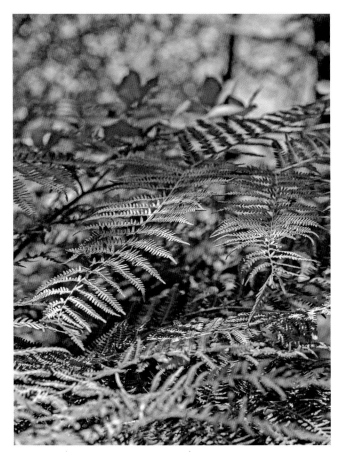

Bracken (*Pteridinium aquilinum*) can be wilted and composted

and have several true leaves, they need to be moved on in order to develop good root structures. The seedlings can be replanted in well-drained compost with more nutrients where they can stay until ready to be planted outdoors. Less hardy plants such as purple coneflower (*Echinacea* species) need to be grown on in frost-free conditions until they can be placed outside after frosts, usually from the end of May in the UK. This works well for some of the less hardy trees and shrubs such as eucalyptus or myrtle.

Whilst many herbs may grow rapidly for planting out in the same season, shrubs and trees may be kept in a seedbed or container for several years to establish well before planting out. Many tree seedlings are able to survive with very little additional nutrition; they 'persist under adverse conditions, making little growth, but slowly developing.'[6] As it might do in a forest with a canopy, a tree seedling can do with remarkably little for many years, and then when it receives light, water, nutrients and warmth, it will shoot up. An increased proportion of compost can be used in the planting mix plus a small amount of long-term fertiliser granules (approximately 1g per litre of compost) if a plant is likely to remain in a pot for a long time, or add sieved worm compost which is rich in nutrients. Grit can be incorporated to ensure good drainage. As seedlings are moved they will benefit from mycorrhizal inoculation by incorporating a small amount of mycorrhizal granules into the potting-on compost, at the rate of about 1g per litre of planting mix, or lightly dusting the planting holes.

Propagating with cuttings

Taking cuttings is an ideal method for reproducing many plants, and can provide a head start compared to seed for some shrubs and trees. See the following page for examples of propagation by cuttings of medicinal trees and shrubs. Cuttings will have the same genetic make-up as the parent plant and this may be desirable if the same medicinal qualities are wanted. A sharp knife or a pair of good quality secateurs is needed to remove woody stems cleanly from plants. Softwood cuttings are usually taken in the late summer when the plants are still growing, hardwood cuttings are taken later in the year during the autumn and overwintered till the following spring. If you want to propagate your own existing woody plants then you will benefit from keeping a bush or tree heavily pruned in order to ensure that shoots of younger wood are produced for cuttings.

Cuttings can be trimmed to reduce leaf surface area, and then trimmed at the bottom of the stem just below a leaf node. Some plant cuttings do best with a heel from the attachment point to the larger stem of the plant. This exposes part of the cambium layer below the bark which has cells that can develop roots. Cuttings do well in free-draining compost so long as they are provided with sufficient moisture, even producing roots in grit/perlite mixtures. Place the cuttings in a pot of compost, firm soil around the sides and water. Moisture can be conserved by putting the pot into a propagator, or by

enclosing in a clear plastic bag. Once roots begin to grow then you can move the cuttings on into a longer term growing medium with more nutrients. Hardwood cuttings can also be placed in outdoor beds in the winter, to be lifted the following autumn and planted out.

Vigorously growing plants, such as willow (*Salix* species) and fig (*Ficus communis*) may be successfully grown from cuttings taken in spring. Young stems of willow will readily grow on when placed in soil, or even produce roots when stood in water. The establishment of cuttings may be helped by dipping them in a hormone rooting powder. Although commercial versions of hormone rooting extract can be purchased, a naturally derived version can be made from young willow stems and tips, which contain plant hormones, indolebutyric and salicylic acids. To make willow hormone rooting extract, the leaves are removed from one-year-old willow shoots (almost any vigorously growing *Salix* species can be used) and the stems are chopped into 2-3cm length pieces. These stem pieces are placed in a container, covered with boiling water, and allowed to stand for 24 hours. The liquid is then strained off, bottled, labelled and can be kept refrigerated for several months. Stand plant cuttings in the liquid willow extract for 2-3 hours before placing in compost or a seedbed, or water them several times with the liquid willow extract.

Other methods of propagation

Both layering and root division are useful techniques for producing well-rooted plants. Shrubs can often be propagated by layering, which involves taking a flexible branch down to the soil where it can produce roots over a 12-18 month period. To layer a plant, clear a soil area around it and use several tent pegs to hold a branch down to the soil level; you need to ensure that the branch has good contact with the soil. Nick the branch in the area below a node and heap up a little soil around. This approach can be used with chaste tree (*Vitex agnus-castus*), cramp bark (*Viburnum opulus*), rosemary (*Rosmarinus officinalis*) and witch hazel (*Hamamelis virginiana*). An advantage is that a new plant is formed which is well advanced with root growth. However, the main difficulty with

Propagation of medicinal plants by cuttings

Latin name	Common name	Type of cutting	Time
Aronia melanocarpa	Black chokeberry	Softwood	July
Berberis aquifolium	Oregon grape	Bud	Feb-Mar
Betula pendula	Silver birch	Softwood	May-Jun
Ceanothus americanus	Red root	Softwood	Jun-Aug
Cytisus scoparius	Broom	Softwood	Jul-Aug
Elaeagnus rhamnoides	Sea buckthorn	Softwood	Jul-Aug
Forsythia suspensa	Forsythia	Softwood	Jun-Sept
Humulus lupulus	Hops	Basal	Apr-May
Juniperus communis	Juniper	Softwood	Jun-Jul
Laurus nobilis	Bay	Hardwood	Nov-Dec
Morus nigra	Mulberry	Softwood	Jul-Aug
Myrtus communis	Myrtle	Softwood	Jun-Aug
Passiflora incarnata	Passionflower	Softwood	Jul
Prunus padus	Bird cherry	Softwood	Jul-Aug
Ribes nigrum	Blackcurrant	Softwood	Jun-Sept
Rosa canina	Rose	Softwood	Jul-Aug
Rosmarinus officinalis	Rosemary	Softwood	Jul-Sept
Rubus idaeus	Raspberry	Softwood	Jun-Jul
Salix daphnoides	Willow	Hardwood	Nov-Mar
Salvia officinalis	Sage	Softwood	Jun-Sept
Sambucus nigra	Elder	Softwood	Jul-Aug
Schisandra chinensis	Schisandra	Softwood	Aug
Scrophularia nodosa	Figwort	Basal	Apr-May
Solidago virgaurea	Goldenrod	Basal	Apr-May
Thuja occidentalis	Arbor vitae	Softwood	Apr-May
Vaccinium myrtillus	Bilberry	Hardwood	April or Sept
Viburnum opulus	Cramp bark	Softwood	Jul-Sept
Zanthoxylum americanum	Prickly ash	Softwood	Jul-Aug

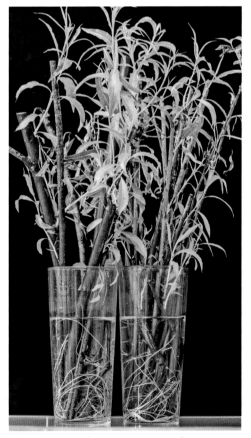

Violet willow (*Salix daphnoides*) cuttings readily produce roots in water layering is keeping the area sufficiently moist yet weed-free to allow for new plant growth. A similar layering technique is the kind of approach used to restock coppice stools – known as 'plashing' or cutting three-quarters of the way through a stem and then pegging it down to the ground. Another way is to mound over a coppice stool with soil, so that additional roots form on the stool stems, and and then split off new plants with roots.

Root clumps that can be readily divided include lemon balm (*Melissa officinalis*), mints (*Mentha* species) and meadowsweet (*Filipendula ulmaria*). This is a good way to produce larger numbers of well-grown plants in the shortest possible time. Root division often works well with plants that have chunky roots bearing additional buds. Root division is best in autumn or winter, and this can coincide with harvesting roots for medicinal use. For example, comfrey (*Symphytum officinale*) roots can be readily separated and each portion replanted in pots or in the soil with the buds pointing upwards to grow on into new plants. Other plants that can be divided in a similar way include elecampane (*Inula helenium*) and paeony (*Paeonia lactiflora*).

Sourcing seeds and plants externally

Commercial garden centres are not always ideal seed sources since seeds on sale are likely to be for popular flower varieties for the garden. For example, seed of Californian poppies (*Eschscholtzia californica*) and marigold (*Calendula officinalis*) are often sold as mixed colours. Such plants may have a limited medicinal activity but there may be native wild flower species available, unless there is a key reason for selecting a cultivar. Similarly, the range of trees and shrubs available in garden centres is largely based on consumer demand for ornamental plants. For example, in the UK, most garden centre witch hazel shrubs are varieties of an Asian species (*Hamamelis mollis*) designed to produce larger and colourful flowers. It is usually best to try to obtain the medicinal species rather than such cultivars. The exception to this general rule may be for woody plants where a species variety has been bred to produce more flowers, leaves or fruits with medicinal qualities, as in the commercial production of various rosemary (*Rosmarinus officinalis*) cultivars for essential oils, or for more flowers and fruits, such as elder (*Sambucus* species) cultivars. Developments in

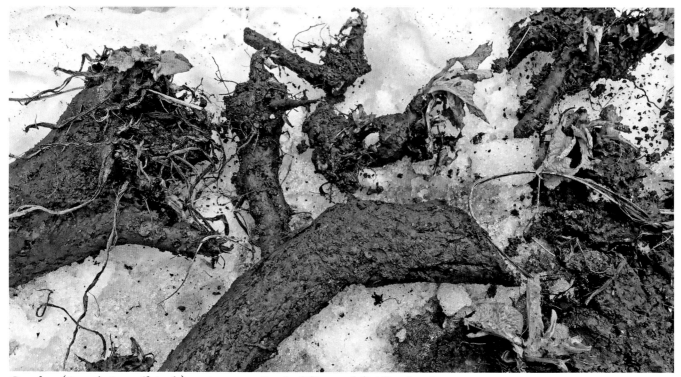

Comfrey (*Symphytum officinale*) root propagation by lifting and dividing in winter

The Agroforestry Research Trust website

Agroforestry
research trust

Shop ∨   Courses ∨   Tours ∨   About Agroforestry ∨   The Trust ∨   🛒   🔍

About Agroforestry

Agroforestry is the growing of both trees and agricultural / horticultural crops on the same piece of land. They are designed to provide tree and other crop products and at the same time protect, conserve, diversify and sustain vital economic, environmental, human and natural resources. Agroforestry differs from traditional forestry and agriculture by its focus on the interactions amoungst components rather than just on the individual components themselves.

Research over the past 20 years has confirmed that agroforestry can be more biologically productive, more profitable, and be more sustainable than forestry or agricultural monocultures. Many other benefits have been shown. Temperate agroforestry systems are already widespread in many parts of the world and are central to production in some regions.

Success of agroforestry is largely determined by the extent to which individual forest and agricultural components can be integrated to help rather than hinder each other. The choice of tree and crop species combinations is critically important when setting up systems.

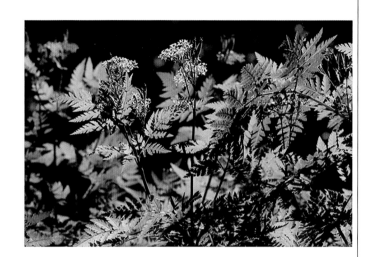

SUCCESSFUL FOREST GARDENING NEEDS RESEARCH

NAME: Agroforestry Research Trust

LOCATION: The Agroforestry Research Trust is based in Devon, UK.

ACTIVITY: Since 1994, when a demonstration project was first established by Martin Crawford in Devon, there has been much development of forest gardens providing foods, medicinal and other useful products. Research and experimentation through the Agroforestry Research Trust has helped to identify new plant species and techniques of managing a forest garden. The useful knowledge gained is crucial in anticipating changes in climate through supporting the development of resilient forest garden planting. Martin's forest garden is now well established as a

venue for training events, and a wide range of plants and seeds are available to purchase online, including many with medicinal uses. Martin is the celebrated author of numerous books on forest gardening and has supported further networking of agroforestry and related projects. The addition of an online forest gardening course will make information available to a wider range of people. Overall, the ongoing research has supported the development of agroforestry systems and forest gardens and identified further possibilities to be explored.

KEY POINT: Research has played an important role in the successful development of forest gardens.

INFO: www.agroforestry.co.uk

agroforestry and agroecology are encouraging more nursery suppliers of plants for functional uses, and the best established is the Agroforestry Research Trust (p.65).

Another source worth considering is the garden centre that provides hedging supplies, since these may often provide low cost and easily established young trees and shrubs. Further afield, online specialist suppliers for both seeds and plants may be found by Internet search, and some suppliers of medicinal plants are identified in Appendix 6(F).[7] See Poyntzfield Herbs (opposite), a well-established herb nursery based in Scotland, growing a wide range of hardy and half-hardy plants from native and introduced sources.

Some plant centres and nurseries specialise in the supply of trees and shrubs of different sizes. With regard to medicinal trees and shrubs, the choice of nursery stock is influenced by numbers required and budget available. Nursery stock of trees can be classified as seedlings, seedling transplants, whips, feathered whips, feathered trees, standard trees, and the form of production might vary from seedlings to grafts, budded plants,

layers, root cuttings and stem cuttings. The table below describes this range of possible types of nursery stock. If you have a choice, then the smaller the size at planting the better the chance of establishment and the less the cost of replacement if a plant fails to thrive.

Mass woodland planting schemes usually opt for smaller stock using bare-root plants as this results in lower cost and easier establishment, and these plantings can be thinned at a later stage. Most suppliers will usually only send out bare-rooted plants in the dormant season suitable for planting, and the roots must be kept covered to prevent desiccation. Trees and shrubs should always be checked on arrival or collection from a supplier, looking for pests, disease, any substitutions or constricted roots if containerised. They can be heeled in by laying in a soil trench to keep moist if need be, and protected in frosty weather with straw or hessian in a frost-free location.[8] Container-grown plants are more expensive and suffer little root disturbance when planting so can establish quickly even out of normal planting season. However, the container-grown plant does need watering in dry periods.

Types of tree nursery stock

Name	Description
Seedling	Young tree raised from seed, usually under 100cm, likely to be one or two years old
	1+0 indicates one year in the seedbed
	1+1 indicates one year in seedbed and one year transplanted
	1u1 indicates one year in seedbed and then roots undercut* before transplanting for one year
	2+0 indicates two years in the seedbed (less desirable than above)
Whip	Next size up from a seedling, could be 100-150cm tall, likely to be 2-3 or more years old and may be feathered with some lateral branches
Standard	Has a single stem up to 1.8m
	Short standard, half standard, garden standard, light, selected, heavy standards

Adapted from Watson B. (2006) *Trees: Their Use, Management, Cultivation and Biology*, Marlborough, Wilts: Crowood Press, p.328
* Undercutting encourages the growth of lateral roots which improves survival on planting out.

Seed saving – gathering, processing and storage

You may wish to collect and save your own seed to produce additional plants, or to sell or give away, whether herbaceous or woody medicinal plants. Seed reflects the genetic material of parents and is often produced in large numbers. Mixing of genes is generally advantageous, as the variability of outcomes can enable plants to adapt to changing conditions. Thus, plants grown from seed have the potential to develop traits conferring more resistance to environmental damage and stress.

A rather startling analysis of the global seed industry reveals how the sale of seeds has become dominated by just a few major pharmaceutical/chemical companies.[9] Previously, the commercial seed industry was composed mainly of small family-owned firms, and there was a widespread culture of seed saving amongst growers. There is a danger that increased patenting and cross-licensing will particularly affect renewable agricultural practices, since access to non-patented varieties will

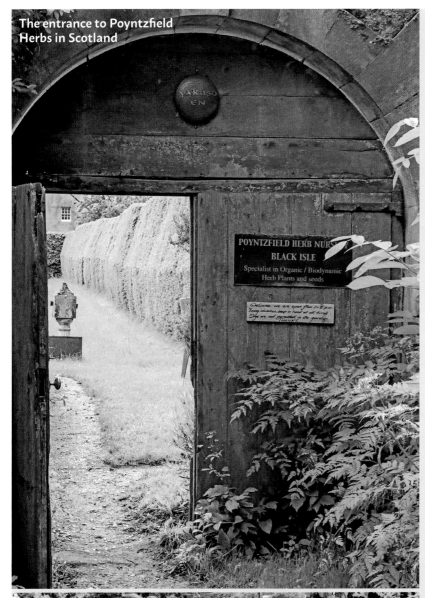
The entrance to Poyntzfield Herbs in Scotland

POYNTZFIELD HERB NURS
BLACK ISLE
Specialist in Organic / Biodynamic
Herb Plants and seeds

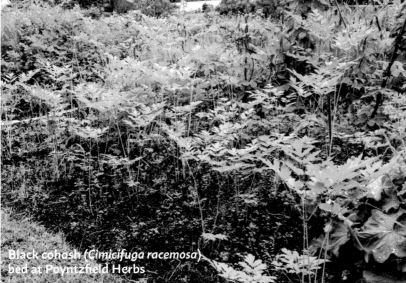
Black cohash (Cimicifuga racemosa) bed at Poyntzfield Herbs

OBTAINING HARDY MEDICINAL PLANTS

NAME: Poyntzfield Herbs

LOCATION: Based in Scotland, on the east coast of the Scottish highlands.

ACTIVITY: Established in 1976 by Duncan Ross on the Black Isle in Scotland, in an area known for its relatively mild climate, Poyntzfield Herbs is one of very few sources of biodynamically grown medicinal plants in the UK. Over 400 varieties of plants and 100 species of seeds are offered which are either hardy in the British Isles, or at least can be readily grown in protected conditions. A wide range of medicinal plants from all over the world, including trees and shrubs, are grown to a high standard. Most plants are lifted to order in the winter season and sent through the post, carefully wrapped in moss. Herbs for other aromatic, culinary and wildlife uses are also offered with guidance on cultivation. New introductions from a range of sources such as South America are constantly being added to the available stock. An informative catalogue is available online and in print, while eight more detailed grower guides and a further design and advisory service can also be obtained. Visitors are welcome from April-September; details are on the website.

KEY POINT: Having committed growers with lengthy experience like Poyntzfield Herbs as a source of herbs makes a vital contribution to confidence in obtaining and cultivating medicinal plants.

INFO: www.poyntzfieldherbs.co.uk

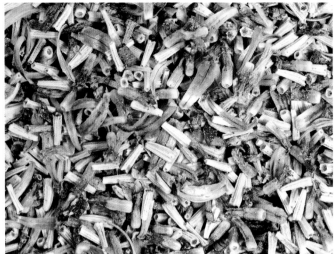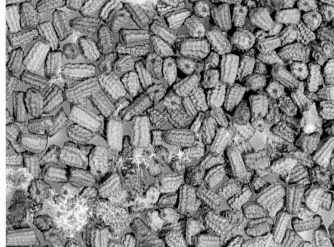

Seed saving: feverfew (*Tanacetum parthenium*) and mullein (*Verbascum thapsus*)

decrease, and available seeds will be increasingly tied to unsustainable agricultural practices. The skills of seed saving are relatively simple to learn, and by saving and sharing seed effectively you can help join in a movement to restore independence to growers on a wider scale. Fortunately there are further initiatives to encourage seed saving, including online guidance.[10] Some outline suggestions are given here on collection and storage.

Seed collection

Seed quality is key, thus the importance of good practice at every step of collection, extraction, processing, drying and storage. Many herbaceous medicinal plants can be readily harvested for seed. By observing plants that are growing, you can identify ones that look healthy and are productive. Generally flower formation is increased if temperature and light intensity are higher, although in fertile soils this may result in plenty of leafy growth rather than flower production. As seeds ripen they increase in size and develop essential structures for reproduction, then they undergo a loss of moisture and reduce in size. So it is best not to select plants that are ripening seed early. Allow the plants to mature and flower, then let the seeds ripen on the plant as long as possible. As seed capsules begin to brown you will need to remove the stems or branches and put into paper bags to capture the seed if it starts shaking loose from the capsules. Herbaceous plants that can be readily harvested in this way for seed include

St John's wort (*Hypericum perforatum*), feverfew (*Tanacetum parthenium*), mullein (*Verbascum thapsus*) and vervain (*Verbena officinalis*). These are bountiful plants that provide seed mixes to use as additional ground cover – some grow tall and will need cutting back.

The age at which trees achieve maturity in terms of seed production appears to vary. Ideally, seed should be collected from healthy trees of middle to mature age.[11] Willow produces seed only five years after striking from a cutting, birch and rowan within 10 years, sweet chestnut and hazel coppice carry nuts 12 years after cutting back, ash will seed after 15 years, Scots pine will seed after 20 years and ginkgo produces nuts when over 30 years of age. In general, many trees will seed after 15 years given a good site and sunlight.[12] Most native trees will produce viable seed at least every other year, whereas introduced trees and shrubs may be far less reliable to propagate by seed. For example, the seed of *Hamamelis virginiana* may be produced in the UK but may not mature to become viable. In the North American native environment, the witch hazel seed capsule sits on the tree for at least a year before it dehisces (explodes due to moisture reduction) and ejects seed some distance away.[13]

Many trees show periodicity in seed production, having years of abundance every other year or less often. Thus trees produce seed in variable quantities each year, and some have large seed crops in 'mast' years. One possible reason for the 'barren' years is that a fall in seed

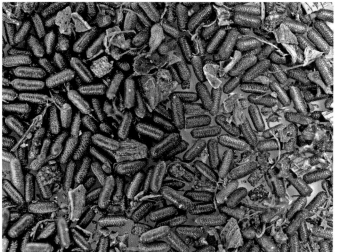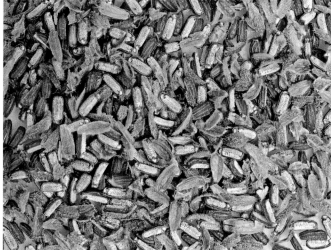

St John's wort (*Hypericum perforatum*) and vervain (*Verbena officinalis*)

production causes predator populations to drop, so that in a subsequent year more seeds will survive. Alternatively there may be variation in weather from year to year. Whatever the reason, you should try to collect in a good year.[14] Seed from most temperate tree and shrub species is usually gathered in the autumn when it is fully ripe. By gathering your own seed, you will be using plants which are better adapted to the location, and this local provenance is advised for subsequent plants to flourish. If you are gathering from further afield then remember to check if the landowner agrees and choose areas away from busy roads or industrial activity. It is better not to gather seed and fruit that have fallen on to the ground but to collect from tarpaulins placed on the ground. If fruits are likely to be taken by birds and animals as soon as they are ripe then it may be necessary to harvest them several weeks before seeds are fully ripe, allowing ripening to complete indoors. Ensure that the seed collected is labelled with name of species and date and location of collection.

Processing seed

For dry seed in capsules or husks, you will need to separate the seed out, and this can be done using a mesh screen and winnowing. The dried seed-containing material is rubbed gently across a screen to loosen the seeds and allow them to fall through into a container, capturing the larger chaffy parts for removal. The remaining mix of seeds and husks can then be winnowed or 'poured' from one container to another so that the heavier seed is collected and the lighter husks are blown away. Fleshy tree and shrub fruits, like myrtle seeds, can be rubbed in a bag of grit to help separate the seed from the flesh. The mixture can then be put in water so that the grit and viable seed drop to the bottom while the pulp and empty seeds float and can be scooped away.[15] More water is added and swirled around to lift the viable seed from the grit to be poured off into a sieve. Repeat as often as needed until the grit remains in the container with the cleaned seeds in the sieve.

Seeds of some species, especially in the tropics, are 'recalcitrant' (temperate examples are *Acer*, *Aesculus*, *Castanea*, *Populus*, *Quercus*, *Salix* species), which means that they do not survive for long, and they die if dried out below a level of 40% moisture. These recalcitrant seeds must generally be sown immediately. However, the vast majority of seeds are 'orthodox' which means that they can be collected and dried for storage, remaining viable for future sowing. Once orthodox seeds are dry, effectively down to 10-15% of moisture content, they can be stored with every prospect of survival. They are best kept in a tightly tied polythene bag at 3-5°C (37-41°F) in a refrigerator, and can last as long as 5-15 years or even longer if kept in a colder temperature range in a freezer.[16]

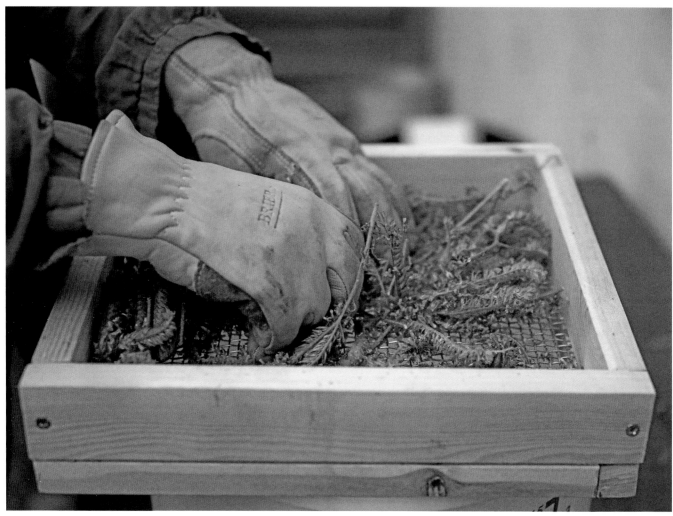

Rubbing ripe seed on a screen to separate seed and husks

Provenance and climate breakdown

Careful selection of seed or plants is important for planning the medicinal forest garden as changes in the climate increasingly affect the environment.[17] Provenance is the term used to describe the location of the source from which plant material, such as seed or cuttings, has been collected. This may be the location in which plants are native and within which their genetic characteristics have been developed through natural selection. For the UK, it may be appropriate to seek out more southern European species for planting. A range of adaptation measures, including use of non-native species matched from similar climates, have been suggested.[18] There are also indigenous species that may have the capability to adapt to changing climate conditions, and some of these species are of medicinal use, such as small-leaved lime (*Tilia cordata*) and black poplar (*Populus nigra*) in the UK.[19]

How variations in provenance and growing conditions can affect the medicinal potential of a tree is a hugely under-researched area. One study looked at various mountain ash species (*S. americana* and *S. decora*) in different latitudes of Canada, to compare anti-oxidant content. The study findings were that gene expression of a flavonoid, flavonol synthase, increased in the most northern latitudes. This medicinal flavonoid constituent helps the plant to defend leaves against oxidative damage from ultraviolet radiation and insect

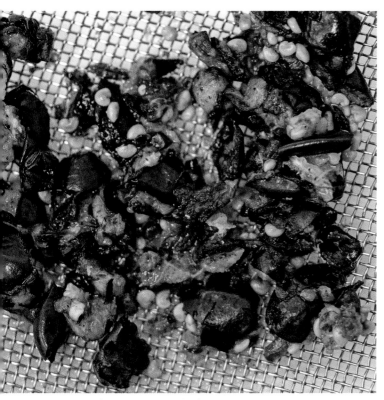

Myrtle (*Myrtus communis*) berries while cleaning seed

attached to plants that have spent a 'considerable time' growing in a UK nursery, even though the original seed or cuttings may have been imported. Many cuttings used as sources for UK-grown plants originate from another country such as Holland or Africa. At the time of writing, EU plant passports were not issued to everyday customers buying plants but were used by authorised suppliers to the horticultural trade. They were required for possible host plants of *Xylella fastidiosa* including important commercial fruiting and ornamental plants (such as almonds, lavenders, oleanders and olives). It is likely that this form of regulation will be extended to all plant sales, and this will help to identify imported plant sources. Some responsible plant retailers have already switched to propagation with domestically sourced plants, where possible using their own stock, such as Wyevale Nurseries, Hereford, UK.

Conclusion

As more and more growers see the potential of medicinal plants, there is likely to be more demand for them. This may open up some interesting avenues for entrepreneurs who like to propagate.[21] A particular shortage at the time of writing is of organically certified seed or nursery-grown stock. Setting up your own tree nursery may be appropriate if you want to propagate large numbers of trees and shrubs, for your own use or for commercial gain.[22] Meanwhile, there is a need for more research to help us understand which medicinal varieties and cultivars could be worth further exploration. Sharing seed and cuttings, as well as our experiences in propagation, both successes and failures, will help to spread diversity and accumulate techniques of propagation that work well.

predation.[20] Interestingly, the experimental results corroborated traditional reports gained from Cree healers that northern latitudes and coastal regions were better for harvesting material from the mountain ash. Thus, we need to ensure that traditional methods of harvesting plant medicine are properly recorded since they may help us to identify better approaches to choosing and locating plants.

Bear in mind that not all plants from garden centres and nurseries are fully labelled with regard to their origin, so their true provenance may be unknown. There is a Home Grown scheme label in the UK which can be

CHAPTER 5

Harvesting

There is great satisfaction to be had in harvesting healing plants of the best quality, knowing that they will regenerate for further harvests. Above all, a good herbal harvest is such a pleasure, as Robert Hart described in *Forest Gardening* back in 1991:

> My living room is adorned with a herb-rack hanging from the ceiling and every autumn it is filled with aromatic herbs which are left throughout the winter to dry.... These drying herbs give a delicious and healthful atmosphere to the room.[1]

For our own satisfaction, we want to maximise active ingredients and the best quality. And, ideally, we want to preserve these wonderful medicinal plants well for later use. For these reasons it is important to have a good understanding of principles and practice involved in harvesting, drying and processing medicinal plant parts from roots to bark, flowers, fruit and leaves. This chapter covers sustainable harvesting on a small scale with pointers towards dealing with larger harvests having more commercial potential. Key aspects of planning seasonal harvesting arrangements are identified for bark, leaves, flowers, seeds and roots. Good practices for harvesting of cultivated medicinal plants are described, with subsequent drying and processing techniques. Storage matters are discussed, including the shelf life of preserved plant material. The importance of monitoring, labelling and recording outputs is emphasised. For further detail on harvesting of individual trees and shrubs you can also view the plant profiles in the Part 2 Directory.

Good harvesting practice

Harvesting right is critical to the whole process of producing quality materials from medicinal plants. Good harvesting is sustainable and ensures consideration of future years of supply. The highest quality of harvested products is essential for users and producers of medicinal plants, whether intended for domestic use or for commercial markets. Ideally, an end product is required that is the correct plant, the relevant part, with a maximum of active constituents, deriving from material without contamination or degradation, and obtained without ruining the environment or affecting biodiversity. Getting this right means applying some general principles to harvesting of medicinal plants whether in cultivation or in the wild:[2]

- Planning of harvesting
- Harvest should be carried out in appropriate conditions
- Clear instructions on safety and procedures for those harvesting
- Ensure accurate identification of plants
- Caring for the environment
- Minimise damage and contamination
- Ensure labelling of harvested material
- Keep records to allow traceability and monitoring.

Planning the harvest

Planning of harvests involves an estimation of timing, location, personnel and resources needed. Traditional approaches base the appropriate time for harvest on seasons when the best outcomes have been observed in practice (see table below). Bark harvests can be carried out all year round, though probably the best time for collecting bark with the maximum active ingredients is early spring, just before active growth is seen.[3] Roots are thought to have most active ingredients in the dormant season, based on their stored materials. Many of the medicinally active ingredients in plants are secondary metabolites intended to protect from insect attack or to help limit damage. Thus leaves and 'tops' are usually thought to be at their best in spring shortly before flower buds open. Aromatic herbs, such as mint, appear to have their maximum content of essential oils in summer.[4] The period for harvesting flowers may be limited since these can reach their best for a short period, sometimes just a matter of days. There are always exceptions, for example the leaves of the ginkgo (*Ginkgo biloba*) are reputed to be highest in flavonoid active constituents just as they begin to yellow in the autumn. The level of active constituents in healing plants is surprisingly variable and research may not always provide conclusive advice. For example, isoflavonoids in a Chinese root herb were found to be most concentrated at the age of three years old if harvested in winter,[5] but another investigation found that phenolic ingredients were highest during spring harvesting.[6] Thus, different key constituents in medicinal plants can vary in their proportions throughout the year. More research is needed on the most appropriate periods for harvesting in order to maximise the most useful plant constituents.

Appropriate conditions

Having the right conditions for harvesting medicinal plants helps to ensure that there is minimum deterioration before transport and further processing takes place. In general, dry and cool conditions are preferable for

Seasonal harvests

SPRING BARK AND BUDS

Alder (*Alnus glutinosa*)
Alder buckthorn (*Frangula alnus*)
Birch (*Betula pendula*) buds and sap
Blackcurrant (*Ribes nigrum*) buds
Cherry (*Prunus avium* and *P. padus*)
Cramp bark (*Viburnum opulus*)
Prickly ash (*Zanthoxylum americanum*)
Willow (*Salix daphnoides* and *S. alba*)

SUMMER LEAVES AND FLOWERS

Elder (*Sambucus nigra*)
Lavender (*Lavandula angustifolia*)
Limeflower (*Tilia* species)
Marigold (*Calendula officinalis*)
Mint (*Mentha* species)
Mugwort (*Artemisia vulgaris*)
Nettle (*Urtica dioica*)
Purple coneflower (*Echinacea purpurea*)
Raspberry (*Rubus idaeus*)
Rose (*Rosa* species) flowers
St John's wort (*Hypericum perforatum*)

AUTUMN FRUITS AND SEEDS

Blackberry (*Rubus fruticosus*)
Blackcurrant (*Ribes nigrum*)
Chokeberry (*Aronia melanocarpa*)
Hawthorn (*Crataegus monogyna*)
Hops (*Humulus lupulus*) strobiles
Prickly ash (*Zanthoxylum americanum*) berries
Rose (*Rosa canina*) hips

WINTER ROOTS

Comfrey (*Symphytum officinale*)
Elecampane (*Inula helenium*)
Mallow (*Althaea officinalis*)
Oregon grape (*Berberis aquifolium*)
Paeony (*Paeonia lactiflora*)

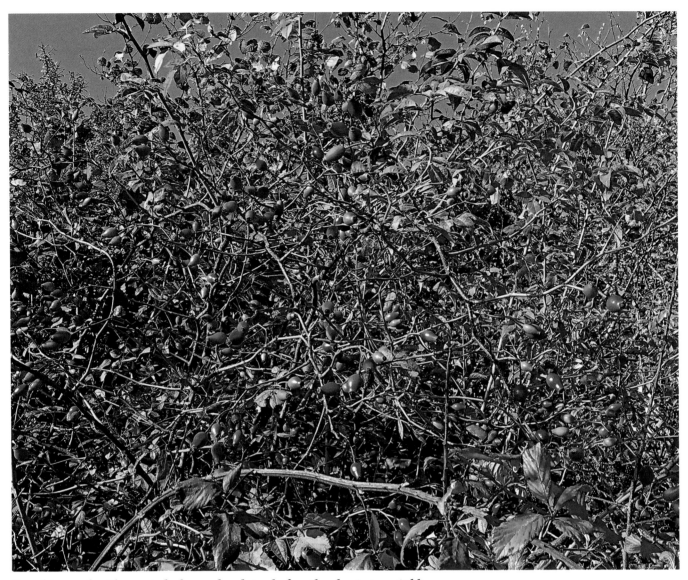

Rose hips are best harvested when red and ripe before they begin to wrinkle

harvest. For any material harvested above ground, it is important to avoid wet conditions, as any moisture will contribute towards rapid deterioration. It is better to wait until conditions improve, but if there is no alternative then there must be a plan to dry the harvested materials effectively. Suitable equipment for harvesting includes sharpened tools (secateurs, loppers, pruning saw, spade), collecting bags (at Holt Wood we find that cotton pillowcases are excellent), pen and labels (string is useful to tie labels to bags). Health and safety precautions should be considered, with identification of any risks arising from harvesting, such as uneven ground, using sharp tools or felling tree branches.[7] Depending on the conditions and site, collectors should wear long-sleeved shirts, thick trousers, hats, gloves and boots. The process of carrying out a risk assessment for an activity in the forest garden is covered in Chapter 3.

Accurate identification of plants

In a cultivated environment, it is likely that plants are easily identified if an example is shown and this will help to avoid contamination with the wrong plants. Correct identity may be less easy to spot in a forest garden with diverse planting, and the situation may resemble wild-harvesting. It may be necessary to have on hand some botanically accurate plant descriptions to check the identity of specific plants.[8] If harvest helpers are involved, then they need clear instructions about identification of the correct parts of plants to harvest, to avoid inappropriate material being harvested.[9]

Caring for the environment

Caring for the environment in a sustainable way during harvesting involves thinking ahead to the next harvest, thus ensuring that herbs, trees and shrubs are harvested in a way that allows ongoing production in the future. Some roots can be replaced in the ground to produce new plants; some flowers can be left to form seed. Any harvesting process needs to be considered in terms of disturbance and compaction to the soil which can impact on landscape and wildlife. Ideally there need to be paths of sufficient width to enable access. Use of light wheeled carriers such as a wheelbarrow may be appropriate to avoid repeated trips. Care is needed with removal of large branches or trunks by dragging away from the harvest site as these can also damage surrounding vegetation. Smaller branches and twigs can be bundled up for easier carrying.

Minimise damage and contamination

All harvested material should be inspected for dirt, insects and damaged parts. Flowers may need to be harvested by hand, looking out for insects and shaking them off. To enable further insects to escape, you can spread out flowers and leaves in a thin layer.[10] Fruit must be harvested with care to avoid bruising so that there is less likelihood of deterioration. Roots are best harvested in drier soil conditions to reduce the amount of soil attached, then they can be washed in a bucket or tank of water. Harvesting bark is destructive for a tree if removed around the whole circumference of a tree trunk, and so it is preferable to harvest branches and peel these stems for bark. Many tree and shrub species will regrow from the base as a coppice crop, while others can be pollarded at 2 or 3m height to allow new growth of branches. Care should be taken to leave a clean stump since a damaged stump is likely to rot or die back.[11]

Ensure labelling and keep records

Labelling of the harvest is essential to avoid mixing up batches of plant material as they are moved through to drying, processing and on into storage. It is impossible to remember which plants are which, especially since they will look completely different once chopped up and dried. Labelling avoids waste too, as unidentified plant material cannot be used and, at best, has to be recycled as mulch. Use of both common and Latin names helps to ensure accuracy where there are similar plants being harvested. Other details include the part harvested and location with date of harvest. A label provides the basis for tracking a herb. Record-keeping of dates, locations, personnel and amounts of plants harvested is good practice (and essential for organic or other accreditation).

You may also want to keep plant samples in case of a need for future checks or responding to queries about provenance. Keeping a voucher specimen as a herbarium sample is a way to do this. Voucher specimens can be preserved using a plant press with boards, held together by screws. Typically, a whole plant is collected, or if large then representative parts of leaf and flower, slices of stem and bark. To complete the record, note the collector's name, date, exact location, habitat type and additional details about the plant. The plant material is placed in the press, between blotting paper sheets, which is then placed under a weight or strapped tightly. The plant can be trimmed or rearranged after a few hours. The paper is changed frequently (daily) so that moisture does not allow degradation. The press can be kept in a warm well-ventilated area, and when fully dried the specimen is attached with glue dots or mounting tape to the herbarium sheet, leaving space for a label. Plant fragments such as seeds can be placed in an envelope and this is attached to the sheet.[12] A well-made herbarium can keep indefinitely, providing an excellent record of actual plant source material.

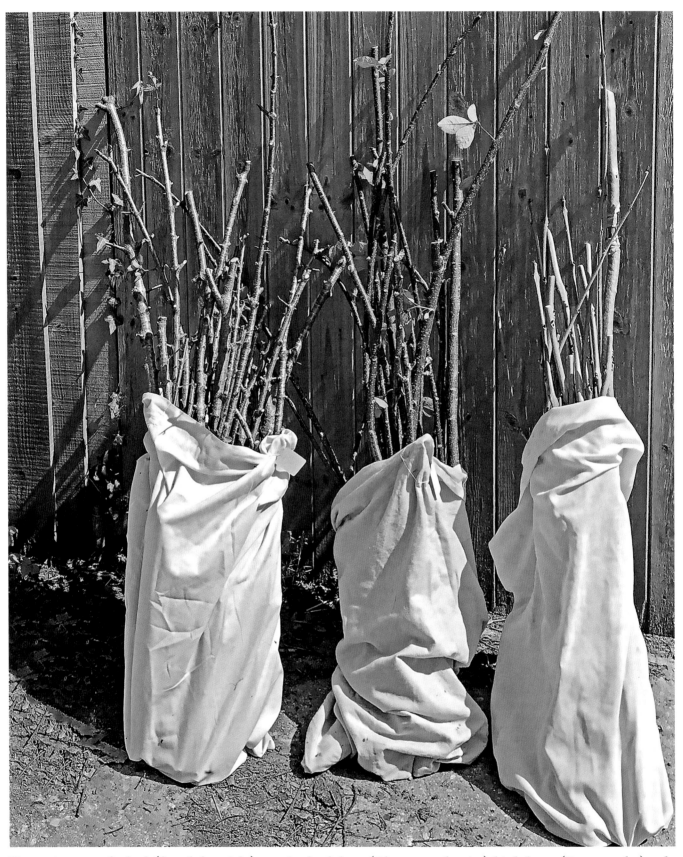

Harvesting stems for bark (from left to right): purging buckthorn (*Rhamnus cathartica*), bird cherry (*Prunus padus*) and ash (*Fraxinus excelsior*)

Drying herbs

As soon as plant material is harvested it will start to deteriorate and drying to remove moisture is essential to prevent or reduce further decomposition. The moisture content of living trees and shrubs averages around 70% with a lesser proportion in woody parts. Effective drying reduces moisture content to maintain the quality and quantity of important healing constituents. A low moisture content of 10-15% enables storage without deterioration until use or sale. Beyond the care for initial drying, we also need to be aware of the purpose for which a plant is intended, so that the most suitable methods of processing are used.

In the nineteenth century, John Skelton gave some advice on the drying of herbs to herb-sellers, much of which is still applicable today (see panel, right), in his popular *Family Medical Adviser*, which was printed in at least 12 editions; Skelton was keen to ensure that herbs were properly dried and presented well. He advised on tidily bunching herbs for sale, tying with coarse grass and trimming the stems evenly, adding 'I should also say be careful to put every herb you bunch, from the first to last, even[ly] at the top. Your bunches then look as if they had been gathered by a true botanist', noting that he hated 'your slovenly gatherers'.[13]

Processing before drying

All plant material should be checked over for insects (leave outdoors for a few hours to allow these creatures to escape) and shaken to remove any loose matter. Washing is not usually necessary unless essential to remove dirt. Smaller quantities of herbs, twigs and stalks with flowers and leaves can be bundled up, tied with a rubber band and hung from rafters in an airy space indoors. Hanging the bundle inside a large paper bag is a way to protect the material from dust and insects. Once dry, flowers or leaves can then be readily rubbed off stalks, bagged and labelled. Plant parts that are more dense or substantial need to be chopped before drying in order to ensure a more even process of water loss. Fruits, such as berries, may need substantially longer to become thoroughly dried, and other processes than drying such as making syrups and fruit leathers may be

Advice on drying herbs

Directions for gathering and preserving

'Roots. A very great number of our medicinal plants have their virtues in the roots, and unless they are gathered in proper season and carefully prepared, much, if not all that is truly valuable, may be entirely lost. The best time for gathering roots is in the spring, just before the leaves begin to shoot, for then they have their juices rich and full, and consequently their strength is the greatest. About the latter end of December, January, throughout February, and even at the beginning of March, are the best times when they should be sought for.'

'Barks. Should be gathered in the spring, before the leaves begin to bud; they may then be peeled from the trees easily. The outside part or thin skin should be taken off. The bark should be broken into proper sizes, and hung to dry, in the same manner as roots.'

'Herbs. Should be gathered when ripe, as soon as the leaves are in perfection, and when the sun is up, just as the flowers are ready to put forth their bloom. They should not be gathered when wet, either with the dew or by the rain. They should be tied loosely in small bunches, and hung up exposed to a free current of air. Press bunches into a strong box for several days, ensure the lid and side are removable so herbs can be taken out without breaking, pack in brown paper.'

'Seeds. Require to be carefully gathered when perfectly ripe, to be carefully separated from the husks, spread upon a clean cloth on the floor, and exposed to a full current of air, until they are perfectly dry, after which they should be put into bags ... inspect them occasionally to see that they are not getting mouldy ... the least damp will destroy their virtues.'

Text extracted from Skelton J. (1878) *Family Medical Adviser: A Treatise on Scientific or Botanic Medicine*, 11th edition. Plymouth: Published by the author, pp.237-9.

worth considering (see Chapter 6 for sample recipes). Mushrooms can be dried whole unless large in which case they should be chopped into smaller similar-sized pieces of 1-2cm across. Roots should be trimmed to remove any damaged sections, then chopped into pieces of 1cm or less using a sharp knife, and the pieces placed in a single layer. It is also helpful to chop up bark into sections of less than 1-2cm long as they will be easier to handle at a later stage.

Best drying arrangements

Shaded, dry warmth with good air circulation creates the most favourable conditions for dehydrating fresh herbs. Airflow is crucial to the effective removal of water from plant material, and it can be increased by spreading herbs in thin layers, or using fans to move the air. Drying herbs must be kept in the shade and out of direct contact with sunlight. Different drying regimes can have a significant effect on medicinal constituents, particularly with regard to the temperatures used in drying.[14] The optimal temperature for faster drying is generally thought to be between 30-40°C (86-104°F), requiring some additional heat beyond room temperature of around 20°C (68°F). In some cases a higher temperature may be justified. For example, fresh willow bark can be dried at 48°C (118°F) for 8-16 hours to reduce losses of phenolic content.[15] Drying herbs should be protected at night from moist air which can rehydrate the herb and affect quality.[16] Once dry, leaves should break up easily when rubbed in the hands or through a screen – stems and roots should be brittle enough to snap with a 'crack'.[17] When fully dried, the plant material can be bagged and labelled.

Drying equipment

For home production, with harvests of less than a kilogram, little is needed beyond general kitchen equipment including a sharp knife for chopping up bulkier items and a rack or screen for allowing herbs to dry. Homemade screens are ideal for spreading out herb material in thin layers, and can be constructed so that they stack easily. Larger quantities of herbs, such as 1-2kg or more in fresh weight, can be dried by spreading out on trays and placed in a shaded and well-ventilated area for 1-2 weeks. Overall the number of racks needed depends on weather, yields, speed of drying and number of crops being harvested. For more controlled drying, a dehydrator can be used which offers both a temperature setting and a timer. For commercial production there is a need to consider practical and economic aspects of providing a dryer system able to cope with larger quantities in adverse weather.[18]

At Holt Wood Herbs we have experimented with a number of arrangements for drying. A starting point was adapting a portable greenhouse with wire mesh shelves using a plastic cover painted black to attract heat and mesh-covered holes to encourage airflow. The design of our most effective dryer to date involves stacked catering trays on a moveable trolley with a fan and heating pad below, all surrounded by a plastic cover held in place with velcro. The drying effect appears to be improved with the plastic cover, which helps to funnel air up through and around the trays, and also serves to protect the crop in the trays. Development of further designs which make use of solar energy and wind power is desirable for drying plants.[19]

Further processing of herbs

Once a medicinal plant is dried, it can be stored whole, or processed into smaller pieces known as 'cut herb' in the trade, or powdered. This additional processing largely depends on whether the herb is to be used for alcohol or water extracts, or for other purposes such as filling capsules. The reduced size of plant particles can have a significant influence on the amounts of active constituents that are available in extracts. For example, a study of powdered particles of ginger ranging from 0.425-1.180mm in size found that the finer particles released the most anti-oxidants in an infusion.[20] If herbs are grown for a manufacturer making medicinal products, then these supplies are usually provided in whole or coarser cut form (such as pieces 25-50mm), enabling the manufacturer to check identification and quality and then apply their own processing methods. For domestic culinary or herb tea uses the herb particles may need to be smaller, such as in a fine cut form up to 3mm in size.[21]

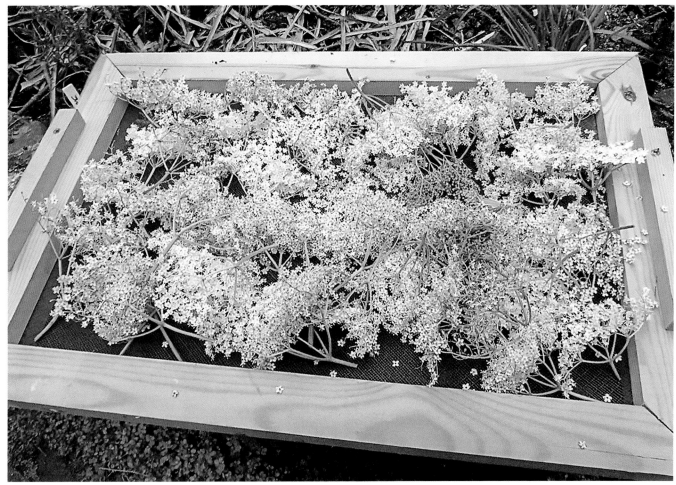

A drying rack with a layer of elder (*Sambucus nigra*) flowers

Crumbling and shredding

Small quantities of dried plants may be roughly crumbled by hand or broken up with a pestle and mortar. Screening is a method of separating a mixture of pieces into two or more size fractions, the over-sized materials are trapped above the screen, while undersized materials can pass through the screen. A simple but effective form of processing is to rub dried plant material through screens of wire mesh of different sizes. A number of scales are used to classify screens or sieves and particle sizes including the US sieve series and Tyler mesh size (based on number of openings in the width of one inch). Larger mesh sizes may be given as the size of opening in millimetres or inches. Some sizes of mesh opening are given on the right and screens at some of these sizes may be available

Comparative sieve sizes for screening herbs

US sieve size	Tyler equivalent	Opening size mm	inches	Ideal for
5/8 inch	–	16.00	0.625	Coarse cut
5/16 inch	2.5 Mesh	8.00	0.312	
No.5	5 Mesh	4.00	0.157	
No.10	9 Mesh	2.00	0.787	
No.20	20 Mesh	0.841	0.0331	Coarse powder
No.40	35 Mesh	0.42	0.0165	Coarse powder
No.60	60 Mesh	0.25	0.0098	Fine powder
No.120	115 Mesh	0.125	0.0049	Fine powder

Adapted from Wikipedia, http://en.wikipedia.org/wiki/Mesh_%28scale%29#Sieve_sizing_and_conversion_charts and US Pharmacopoeia, www.pharmacopeia.cn/usp.asp (accessed 25 March 2019).

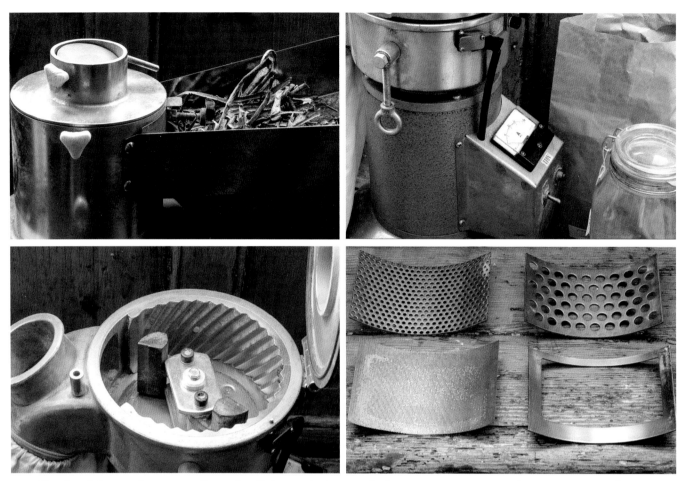

Dried bark is fed into a hammermill grinder (left to right from top): feed tray with dried ash (*Fraxinus excelsior*) bark; controls; chamber where bark is ground; screens used to reduce particle size

at beekeeper suppliers. If using a rubbing screen it is helpful to set up a frame with a tray or sheet below to catch the material. A chaffcutter may be considered for larger quantities of plant material, and can be hand-operated or sometimes can be mechanised with the addition of an electric motor. An alternative to the chaffcutter is an electric shredder dedicated for use with dried herbs. This is what we use at Holt Wood, and we deliberately selected a model which can be readily taken apart for cleaning between batches of herb.[22]

Powdering

Once the pieces of a dried medicinal plant are reduced in size, then they can be further processed by powdering. Processing to particle size suitable for use as a coarse or fine powder can add considerable value to herbs, as they then have a range of uses including percolation as a fluid extract or filling capsules. At Holt Wood we harvest cramp bark and after drying it is powdered for making capsules or tincture (see p.81, opposite). However, it should be noted that powdering does reduce the length of storage time possible for the herb material. For small quantities, hand powdering of dried herb can be done using a pestle and mortar or a coffee bean grinder, with repeated sieving to remove fibrous material. A hand-operated grain grinder also provides an effective way of grinding dried plant material, and can be adjusted to provide coarse or fine particles.

For larger quantities of herbs, a hammermill grinder can process cut herbs into pharmacy grade powder by using metal screens, and is suitable for long runs with a continuous feed for powdering dried bark, leaves,

HARVESTING CRAMP BARK

NAME: Holt Wood Herbs

LOCATION: Devon

ACTIVITY: Cramp bark (*Viburnum opulus*) is an anti-spasmodic remedy, also known as guelder rose or snowball tree. It is ideal for use in reducing menstrual cramps and other colicky complaints. In Holt Wood we planted cramp bark whips, 40-60cm, at the edge of

newly planted woodland areas prone to flooding. Apart from fencing for deer protection, and bi-annual strimming around the shrubs, no other special measures were taken. Spacing of the plants varied but averaged approximately 1.5-2m apart. After several years, each shrub, having reached a height of approximately 2m, provided five to six stems. In early spring the stems were cut off at a height of 10-20cm from the ground. Leaves and twigs less than a pencil in thickness were removed, and this material was used for compost or mulching elsewhere on the site. The cleaned branches were then stripped of bark using a curved blade (a boning knife was found to be ideal). These bark pieces were dried at 20°C (68°F) for three weeks and then cut and ground to powder. Quantity of fresh stem bark per plant averaged 350g which meant that, after drying, 1kg of dried powdered bark could be gained from six shrubs (this would be the equivalent of 2500 capsules containing 400mg powder per capsule). The remaining branches, having been stripped of bark, were chipped for mulching paths. The coppiced stumps can be left to regenerate over subsequent years.

KEY POINT: A sustainable harvest of cramp bark can be readily produced using coppicing techniques.

INFO: www.holtwoodherbs.com

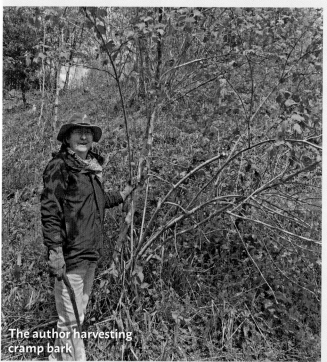

The author harvesting cramp bark

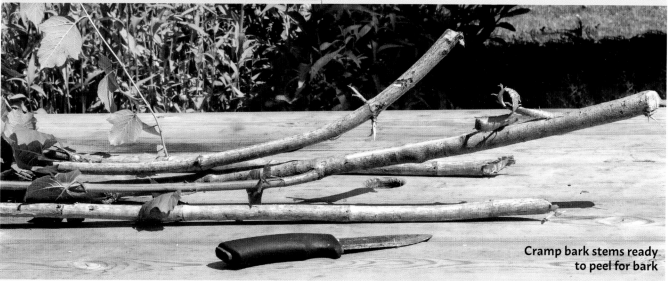

Cramp bark stems ready to peel for bark

roots and twigs.[23] The hammermill screens come with a range of different aperture sizes, so that particle size can be reduced in stages without overheating the plant material.

Powdering of dried herbs can produce a lot of dust! Protective equipment may be necessary for processing of drying herbs, to avoid dust inhalation and irritants to the skin and eyes. Flexible leather gloves with long cuffs are suitable for handling and for rubbing herbs. A dust mask, such as a disposable paper mask used in building and decorating, is probably suitable for working with most dried herbs. Ear protection may be needed if machinery is used.[24] Take particular care with machine use and select a wooden tool rather than fingers to push herbal material through the machine. Powdering of herbs should always be done in a well-ventilated area.

Storage of dried herbs

Dried herbs ideally need to be stored in cool, dark and dry conditions to limit further degradation. They need to be checked regularly in case of mould due to inadequate drying or infestation by insects. Plant material that is beyond its use by date can be recycled in compost or as a mulch on soil. The length of time during which plant materials can be reasonably expected to last without deterioration varies according to the part of plant and the amount of cutting and powdering done (table on the right). Generally, the greater the level of processing, the greater surface area in the herb material for further oxidation and degradation, so powder is most vulnerable. For short-term storage of dried herb material, paper or cotton bags can be used, closed with string or elastic bands, but these will allow in moisture unless they are further packed within moisture-proof bags or containers. For longer-term storage a variety of suitable containers can be used to prevent moisture and insects from getting in, such as large glass jars or plastic bins. Recycled food grade plastic tubs with sealable lids are ideal as containers to prevent dust, insects or vermin. An advantage of glass or clear plastic is that it allows inspection of the material inside. More substantial protection may be needed if the herbs are to be transported and large woven polypropylene sacks with inner liners can be obtained for this purpose.

Storage times for dried plants

Material	Length of storage
Roots, whole	2-5 years
Roots, cut	2 years
Roots, powdered	1 year
Leaves, stems or flowers, whole	2 years
Leaves, stems or flowers, powdered or cut	1 year
Bark, cut	2 years
Bark, powdered	1 year
Seeds, whole	up to 10 years in cold conditions < 10°C
Seeds, powdered	1 year
Fruits, whole	2 years

Insect contamination

Freezing can be used to doublecheck that plant material is not contaminated by insects. Herb material can be frozen in a domestic freezer at between -18 and -20°C (0 to -4°F) to ensure that no viable insects or their eggs are present. To do this, place the dried herb material in a plastic bag and seal at room temperature. Then put the bag in a freezer and enable the fast freeze option if available. The purpose of freezing rapidly is to ensure that insects cannot protect themselves against the cold (some insects can produce a natural antifreeze). If a large quantity of material needs to be frozen then it would be best to decant into smaller bags to ensure fast freezing. Keep the plant material in the freezer for 3-7 days. Then remove the bags of material and allow to return to room temperature for 24 hours without opening in order to avoid condensation dampening the herbs. Record the dates that the bags were inserted and removed from the freezer.

Sample label format for harvested plants

Herb Latin name	Herb common name	Part
Weight, fresh	Location	Batch number
Grower name	Telephone/email	Harvest date
Processing (whole/cut/powdered)		

Adapted from Whitten G. (1997) *Herbal Harvest: Commercial Organic Production of Quality Dried Herbs*, Hawthorn, Victoria, Australia: Bloomings Books, p.221.

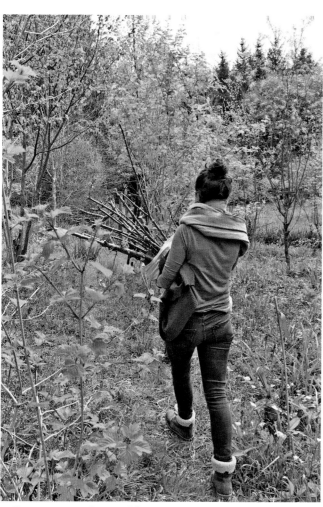

Pillowcases can be used for carrying the harvest

Keeping records of the harvest

Our experience at Holt Wood has been that there is an abundance of healing plants growing. We have needed to find efficient ways of processing the harvest to maximise quality and keep it well. We have found that it is vital to label (see the label format in the example above) and keep records of harvests as a good practice measure. Our harvest record book provides batch numbers which can be used to trace particular plants from harvest to use in preparations. The date of harvest is noted alongside the plant name and part, as well as the person who confirmed the plant's identity. Further useful information recorded is the fresh weight of the plant harvested and any particular key details about the source – for example, for trees this could be the location and/or the size measured as diameter at breast height. Additional details are added at a later stage of how the batch is processed, for example giving dried weight and quality. Measurements like this for agriculture and timber production are well established, but much less so for herbal plant cultivation or non-timber forest products.[25] Keeping such records of harvests will go a long way towards providing a set of data which builds up year by year. In the future we hope to compare yields between sites, and to relate them to environmental and other changes.

CHAPTER 6

Herbal Preparations

What a delight it is to grow and make your own herbal preparations for home use! Herbal remedies can be made from plants throughout the seasons of the year. Even better, the added value of handmade artisan products based on healing plants means that some items can be used as gifts or marketed more widely. In this chapter I look at examples of preparations using materials harvested from the medicinal forest garden. Sample recipes using bark, leaves, flowers, fruits and roots are given here, with indications of how they might be used, internally or externally, for a variety of common ailments and body care. Many of the recipes can be readily adapted for use with other plant species. The range of possibilities is great and this chapter gives some ideas intended to get you started. All of the suggested uses and doses advised in this chapter are based on adult use.[1]

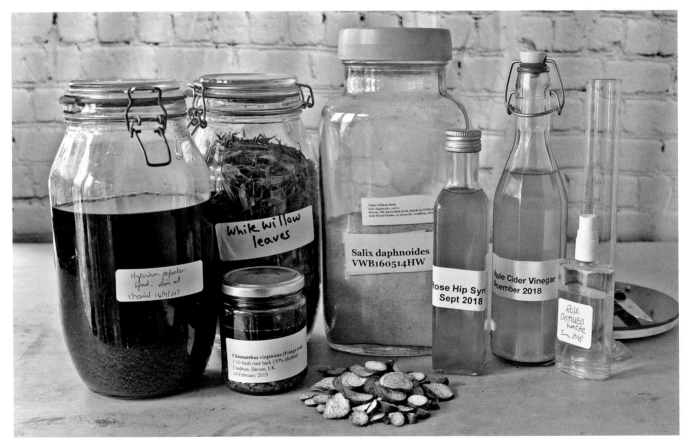

Herbal remedies can be made throughout the year

About sourcing plant ingredients

You may be keen to be self-sufficient and grow all of the ingredients used in herbal preparations for your home or business. At Holt Wood in the UK, we have not taken this route, partly for practical reasons of availability of time, effort and space. We suggest that instead of trying to be completely self-sufficient it is better to develop co-operative links with other grower and supplier enterprises using sustainable approaches. Our beeswax is obtained locally and we aim to support friendly beekeepers who can also provide honey. Our alcohol for tincture making is purchased from a UK manufacturer, and is derived from organically grown wheat. Some of our carrier oils (olive, sweet almond etc.) are based on imported organic supplies although we would like to promote more alternatives grown in the UK such as hemp seed, rapeseed and poppy seed oil.[2] For ointments and balms, we use cocoa butter and shea butter which are sourced from organic and Fairtrade suppliers. However, if you wish to be more self-sufficient in ingredients then you could focus on infusions, decoctions and poultices which are all water based, alongside fruit leathers, syrups, pills and vinegars which can be made using fruits and honey. Foraging may also be a way forward to gather a wider range of herbal ingredients than those cultivated, and can reflect a seasonal focus, developing an awareness of the local native plants that can contribute to wellbeing.[3]

Herbal preparations for internal use

A wide range of preparations for internal consumption can be made with medicinal plants, from alcoholic tinctures to sweet syrups, providing palatable remedies. In this section there are outline details of different types of plant extracts with different liquid vehicles, such as tinctures with alcohol/water, syrups with sugar and honey, and glycerin and vinegar-based extracts (see table on next page). Some more solid preparations can also be made and examples are fruit leather and honey-based pills and capsules.

Dosage and indications

For minor ailments and common complaints, there are many herbal preparations that can be of benefit in helping to allay symptoms such as pain and inflammation. In the recipes that follow, and in the plant profiles in the Directory in Part 2, there are sample indications and dosages for medicinal use. However, these are given only to provide an idea of possible uses and they must not be taken as claims to cure or as suitable medications for every situation. The choice of plant(s), preparation and dose should always be based on an accurate assessment of the person concerned and their medical complaint, and professional advice and diagnosis should always be sought in cases of doubt. Be aware that many herbal remedies can interact with other medicinal prescriptions, sometimes having a potentially adverse effect. Many plant remedies have a wide range of safe therapeutic dosing but there are some that can be toxic or unsuitable and the advice of a clinical herbal practitioner is essential. None of these remedies are suitable for children without professional advice.

Making alcohol-based extracts – tinctures

Fresh plant material can be used to make a tincture extract by steeping or macerating the herb in a liquid mixture of alcohol (ethanol) and water. Tincture strength can vary from 1:3 (one part of herb by weight to three parts liquid by volume) to 1:10 (one part herb to 10 parts of liquid). Fluid extracts are stronger, having a strength of 1:1 or 1:2 and are usually made with specialised equipment on a commercial scale. Use of alcohol with various proportions of water enables a good range of plant constituents to be extracted. Most simple tinctures made at home will have about 25% alcohol content, which is the minimum proportion of alcohol needed to extract active constituents and to prevent significant deterioration over time. Use of a spirit like vodka is ideal as it is largely flavourless and contains about 40% alcohol and, allowing for the water content in the fresh plant, it is likely that the final product will contain about 25% alcohol and be well preserved. Some plants, especially those with resinous constituents, can be better extracted in a mixture containing up to

Range of herbal preparations for internal use

Herbal preparation	Characteristics of preparation and shelf life	Examples
Decoction	Plant material is boiled in water, and then strained. Suitable for woodier parts such as bark, seeds or roots. Must be used within 24 hours or, if refrigerated, several days.	Willow bark Cramp bark Oregon grape root
Infusion or tea	Plant material is allowed to stand in boiling hot water for a few minutes or longer, and then strained. Used mainly for cut leaves and flowers and these can be fresh or dried. Used as tea or gargle. Must be used within 24 hours or, if refrigerated, several days.	Bilberry leaves Birch leaves Forsythia flowers Lime flowers Magnolia flowers Myrtle leaves Raspberry leaves Sweet chestnut leaves
Capsules and pills	Finely ground dried plant material pressed into capsules or mixed with honey to form stiff paste.	Cramp bark Ginkgo leaves Willow bark
Tincture or liquid extract	Fresh or dried plant material is mixed with alcohol and water and then pressed out to leave the tincture. Alcohol strength must be at least 25%. Alternatively a liquid extract is based on percolation through a column of finely powdered herb. Long shelf-life and good keeping qualities for at least three years.	Chaste tree leaves and berries Cramp bark Ginkgo leaves Hawthorn berries Prickly ash bark or berries Willow bark
Glycerin extract	Glycerites are made by infusion of plant material in glycerin. Keeps 1-2 years.	Blackcurrant buds Birch buds
Syrup	Plant material is infused or decocted, then strained, and sugar is added and dissolved in the liquid. Keeping qualities similar to jam, for several years.	Cherry bark Elderberries Marshmallow root Rose hips
Vinegar and oxymel	Plant material is dried and infused in apple or wine vinegar, can keep 1-2 years. Addition of honey to make the oxymel.	Alder bark Elderflowers Raspberry leaves
Fruit leather	Fruit is cooked gently to a firm paste and then spread out thinly to dry. Can be frozen and keeps well.	Blackcurrant fruit Fig fruit Chokeberry fruit

60% alcohol. Determining the ideal strength of alcohol to use for individual plants can be done by looking at manufacturers catalogues. If large quantities of alcohol are to be used for medicinal or manufacturing purposes then application for a licence to purchase duty-free alcohol (96% alcohol) may be considered.[4]

The process of tincture making, whether from fresh or dry plant material, is an effective way of extracting and preserving the active healing components of a medicinal plant. Tinctures have good keeping qualities. The recipes below will make a tincture of approximately 1:5 strength, which is a proportion of 1g weight of the herb to 5ml volume of the liquid, so that a 5ml teaspoon dose of the tincture provides the equivalent of 1g of the medicinal plant.

The use of fresh plant material for making tinctures involves some uncertainty about the alcohol strength of the final extract, since the volume of water in fresh leaves or other plant parts can only be estimated. The moisture content in plant material can vary considerably from

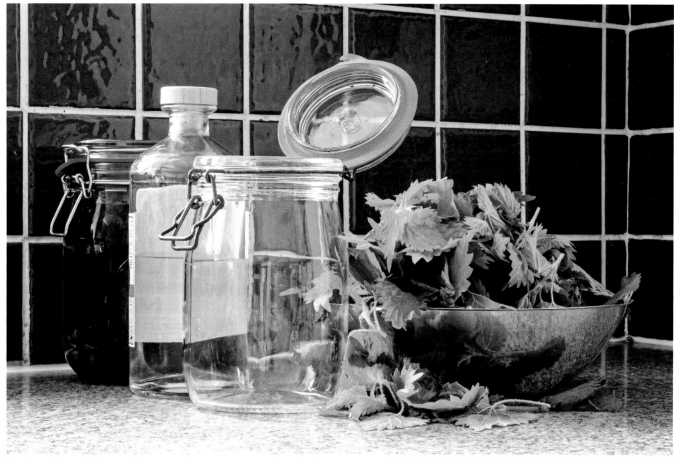

Making a fresh plant leaf tincture

Fresh nettle leaf tincture

You need:

Several handfuls of freshly picked young nettle tops (use gloves!)

About 300ml spirit such as vodka or gin which is 40% alcohol by volume

A glass jam jar or preserving jar with an airtight lid

1. Do not wash the leaves but pick off any damaged parts, dirt or insects.

2. Cut the leaves into smaller pieces, discarding any tough stems or roots.

3. Press the leafy material down in the glass jar, up to 5-10cm below the top, and cover with the spirit. Use a weight (small glass or preserving weights are ideal) to ensure that the plant material stays under the surface of the liquid. Add more spirit if necessary.

4. Close the top and label the jar with plant name and date. Stand on a windowsill and turn and stir the mixture daily for 3-4 weeks.

5. Strain the mixture through a muslin cloth and discard the solid plant material in the compost.

6. Store in a labelled glass bottle, in a dark place.

7. Nettle tincture can be taken at 1 tsp per day in a cup of water up to three times daily for arthritis or urinary complaints.

Note: This tincture recipe can be used with other fresh plant material such as bilberry or birch leaves, elder or hawthorn flowers, as well as other plant parts such as chopped fresh cramp bark or Oregon grape roots.

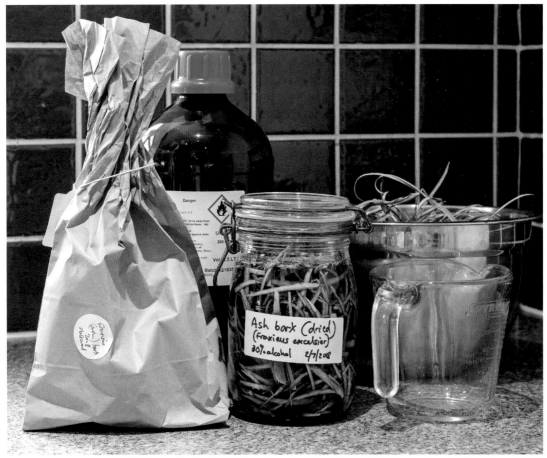

Making a tincture with dried bark

Dried ash bark tincture

Dried ash bark, 100g
Spirit 40% alcohol by volume, 300ml
White wine 10-12%, 300ml

1. Place the dried bark in a glass jar.

2. Mix the wine and spirit and pour over the bark in the jar, making sure the bark is fully covered.

3. Stir well, screw on the top and leave to stand for four to six weeks, shaking every other day or so.

4. Press and strain off the liquid, discard the spent bark in the compost, and bottle and label.

5. This tincture is taken at 20 drops (1ml) up to three times per day before meals as a bitter tonic providing a digestive stimulant helping to regulate blood sugar levels.

Note: This recipe for making a tincture based on dried plant material can be used with a wide range of plants. If a harvest has been exceptionally large then some plant material can be dried for later use, and this method of making a tincture can be used.

30-90%, depending on the species and part of plant used. Fresh leaves and flowers are also fairly bulky and so there is a risk that some plant material may not be fully covered by the liquid inside a jar and spoilage can occur. One way around this is to dry the plant material before making a tincture. The process is then somewhat similar to making a fresh tincture, except that a lower level of alcohol percentage by volume is needed. This is a more accurate method and an economical mixture of equal parts of white wine and spirit can be used which gives an alcohol content of around 25-30% by volume.

Making water-based extracts – infusions and decoctions

Infusions and decoctions are water-based extracts of plants. The term 'infusion' generally refers to extraction in hot water though sometimes a cold infusion is made. When hot water is used, the infusion is more commonly known as herb tea. Fresh or dry plant material is put into a vessel with water that has just boiled, and the mixture is allowed to steep, usually for 5-10 minutes. An infusion is best made in glass or china pots rather than metal containers. A good guide as to when the infusion is ready to use is that the leaves or other

Fresh woodland tonic infusion

Young shoots and leaves from a variety of trees and shrubs including birch, Douglas fir, bramble, approximately 50g weight altogether (if dried then use half the quantity, about 25g)
Water, 500ml

1. Chop or bruise the plant materials and place in a teapot.
2. Heat the water to boiling and add to the teapot, cover with lid.
3. Allow to stand for 5-10 mins and then strain.
4. Drink immediately or store in a labelled bottle in the refrigerator for 1-2 days.

Note: This infusion recipe can be used with individual plants or combinations of 2-5 plants. We have found that the inclusion of at least one aromatic herb (such as pine or mint leaves) and at least one astringent herb (rose or bramble flower or leaf) often makes a good combination. Adding a bitter warming herb (such as yarrow) makes a more stimulating and invigorating tea, whereas adding a demulcent and cooling herb (such as lime flower or leaf) makes a calming and relaxing tea.

Making a herbal infusion

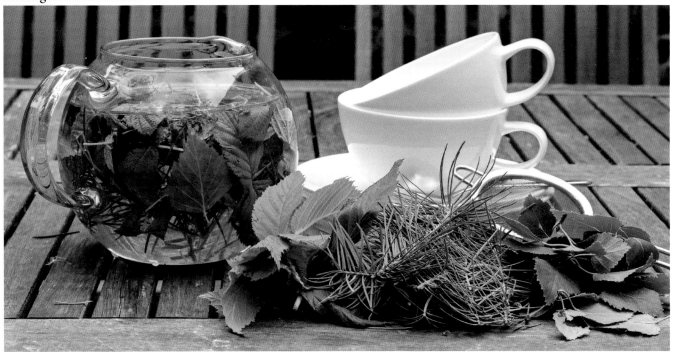

material sink to the bottom of the container. Hot infusions are suitable for soft herbal material such as flowers and leaves, helping to release aromas from essential oils and other constituents. Quantities are not exact and can be adjusted according to taste, although it is commonly recommended to use 25g of dried material in 500ml of hot water for medicinal use. If fresh plant material is used then the quantity can be doubled to 50g. A cold water infusion is preferred if you do not want to lose aromatic components through evaporation, or if there are plant constituents such as mucilage which can be easily destroyed by heat. Usually a cold water infusion involves standing the plant material in water for a period of 8-12 hours or overnight and then straining off the liquid for use. Water extracts based on an infusion are rather short-lived and best used straight away, or kept for just 1-2 days in a refrigerator. In addition to being drunk as a tea, an infusion can be used to provide an inhalation or a mouthwash.

Placing plant materials with aromatic properties into hot water helps to release their essential oils, often with positive anti-inflammatory and antiseptic effects. In addition to drinking as tea, another way to benefit is to inhale the steam.

The term 'decoction' refers to placing plant material in water and applying heat to raise the temperature to boiling and then continuing to heat for a period of 20-30 minutes or even longer. Once made, a decoction can be used in much the same way as an infusion. The decoction process is suited to tougher plant material, such as bark, dried mushrooms and roots. Decoctions can be made into more concentrated extracts by continuing the simmering process until at least half of the water is boiled off.

Making sugar-based extracts – syrups, fruit leathers, glycerites, oxymels

Sugar-based extracts of plants range through syrups and cordials to glycerin or honey preparations. Sugar acts as a reasonably effective preservative and so herbal syrups can provide another way to keep plant materials for later use. The advantages of syrups are that they are palatable to children, can disguise horrible-tasting herbs, and are fairly easy to make. An equal amount of sugar to liquid is generally needed. The usual method is to make an infusion or decoction from bark, fruits or roots and then add at least 500g of sugar per 500ml of liquid and heat while

Inhalation of sweet gum leaf

Young leaves of sweet gum, about two handfuls
Water, 1000ml
A large bowl and a towel

1. Crush up the leaves and place in a large bowl.

2. Heat the water to boiling and pour onto the leaves, taking care not to get splashed.

3. Lean over the bowl carefully, as the steam will be hot, and place a towel over head and bowl.

4. Gently breathe in the aromatic steam for a few minutes, taking a break if the warmth is excessive. Repeat as needed in cases of colds and sinusitis.

Note: This recipe for steam inhalation can be used with other aromatic and antiseptic plants such as Scots pine and eucalyptus.

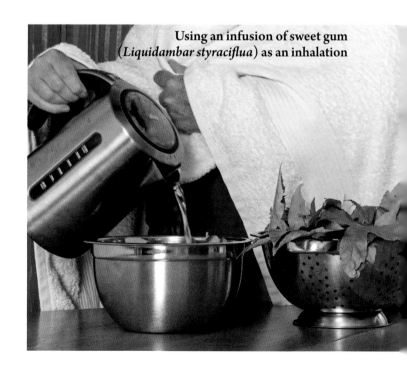

Using an infusion of sweet gum (*Liquidambar styraciflua*) as an inhalation

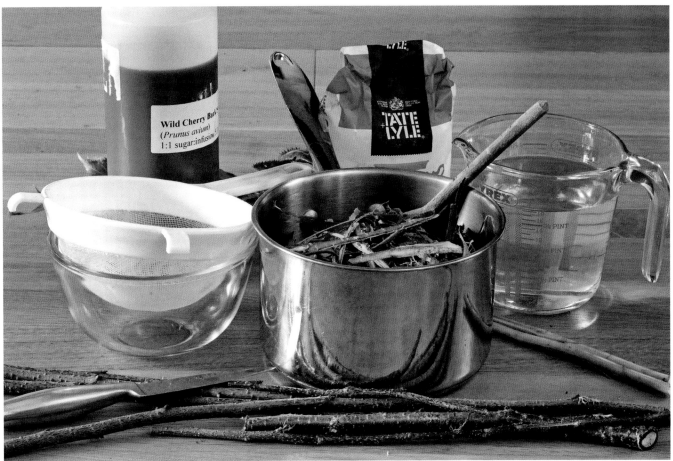

Making a herbal syrup with fresh cherry bark

Cherry bark syrup

Fresh cherry bark, approximately 50g weight (from bird cherry (*Prunus padus*) or wild cherry (*P. avium*))
Water, 500ml
Sugar
Glass sauce bottles with lids

1. Check that the bark is clean, removing debris and damaged parts, then shred the bark coarsely and place in a saucepan.

2. Add the cold water to the bark and stand for 8-12 hours.

3. Gently bring to the boil and simmer covered for 15-20 minutes.

4. Remove from the heat and allow to cool till lukewarm.

5. Strain off the liquid and allow to cool, discarding the bark to compost.

6. Use this decoction to make a syrup by adding 500g of sugar per 500ml of liquid, warming and stirring until fully dissolved.

7. Allow to cool and then bottle and label.

8. Take 1 tsp up to three times per day for a dry and irritating cough.

Note: This recipe requires both cold infusion and a hot decoction to maximise the cherry bark extract constituents. Note that cherry bark syrup is used to suppress an irritating cough and should not be used where a cough is productive. If using dried bark then you can halve the weight of bark. Other tree barks can be decocted in water and made into a syrup including aged alder buckthorn (*Frangula alnus*) bark as a laxative remedy. Infused flowers (elderflower) and fruit (sea buckthorn) juice also make good syrups.

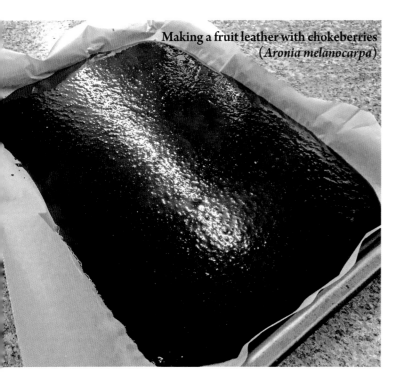

Making a fruit leather with chokeberries
(*Aronia melanocarpa*)

stirring to dissolve the sugar. The syrup can be given neat or further diluted with water to make a pleasant drink, like a cordial. Similarly to jam preserves, a syrup will keep reasonably well for several years, but if it becomes discoloured or mouldy then it should be discarded.

Making a fruit leather

The preserving quality of sugar is also helpful in making fruit leathers, since the natural sugar content in a fruit purée is readily concentrated. Additional sugar may be needed for fruits that are somewhat sour in nature. The fruit purée is heated and water is evaporated until the purée is fairly stiff and can be spread out on a sheet of greaseproof paper to further dry. The dried fruit leather can be cut into squares or rolled up and also freezes well.

Making a glycerite

Another vehicle of a sweet nature is glycerin, which can be vegetable derived and has the advantage of being non-alcoholic and more appropriate for use with those who cannot take alcohol. Glycerin and water together provide a reasonable solvent for plant constituents such as tannins but not aromatic resins or fixed oils. Glycerin tends to absorb water from the air, and so even when pure is likely to contain 5% water by volume.[5] A glycerin/water mixture strength of 60-75% glycerin is regarded as an adequate preservative, the lower level for dry plant material, and the higher level for fresh plant material, although up to 90% may be needed for very juicy plant material. A glycerin extract is made in a similar way to the fresh plant tincture which is made with alcohol/water. Glycerites should be kept in a cool dark place or refrigerated in an airtight container.

Chokeberry fruit leather

Fresh ripe chokeberries, approximately 500g weight
Cold water, 100ml
Tray and greaseproof paper

1. Check the fruit is clean, wash if necessary and place in a saucepan.

2. Add the cold water and heat gently for 15-20 minutes, stirring to break up the fruit.

3. Using a wooden spoon, stir and press the fruit through a sieve to make a purée.

4. Re-heat the purée, driving off water until it is fairly stiff.

5. Spread the purée thinly on the greaseproof paper on a tray, up to 5mm thick.

6. Allow to dry, either in a warm and airy place or at the lowest possible oven setting.

7. Cut into squares or roll up pieces into tubes. This fruit leather can be used as a regular snack for anti-oxidant effects and to help regulate cholesterol and blood sugar.

Note: A fruit leather can be frozen if not eaten straight away. Honey can be used as an alternative to sugar, it contains around 20% water but has other constituents which are antibacterial.

Making vinegars and oxymels

Historically, more use may have been made of herbal vinegars, although they seem to be coming back into fashion nowadays. A vinegar with elderflowers was described by Richard Bradley in 1732, advising to gather the flowers when dry in the month of May, and to 'pick them from the Stalks; let them dry in the Shade, and then put an Ounce to each Quart of White-Wine Vinegar to stand in the Vinegar for two Monthes, then

Blackcurrant bud glycerite

Fresh blackcurrant buds, 50g (if dried then use half the quantity, about 25g)
Vegetable glycerin, 150 ml
Water, 50 ml
Jam jar

1. Chop the buds and place in a small glass jar.

2. Combine the glycerin and water.

3. Add the glycerin and water to the jar and stir well. The buds should be fully covered; add more glycerin if not.

4. Tighten the cover and stand for 4-6 weeks, occasionally stirring.

5. Strain through muslin or a tea towel, and squeeze the remaining glycerite out. Bottle the glycerite extract and label. Will keep refrigerated for 1-2 years.

6. The glycerite will be quite strong and is taken in quantities of 10-20 drops per dose up to three times per day for immune support and to help alleviate stress.

Note: Such glycerin extracts are also ideal for small quantities of buds gathered in spring such as those of birch and sweet chestnut.[6]

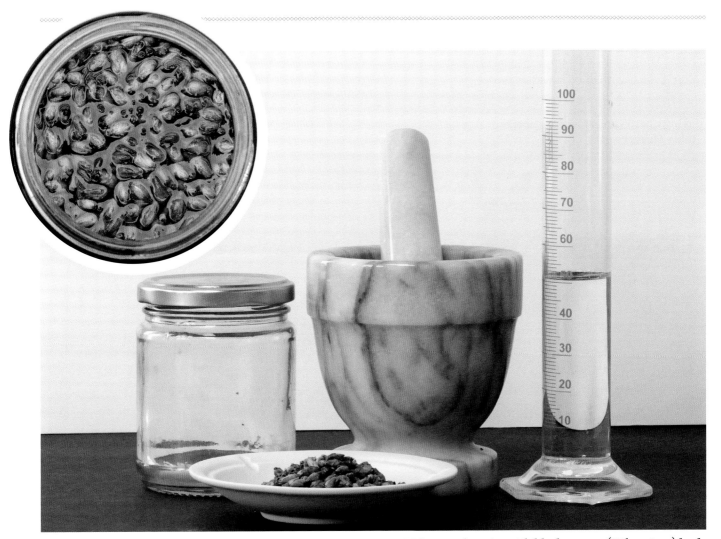

Making a glycerite with blackcurrant (*Ribes nigra*) buds

Raspberry leaf vinegar

Fresh raspberry leaves, 50g (25g if dried)
Apple or wine vinegar, 500ml
Fliptop glass bottles

1. Place the raspberry leaves in a jar and add the vinegar.

2. Stir well, close the lid and stand in a cool dark place for three weeks, shaking daily.

3. Strain, bottle the vinegar extract and label. Use within six months.

4. Take 1 tsp up to three times daily in water (or use in food) to help with digestion or menstrual complaints.

Note: Herbal vinegars of this kind can be made with many healing plants including berries and leaves of chasteberry (*Vitex agnus*) for premenstrual complaints, and sage (*Salvia officinalis*) for menopausal hot flushes. The herb vinegar preparations will keep better if made with dried leaves or berries.

Making a herb vinegar with raspberry (*Rubus idaeus*) leaves

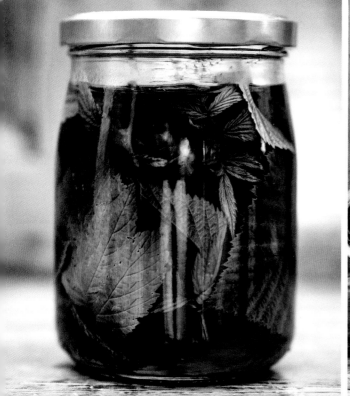

Rosemary and birch oxymel

Fresh birch leaves, 50g
Fresh rosemary leaves, 50g
Apple or wine vinegar, 500ml
Honey, 300g
Kilner or preserving jar

1. Chop and place the leaves in a jar and add the vinegar.

2. Stir well, cover with a non-metal lid and stand in a cool dark place for 3-4 weeks, stirring every few days.

3. Strain the vinegar, discarding the leaves, and heat gently until reduced by a third to about 300ml.

4. Add the honey, stirring well, and when fully mixed, bottle the oxymel and label. Store in the refrigerator and use within 6-12 months.

5. Take 1 tbsp up to three times daily in hot water, to help prevent infections, reduce pain and soothe a sore throat.

Note: Although oxymels have fallen out of use, there could be great benefit in bringing back these complex and tasty concoctions.

Making an oxymel with rosemary (*Rosmarinus officinalis*) and birch (*Betula pendula*) leaves

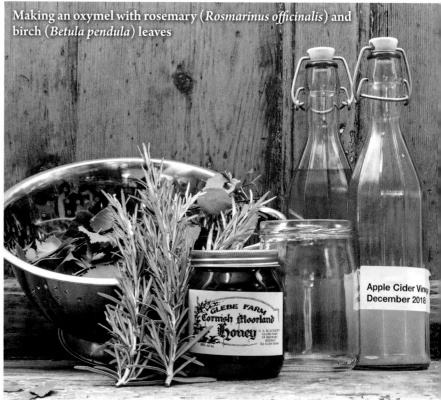

pour the Vinegar from them for use'.[7] This is an old remedy for soothing a sore throat, and can be used in hayfever and sinusitis.

Herbal vinegars are made by infusing plant material directly in vinegar. Vinegar itself is weakly acidic (about 5-10% acetic acid), and is antiseptic and anti-inflammatory, generally having a cooling effect and promoting salivary flow. Homemade vinegar can be made from cider fermented from apples or pears, once you have acquired a 'vinegar mother'.[8] Caution is needed if using fresh plant material as the additional moisture content may dilute the vinegar so that it does not keep well. Use of dried plant material in vinegar preparations avoids any problems arising from diluting vinegar. Coarsely crumbled or powdered dried plant material is placed in the vinegar and allowed to stand for several weeks, shaking daily, then strained and put into sterilised bottles. Herbal vinegar can be taken internally or added to baths.

An oxymel is a traditional preparation made with a combination of vinegar and honey (this is called a shrub if using berries). The proportions of honey and vinegar can vary, and medieval recipes described an oxymel as having four parts: two parts honey, one part vinegar and one part water.[9] In the oxymel recipe given here, the proportions of vinegar and honey are about equal.

Making pills and capsules

Herbs in pill or capsule form are convenient to take. Traditionally, pills and lozenges were made using powdered ingredients mixed with a gum-like thickener. A version of this approach is to use honey to hold the powdered plant material together sufficiently to allow pills to be rolled or cut.

Many plants also lend themselves to filling capsules if dried and finely powdered. A cheaply available handfilling tool can make 50

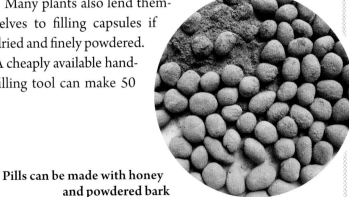

Pills can be made with honey and powdered bark

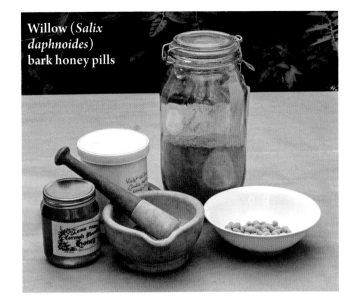

Willow (*Salix daphnoides*) bark honey pills

Willow bark honey pills

Approximately 20g of fine willow bark (*Salix alba* or *S. daphnoides*) powder
Runny honey, 20g
Fine liquorice powder or caster sugar

1. Place the honey in a bowl.

2. Stir in a teaspoon of the willow bark powder using a wooden spoon.

3. Continue adding the powder and stirring it in; the mixture will become almost impossibly stiff, but continue until no more powder can be incorporated. Note that if insufficient powder is used the resulting pills will soon become shapeless and soggy.

4. Roll the mixture into a long pencil-like tube, and cut about 0.5cm width slices off.

5. Roll each slice in the fingers to form a ball and then in powder to coat; liquorice powder is traditionally used because its sweet taste helps to disguise the bitterness of the pills.

6. Label and store in a clean glass jar in a cool dark place.

7. Take two pills up to six times per day. Can be taken to help ease painful complaints such as arthritis.

Note: This method can be used with any finely powdered plant material, and the keeping qualities of the honey pills are good, since the honey acts as a preservative.

Cramp bark capsules

Approximately 25g fine powder of cramp bark
50 vegetarian capsules
Capsule hand-filling kit
Bowls for separating capsule parts

1. Separate the capsules into lower larger and upper smaller parts in two bowls.

2. Adjust the spacers below the capsule-filling tray so that a capsule lower part fits upright with the top edge level with the tray. Place the lower parts of the capsules upright in the remaining holes. Take care that the tray surface and capsules remain level.

3. Spread about half of the bark powder across the tray and fill the lower capsule parts with the powder using a piece of card.

4. Use the tool provided with the kit to tamp down the powder in the capsules.

5. Repeat the addition of powder and tamping down until all of the lower capsule parts are well filled.

6. Carefully remove the spacers so that the tray drops down slightly and so that the edges of the lower capsule parts stand proud above the tray.

7. Place each of the capsule top parts onto the bottom parts, and pressing down gently you should feel a slight click as each capsule top fits securely onto the bottom part.

8. Lift the capsules individually from the tray, inspect to check that they are correctly pushed together, and store in a labelled glass jar out of light.

9. Take 2-3 capsules every four hours for period pains.

Note: This recipe can be used with other powdered herbs such as willow bark (*Salix* spp.) for arthritic pain or aged alder buckthorn (*Frangula alnus*) bark as a laxative. This convenient means of administering herbs enables a combination of the powders to be used.

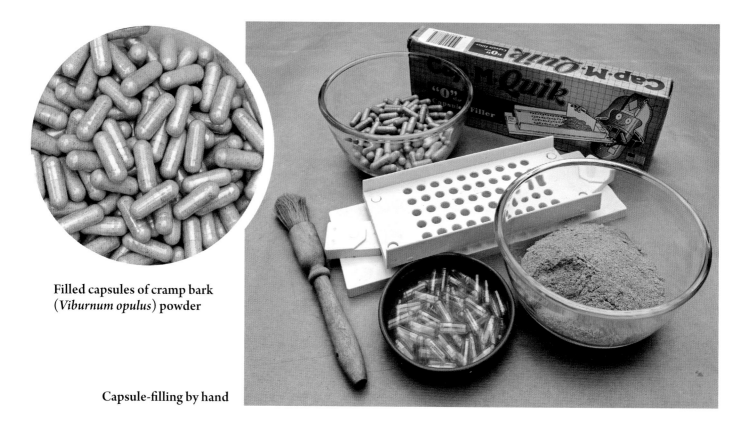

Filled capsules of cramp bark (*Viburnum opulus*) powder

Capsule-filling by hand

capsules (size 0 containing approximately 400mg) at a time. The empty capsules can be obtained in vegetarian gelatine-free form, usually sold in quantities of a thousand. Care must be taken to avoid wetting the capsules as they will readily dissolve and collapse. The shelf life of powdered plant material is relatively short, as it begins to deteriorate after powdering, so these items should be made as close as possible to the time of use.

Herbal preparations for external use

Here are some examples of preparations for external use, from poultices and infused oils to balms and distilled waters or hydrosols. See an overview in the table on the following page.

Making infusions for external use

Plants made up as infusions can provide useful washes for the skin, or rinses for use after a hair wash. Herbal baths are another way in which plants can be used. Making a strong infusion or decoction of plant material, which is then strained, is suitable for adding to the bath, usually around 500ml. Alternatively the plant material can be hung in a muslin bag or a sock under the bath tap, choosing herbs for a relaxing or invigorating bath. Possibilities include limeflowers, eucalyptus leaves, birch leaves, sweet bay, yarrow, willow leaves. Another possibility is a footbath to soak the feet, based on aromatic and soothing herbs such as bergamot, eucalyptus, mint or pine.

Making herb poultices and compresses

In a poultice you process fresh plant material into a paste for direct application to the body. A poultice is usually useful in skin complaints such as superficial burns, splinters, bruises and cuts. You will need to crush, chop or grate herbs into a pulp, and add just enough water to make a paste. You can add flour, clay, bran, honey, soap etc. to make the paste thicker and more drawing of moisture from the skin. The paste is spread evenly on the skin up to 1-2cm thick. Using muslin helps to hold the herb mixture in place. For a small area you can use

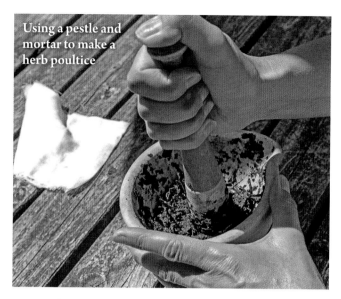

Using a pestle and mortar to make a herb poultice

Making a yarrow poultice

Fresh yarrow herb (a good handful of leaf), 25-50g
Water
A pestle and mortar, muslin and scissors

1. Pick leaves and brush off insects and dirt.

2. Chop or tear the herb coarsely, and place in a pestle.

3. Add a little water and crush and mash herbs into pulp or paste using the pestle and mortar.

4. Cut a piece of muslin about twice the area of skin to be treated, and spread the herb paste onto the layer of muslin. Fold over the muslin onto the herb, like a sandwich.

5. Apply the muslin with herb paste direct to the affected area, tie on with strips of muslin, leave on for 30 minutes and repeat as needed. This recipe is both antiseptic and anti-inflammatory, ideal for applying to bruises, cuts, stings or rashes.

Note: This poultice recipe can be adapted for more specific purposes. Suitable soothing herbs for use as a poultice include plantain (*Plantago* species) especially for insect bites or stings, splinters, boils, also chickweed (*Stellaria media*) or lemon balm (*Melissa officinalis*). Antiseptic marigold (*Calendula officinalis*) flowers and leaves can be used for bruises, burns, cuts, sore and inflamed skin. Comfrey (*Symphytum officinale*) or St John's wort (*Hypericum perforatum*) help in healing superficial wounds, repairing skin damage and recovery from bruises and sprains.

Range of herbal preparations for external use

Herbal preparation	Characteristics of preparation and shelf life	Examples of medicinal trees and shrubs
Infusion or water	Plant material is allowed to stand in boiling hot water for a few minutes or longer, and then strained. Used as a wash for skin, or can be a bath addition. Keeps for 24 hours.	Pine needles Eucalyptus leaf Arbor vitae needles
Infused oil	Fresh or dried plant material is allowed to stand for some days or weeks in a carrier oil (such as olive or sunflower oil) and the oil is then pressed out. Keeping qualities are limited to 6-9 months, much less if fresh herb is used due to moisture content.	Birch leaves Elder leaves Juniper leaves Pine needles
Distilled water and hydrosols	Fresh or dried plant material is boiled and steam condensed to produce small amounts of essential oil and larger amounts of distilled water, known as hydrosols. Essential oils can keep for at least five years but distilled waters and hydrosols may need the addition of alcohol for preservation longer than 6-12 months.	Witch hazel leafy twigs Rosemary leaves Eucalyptus leaves Pine needles Liquidambar leaves Bay leaves Douglas fir
Balms and ointments	Made by adding butters and/or waxes to infused oils. Since these preparations do not contain water they keep better than creams or lotions which are an emulsion of water and oil. Keeps for up to 3-6 months without preservatives.	Birch buds Juniper leaves Pine leaves Rosemary leaves
Poultice or compress	A poultice is based on plant material mashed with water and applied directly to the skin. A compress is a piece of cloth wetted with an infusion or decoction and applied direct. Usually for use immediately though may keep up to 24 hours in the refrigerator.	Birch leaves Yarrow leaves Witch hazel leaves
Incense stick	Partly dried leaves and twigs are tightly bound with string, and then fully dried so that they smoulder when lit. Can keep for 1-2 years before losing aromatic benefits.	Douglas fir leaves Juniper leaves Sage leaves

an empty teabag; for a larger area use a pillowcase to hold the plant paste in place. Leave on for 30 minutes or longer and repeat as needed. It can be helpful to apply a thin layer of oil on the skin first. Larger amounts of plant material can be processed in a blender. Another possibility in poultice-making is use of dried herbs moistened with water, though generally, fresh herbs work best.[10]

A compress is also applied to the skin and is usually based on a piece of cloth soaked in a herbal infusion or decoction. A compress is slightly different to a poultice in that it is based on a strong herbal infusion or decoction, using 5-20g of plant material to 200ml of water. The plant is steeped in hot water for 30 minutes and then strained out of the liquid. A piece of muslin cloth is then dipped into the liquid, squeezed to remove excess liquid, and applied direct to the affected area.

Making infused oils

Fresh plant material can be infused in a carrier oil, and this is ideal for use in external applications. Suitable carrier oils include olive oil, sunflower oil and sweet almond oil. The plant material can be chopped up and placed in a jar, then covered fully with the oil. Rather than replacing the lid, tie a piece of muslin over the top of the jar to protect from dust and insects, and put on a sunny window ledge. The purpose of leaving the jar open is to encourage moisture to escape since any moisture in the mixture will cause deterioration. After 4-6 weeks

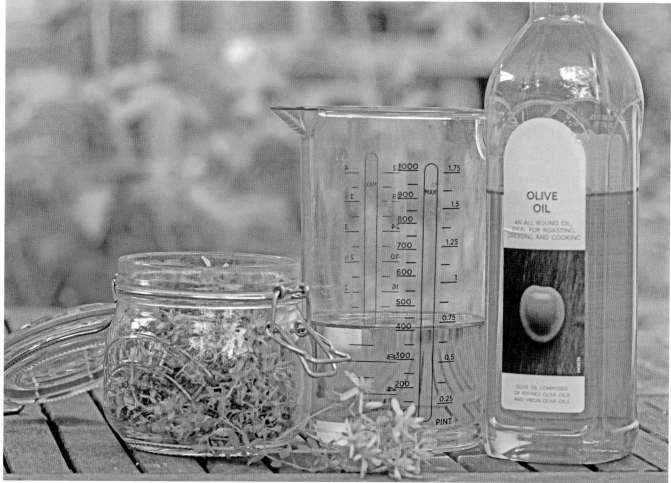

Making an infused oil with St John's wort (*Hypericum perforatum*) flowers

St John's wort infused oil

St John's wort flowers picked over the late summer
Olive oil
Glass jar with muslin cover and string or elastic band

1. Collect St John's wort flowers and tops, picking off insects or damaged parts.

2. Place flowers in a glass jar and cover with good quality oil. Add a weight to stop the plant material sticking out of the oil or it will go mouldy. Cover with muslin or kitchen towel held in place by string or an elastic band.

3. Place on a sunny windowsill and shake gently each day.

4. Continue to add more flowers until the infused oil has a dark red appearance.

5. Strain carefully, leaving behind any sediment and put in a glass bottle and label.

6. Apply sparingly several times a day for skin complaints, such as shingles (but not for use on open wounds).

Note: Many healing plants are suitable for infusing in oil, including leaves of trees such as birch (*Betula pendula*), eucalyptus (*Eucalyptus* species) and juniper (*Juniperus communis*).

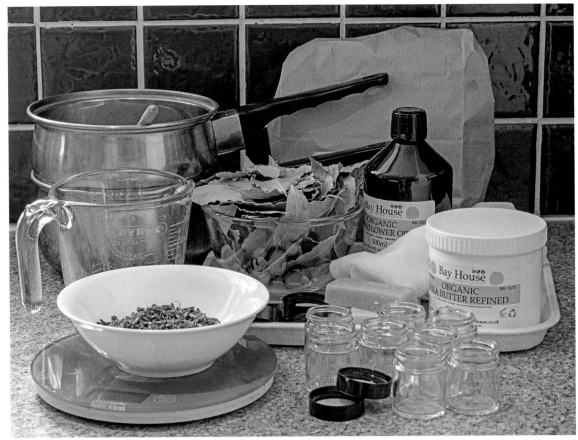

Making a balm with birch (*Betula pendula*) buds and sweet bay (*Laurus nobilis*) leaves

Birch bud and sweet bay balm

Dried birch buds, 20g

Dried sweet bay leaves, crumbled, 20g

Sunflower oil, 200ml

Shea butter, 80g

Beeswax, 20g

A bain marie or double saucepan, muslin, small jars for storage

1. Place the buds and leaves in the oil in the top of the bain marie, or in a pan over a pan of water, and gently warm for 60 minutes.

2. Add the shea butter, stirring to dissolve as it melts.

3. Grate the beeswax and stir into the oil, bud and leaf mixture.

4. Remove from the heat and strain the oil through a muslin cloth into a warmed jug. Discard the used buds and leaves to compost.

5. Pour the oil into small jars, cover and allow to cool and label. Keeps for 1-2 months.

Birch bud and sweet bay balm have antiseptic and anti-inflammatory effects and can be used direct on the skin to help ease insect bites and rashes.

Note: This recipe can be adapted to include other plant ingredients such as eucalyptus or juniper leaves.

decant the oil through a strainer, leaving behind the debris and watery layer at the base of the jar. The process can be sped up by using a bain marie (steam bath), and will take about one hour. This type of preparation does not keep long and should be used within 3-6 months at most. Dried plant material can be used instead of fresh and this will improve keeping qualities as there is less likelihood of introducing moisture into the infused oil.

An infused oil can be used as a base for a lotion, balm or ointment. A lotion is rather like a thin cream and can be made from an infused oil and water mixture shaken up well together to form an emulsion. However, the oil and water will tend to separate without an emulsifier in the mix, and keeping qualities are limited. The balm recipe given here contains no water which makes it more stable and a preparation that will keep better than oil and water mixtures.

Making balms and ointments

Infused oils are ideal as a base for making balms and ointments, a balm being somewhat softer than a waxy ointment. The addition of beeswax and cocoa or shea butter helps to thicken an oil and make a consistency suitable for applying sparingly to the skin. The inclusion of the shea butter in the recipe given here provides a softening effect, melting on contact. For a harder waxy ointment more suitable for a lip wax, the shea butter can be omitted. Essential oils can also be added to help preserve the preparation, for safety usually at a concentration of less than 1%, that is, a maximum of 20 drops for each 100ml made.

Making hydrosols and distilled waters

Distillation is a process suitable for aromatic plant materials, such as the leaves of *Eucalyptus* species or flowering tops of *Lavandula* species. Steam is passed through the plant material or produced by boiling water containing the plant material, and this steam is condensed. The process produces a water known as a hydrosol which is a mixture of both distilled water and essential oil.[11] The end result is often a fairly large quantity of distilled water with a little essential oil floating on top. Considerable plant material is needed for essential oil

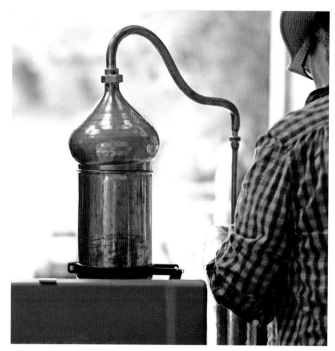
A traditional copper still

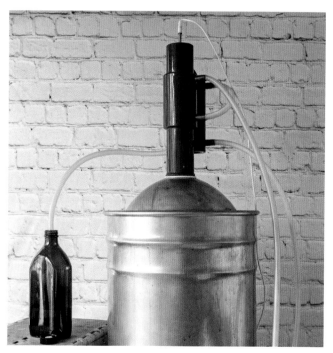
A modern stainless steel still

Making myrtle leaf hydrosol

Fresh myrtle leaves, 100g
Cold water, 1500ml
Ice cubes
A large 3 litre pan, lid, small glass bowl
Spray bottles for storage

1. Remove the leaves from the myrtle stems and chop finely.

2. Place the empty bowl in the centre of the pan with the chopped leaves around in the pan.

3. Add water to the leafy material in the pan (not the bowl). Ensure that the level of liquid does not come too close to the lip of the bowl. Heat until boiling, then set to gently simmer.

4. Place the pan lid upside down over the pan so that steam can collect on its lower surface and cool and condense to drip into the empty bowl below. Place some ice cubes in the top of the upturned lid to increase the cooling effect.

5. Continue collecting the drips into the bowl as long as the steam has some aroma, or until the leafy material is spent.

6. Turn off the heat, pour the liquid from the bowl into a spray bottle and label. Discard the spent leafy material and water to compost.

7. This myrtle hydrosol can be used for acne or irritated skin, or as an antiseptic room spray.

Note: This process of making a hydrosol can be used to distil small amounts of many types of aromatic plant material, including leaves of rosemary, Douglas fir, sweet gum and Scots pine. Keeping qualities for hydrosols in spray bottles are 12-18 months, less if placed in a bottle which admits air when opened. To separate any essential oil from the distilled water, put the hydrosol in a plastic bag in a freezer. Once the water in the hydrosol is frozen it should be possible to squeeze the small amount of essential oil out of the bag.

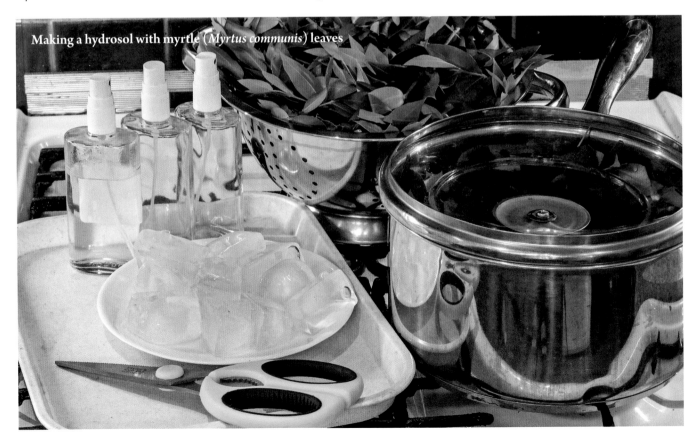

Making a hydrosol with myrtle (*Myrtus communis*) leaves

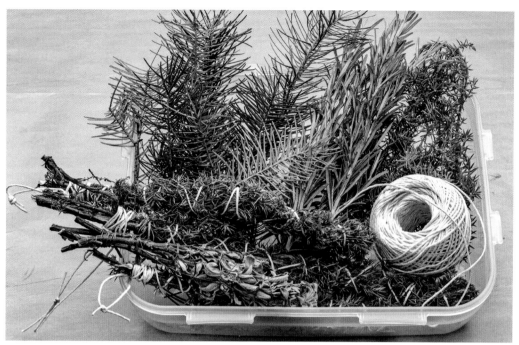

Making incense sticks

Leafy stems of Douglas fir, juniper and rosemary,
3-6 leafy stems about 25cm long
Cotton string, 2m
Scissors

1. Allow the stems to dry for a few days.

2. Bundle the stems together and remove the leaves from the lowest 5cm of stems (use gloves as juniper is prickly).

3. Fold over the very tips at the top of the bundle and tie the top of the bundle with the string in a knot so that two lengths of string are about equal.

4. Wind one length of string tightly around the bundle down to the base. Then wind the other length down to the base and tie the two ends together.

5. Trim the string and loose leaves.

6. Allow to fully dry in an airy place for several weeks.

7. Light the incense stick at the tip and place on a non-flammable surface. Gently blow out the flame and allow to smoulder.

Note: These incense sticks are traditionally made with sage (*Salvia officinalis*) but you can experiment with any aromatic plants.

production, since the amount produced is usually just 1-2% or even less of the starting amount of plant material by weight. With or without the essential oil components, most distilled waters are strongly aromatic and have uses in skin and hair care as well as having household uses. A distilled water lacking essential oils, such as Virginian witch hazel (*Hamamelis virginiana*), may be preserved with the addition of alcohol.[12] In order to carry out distillation, a still is used, which is a specialist piece of equipment consisting of a main body to hold plant material through which steam can be passed and a condenser to enable steam to cool.[13] Smaller quantities of plant materials can be distilled using an upturned lid over a saucepan, as outlined in the recipe given here (opposite) for making a hydrosol.

Making other preparations for external use

Many herbs can be used aromatically, either burnt or warmed in a way that releases active scents. Dried aromatic herbs can be tied up into sachets for drawers of clothes, or tied into smudging sticks for perfuming the home. When making incense sticks allow the herbs to dry a little before wrapping them with string.

Preserving and storing herbal preparations

The shelf life of herbal remedies is an important consideration if they are not to be used straight away. Preparations based on fresh herbs usually contain some moisture and, without preservatives, this means that there will be decomposition and putrefaction. If moisture content is minimised by the use of dried and powdered herbs then keeping qualities of preparations are likely to be better. A good guide to the quality of herbal preparations is your nose, so have a sniff and if anything smells off, rancid or sour then it probably is! Fresh plant material preparations intended for immediate or short-term use must be stored short term in a refrigerator to reduce deterioration but may only last 1-2 days. Well-dried herbs will last much longer, retaining aroma and colour, but should normally be replaced at least every 12-18 months. Alcohol-based plant tinctures and liquid extracts can be kept for a longer period of at least 2-3 years. Even without moisture, most herbal infused oils will tend to oxidise and deteriorate within a year. Extracts from plants containing essential oils may have better keeping potential due to antimicrobial activity. Herbal preparations for external use can be preserved with a rosemary extract which is both antimicrobial and anti-oxidant. Lavender (*Lavandula angustifolia*) in hydrosol form has been proposed as an alternative to water in cosmetics due to its antimicrobial activity against *Staphylococcus* bacteria, *Escherichia coli*, *Candida* species and *Aspergillus niger*.[14] There are further developments in the use of natural approaches, probably driven by consumer interest in more natural preservatives. An extract of American aspen (*Populus tremuloides*) bark has been developed for sale as an additive with anti-oxidant effects for cosmetics.[15] The main constituent appears to be salicylic acid, so there could be more possibilities for plant preservatives based on tree products such as willow, which is also rich in salicin.

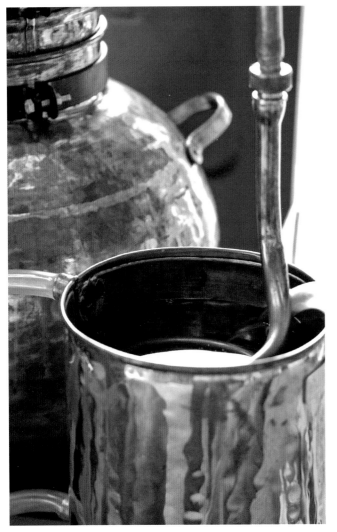

Steam from the still passes through cooling water to condense as a distillate

Conclusion

There are many plant remedies for common complaints and body care which can be prepared at home. They can be used for preventative care and self-help in the family and many preparations are attractive to share as gifts or sell as artisan preparations. In this chapter we have seen a range of sample recipes using healing plants for both internal and external use. Here is an opportunity to get creative, so why not celebrate the bounty of nature by experimenting and designing further possibilities! Of course, these preparations are intended largely for common complaints and it is always advisable to seek professional advice if suffering from a chronic or serious condition or taking prescribed medicines.

CHAPTER 7

Scaling Up the Harvest

A medicinal forest garden can be amazingly productive. You may already be sharing produce with others, or thinking about how to market and sell a surplus of plants and products. So what are the possibilities of scaling up the harvest of healing plants and selling for a profit? Chapter 7 aims to provide an overview of how the cultivation and harvest of medicinal trees and shrubs might be developed as a sustainable commercial operation. Many growers have the facilities to process fresh plant products on a small scale. But what else needs to be thought about in relation to medicinal plants? Key considerations in this chapter include assessing the potential demand and feasibility of supply, legislation and quality matters. First, the potential demand for herbal supplies must be identified, including local opportunities such as community supported agriculture and farmers markets. Second, growing more supplies is likely to involve additional cultivation within, and possibly beyond, the medicinal forest garden. Further cultivation models explored here include agroforestry, wild-harvesting or wild-simulation. Third, there is an overview of relevant regulations for those wishing to grow and sell herbal medicines, foods or cosmetics. A valuable premium can be gained for sales of the products of medicinal trees and shrubs which meet organic and other standards. However, medicinal claims may be problematic. Legal, quality and commercial requirements are outlined with examples of good practice. Lastly, getting started requires investment at the initial stages and needs to be costed, but there are some positive ways of getting ahead, from helpful funding and information sources to co-operative sharing of marketing and techniques.

Herbal trade and demand

The future looks promising for growing healing plants both in field cultivation and in agroforestry projects. Ethical consumption has boomed in recent years as more and more people attempt to make their contribution to planetary health, and as part of movements for social change as well as concerns about the environment. Branding with environmental and ethical connections has become economically attractive in gaining traction in the market. New concepts like agroecology refer to the refocusing of food and farming from monocrop industrial-style solutions to ecosystem awareness and ways of improving soil health and resilience. The rising pressure to plant more trees is likely to promote interest from growers in forestry-related initiatives including those designed to offer health-promoting products. There is potential for non-timber forest products given the large size of the European and US consumer markets for medicinal plants alongside edible and floral products.

As consumers become more aware of the threats to wild-harvested plants, demand for herbal supplies from sustainable sources is likely to increase. But how does this translate into demand for herbal products in your part of the world? After all, you need to be reasonably sure of being able to sell plant materials and products before committing to additional growing and all the associated labour and resources that are needed. An important step is to assess the potential opportunities for sales, based on observation of what has been achieved so far. You may have already identified a unique

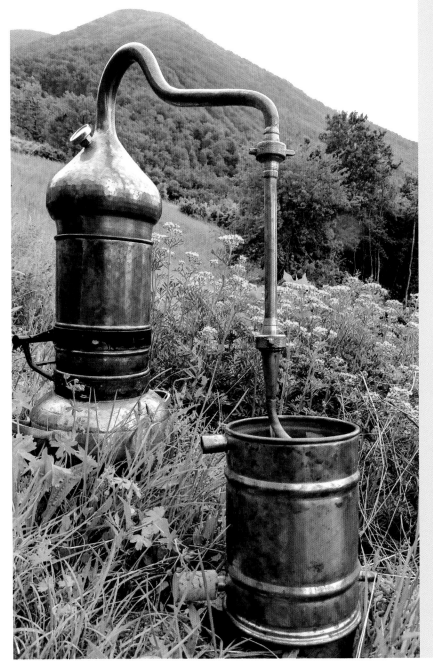

At Mintal Herbal Products in Italy, both wild and cultivated plants are harvested to capture natural flavours and fragrances

NAME: Mintal Herbal Products

LOCATION: Apennines, Italy

ACTIVITY: The Mintal project is a collaboration between artists, herb growers and scientists in Italy and the Netherlands. Raw plant material is harvested from wild and semi-wild plants at the permaculture farm, Trifoglio, in the Apennines in Italy. Some 500 species of plants are available, including elder, juniper, laurel, walnut and willow, as well as aromatic herbs of spearmint, lavender, wild carrot seed, rue, rosemary, savory and others. Handpicked herbs are dried slowly on wooden frames, then cut and packaged in tea blends. The herbal products are unique, varying from season to season. Distilling takes place in both the Netherlands and Italy to produce hydrolats and essential oils that are used to make innovative handmade cosmetics in a small lab in the Netherlands. They are working towards organic certification. Specific hydrolats can be produced on request. For keeping purposes, the hydrolats are stabilised with 10-12% food grade alcohol.

KEY POINT: Collaboration can be creative in combining a range of cultivated and wild plants for teas, distilling and body care products.

INFO: www.mintal.eu

selling point which could attract customers. Through developments such as farm shops and farmers markets, there are increasing opportunities for direct sales of fresh herbs and artisan products to consumers interested in natural cosmetic, health and nutrition benefits.[1] Committed buyers participating in community supported agriculture schemes may be keen to buy regular herb boxes, and this kind of arrangement ensures demand is known and that there is little waste. Additional value can be gained through making handmade and unique herbal products such as botanical tea mixtures, body care preparations, fermented herbal drinks, distilled waters, aromatic incense sticks and other gifts. For example, a collaborative project in the Netherlands and Italy is Mintal Herbs in which new products are created from herbs (see p.106, opposite).

There is now a significant online presence of ethical buyer organisations, and these provide an opportunity to market herbal health products to both a local and a wider audience.[2] Medicinal plants can add diversity to an existing business, for example you may already be using perennial shrubs and trees in floristry[3] or coppice crafts.[4] Further associated possibilities could involve developing local activities with herbal clinical practitioners, gardeners, community and other groups in terms of selling plants, offering short courses and design and consultancy services. If you are able to consider investment to grow and process larger amounts of plant material then the wholesale trade may be worth considering, especially for organically certified plant materials which are in demand from herbal medicine manufacturers, nutritional supplement manufacturers, animal feed suppliers and cosmetic producers. Later in this chapter there are details of certification schemes that may be relevant in your situation.

Upscaling your herbal harvest

If further demand for healing plants and products can be identified, how can you upscale to meet it? Some questions to think about relate to supply levels required, quality standards, and whether ongoing marketing is needed. First, can the level of demand be reasonably identified – are you going to provide added value for a known market such as a community box scheme requiring up to 5kg of fresh herbs, or might you come to an understanding with a manufacturer who would like to purchase a substantial quantity of 50-250kg of dried herb? Second, can you not only grow and supply enough plant materials, but also handle the processing activities after harvesting of cleaning and sorting, finding space in dryers, and providing storage? Third, are you able to meet quality requirements, so that you can charge a premium price? Are you prepared to record everything including batch details, inputs and expenditure etc. to satisfy certification bodies? Lastly, are you going to develop networking and marketing activity to maintain the demand, which means establishing relationships with customers and others interested in your plant supplies? If you can tackle much of the above, then you could be well on the way to starting a viable herbal business!

Having established that there is a demand, more details on the way in which more plants are to be grown can be considered. There are some emerging models that provide extra possibilities for the cultivation of medicinal plants. You might intensify or extend a forest garden, but you could also consider arrangements such as agroforestry and farm woodlands, foraging and rewilding, or wild-simulation forest farming.

(i) Forest garden

Forest gardens are usually diverse plantings designed primarily for production of edible uses. An advantage of these arrangements is that many different plants can co-exist at different levels. This is ideal for a smaller scale of production involving harvests carried out over a lengthy period. The disadvantage is that a relatively small harvest is available at any one time, and a mechanised harvest is unlikely to be possible so labour requirements may be high. The use of forest garden style sources of commercial supplies may involve some compromises in the design process. For example, greater efficiency can derive from grouping plants of the same type together for tending and harvesting.[5] The forest garden approach can certainly provide a wide range of plant materials which may be sufficient for artisan medicinal production in limited batch quantities (see p.108).

HOLT WOOD HERBS

LOCATION: Holt Wood, near Great Torrington, Devon, UK

ACTIVITY: Holt Wood is a medicinal tree and shrub project designed along permaculture principles to provide sustainable supplies of herbs for medicinal and health uses. The project includes native and introduced North American trees and shrubs. Harvests supply ingredients for small batches of artisan handmade body care products. The formulations for these products have been safety assessed and registered with the EU database of cosmetics, in order to be sold. Further testing has been carried out on stability and potential for bacterial growth in water-based items. Products are sold online and directly at events, including distilled witch hazel water based on *Hamamelis virginiana*. Customers are keen to know that these plants are grown in the UK and that purchase of the products can save air miles by reducing imported supplies.

LEARNING POINT: Creating desirable herbal body care products is attracting customers who are especially interested in local provenance.

CONTACT: www.holtwoodherbs.com

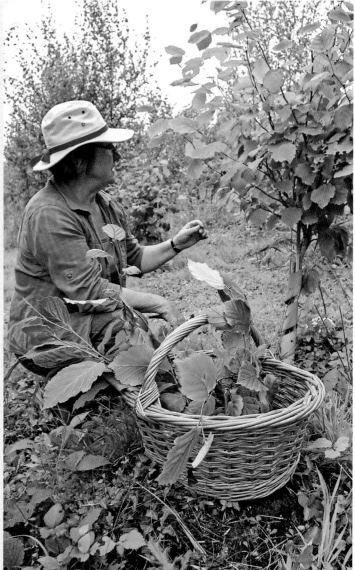

The author harvesting witch hazel (*Hamamelis virginiana*) for Holt Wood Herbs

Witch hazel distilled product packaging

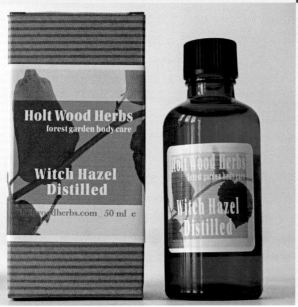

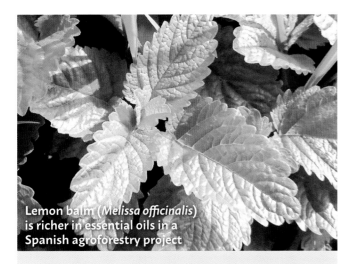

Lemon balm (*Melissa officinalis*) is richer in essential oils in a Spanish agroforestry project

INTERCROPPING MEDICINAL PLANTS WITH CHERRY TREES

LOCATION: Spain

ACTIVITY: The AGFORWARD project in Europe has been exploring innovation in agroforestry systems. Researchers at the University of Santiago de Compostela have shown how cherry trees, a high value timber crop in Spain, have been combined with other crops such as maize. Another crop is the medicinal plant, lemon balm (*Melissa officinalis*) which can be grown in alleys of cherry trees aligned north-south. A gap of 1.5m is kept between the tree and ground crop. The lemon balm plants are planted through mulch mat material to help manage the weeds, and the spacing between rows of plants is 40-70cm. The effects of the lemon balm are to force the cherry roots to penetrate deeper, providing greater resilience of the trees against climate change and weather events. The flowering of the lemon balm is delayed by being grown in the shade and this increases the level of rosmarinic acid in the herb. Harvesting of the lemon balm can continue for 4-5 years before it needs to be replaced, while the cherry trees are harvested after 25 years.

KEY POINT: With planned combinations, plants can increase medicinal constituents in agroforestry, making the tree and crop combination profitable.

INFO: www.agforward.eu

(ii) Agroforestry

Agroforestry refers to a land use system in which trees are grown in association with herbaceous plants or livestock. This could mean silvopasture where animals forage in land with trees, or alley cropping where plants are grown between lines of productive trees, or some other combination with wide spacing to enable access with agricultural machinery. There is now considerable interest in the regenerative benefits of agroforestry developments with a focus on practical examples and sharing best practices.[6] The AGFORWARD project has estimated there are 15.4 million hectares of agroforestry in Europe, about 9% of the agricultural land used.[7] In the US, studies of the economics of agroforestry systems show that silvopasture (combining forage crops, trees and livestock) is comparable or superior in terms of profits to plantations or monocrops.[8] In the UK, some initiatives are being taken to show how agroforestry can work with specialist tree crops such as on the Dartington estate using elderflower trees and Szechuan pepper trees (see p.110). In Spain, an agroforestry approach is in use for harvests of lemon balm (see left).

(iii) Farm woods and hedges

Many small areas of woodland exist on farmland, from hedgerows to copses, often requiring repeated management for little return. Initiatives to encourage the planting of more trees should promote interest in farm woodland projects where trees provide important eco-services in shelter, water management, fuel and supporting biodiversity. Planting schemes could offer additional spin-offs in providing medicinal supplies. For example, there is rising demand for organic hawthorn berry supplies and, since hawthorn trees are widely planted in hedges, there could be a viable harvest from hedgerows on organic farms. Feasibility studies on this kind of development have yet to be carried out.

(iv) Foraging and rewilding projects

Some non-timber forest products such as elder flowers, hawthorn berries, wild garlic, etc. could be harvested on a wide scale in parks, plantations, estates and woodlands. Provided the landowner gives permission,

AGROFORESTRY AND SPECIALIST TREE CROPS

LOCATION: Dartington estate in Devon

ACTIVITY: An exciting agroforestry project is under way in Devon, UK. The Dartington Hall Trust carried out a land use review and determined that converting a 50 acre field to agroforestry would be included as part of an upcoming farm tenancy. Subsequently, the land owners (The Dartington Hall Trust) and the farm tenants at Old Parsonage Farm subcontracted with a number of tree licence holders to deliver the agroforestry. This has resulted in an innovative development providing long-term access to land for tree crops to be planted, grown and harvested within a farm field by three different businesses. The tree crops will be maintained in alleys and harvested for elderflowers (1600 trees), apples (600 trees) and Szechuan peppers (150 trees). Planting commenced in 2017, and it is planned that between the alleys there will be a rotation of arable/silage crops by the main farm tenant. Although not producing specifically medicinal crops, the possibility of further agroforestry plantings for specialist tree crops is enticing. And this project has produced much information about developments, ably written up by Harriet Bell, the Community Resilience (Food and Farming) Manager at Dartington estate.

KEY POINT: Enabling lease of land for long-term access in an agroforestry project is an important component of specialist tree crop developments.

INFO: www.dartington.org

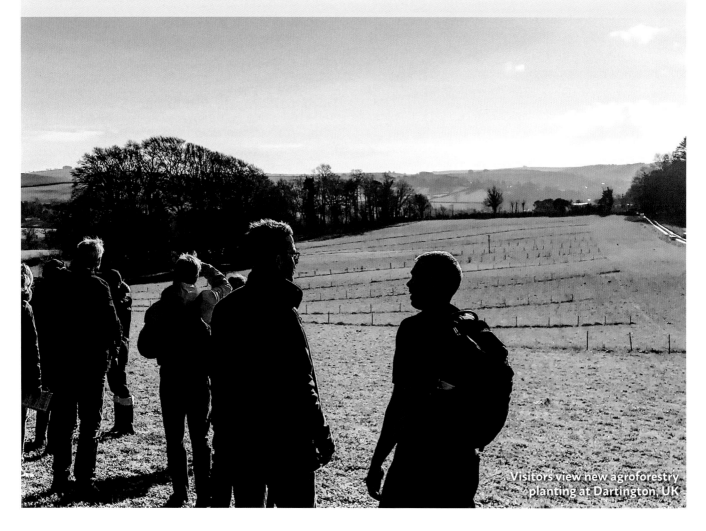

Visitors view new agroforestry planting at Dartington, UK

you may be able to harvest sustainable amounts. This may be a suitable approach for developing a market for a specific tree. For example, Priestlands Birch (p.112) have developed a market for products from birch harvested in Exmoor National Park. More recently there has been interest in rewilding possibilities in agricultural circles, so that wild-harvesting opportunities may become more widespread.[9]

(v) Wild-simulated forest farming

Landowners and farmers in the US are being encouraged to consider sustainable woodland cultivation of threatened plants.[10] In the Introduction we saw that United Plant Savers have established a botanical sanctuary. Further work has shown how valuable plants and mushrooms can be grown in simulated forest environments, or re-introduced into existing woodland.[11] The Association for Temperate Agroforestry has highlighted the possibilities for forest production – roots or rhizomes are harvested and sold for their medicinal properties. These plants include black cohosh (*Cimicifuga racemosa*), bloodroot (*Sanguinaria canadensis*), ginseng (*Panax quinquefolius*) and goldenseal (*Hydrastis canadensis*), the latter two commanding high prices.[12]

Regulations and quality matters

Plant remedies may be sold over the counter to the wider public for a variety of purposes related to health and wellbeing, ranging from cosmetic to culinary and medicinal uses – but there are regulations affecting these sales in most countries. Apart from general requirements to do with good manufacturing practice, there are some specific regulations in the UK, European Union and US which concern sales to the public.

(i) Medicinal herb sales

In the UK, most dried and fresh plants can be sold direct to the public provided no specific medicinal claims are made on the product label or in associated information. Certain plants are legally prohibited from sale to the public, particularly those classified as psychoactive drugs,
poisons or for restricted use. Medicinal claims for herbal products can only be made by manufacturers who have obtained authorisation or a traditional medicines licence. Within the European Union, the European Medicines Agency has a Committee on Herbal Medicinal Products which is responsible for compiling data on traditional herbal preparations. There is a procedure for registering traditional herbal medicines which requires evidence of longstanding use.[13] In the US, herbs are classified as a subcategory of food, dietary supplements, and these items can be sold to the public. However, if sales material or labelling contains specific medicinal claims for a herbal product then it is likely to be considered under the regulations for medicines and require costly authorisation or licensing. So, the marketing of herbs to the public is a somewhat fraught area as you have to be cautious about making claims for medicinal use, to avoid concerns about misrepresentation or illegal practices. However, herbs can be grown and sold to clinical herbal practitioners for individual prescribing to their patients or sold wholesale to producers who manufacture licensed herbal medicines.

(ii) Food sales

Many plants with healing actions are sold as edible products or drinks such as teas, and are included in the general category of food products. There are varied arrangements covering food regulations and food supplements, depending on the country or state. For example, in the US, the FDA does not regulate herbs directly as foods, but does monitor good manufacturing practice of dietary supplements including herbs.[14] In the UK, the Food Standards Agency provides guidance on food safety and hygiene, and food-related businesses should register with their local authority, which may require an inspection for a food hygiene rating.[15] If sales material includes reasonable health-promoting claims for a food product then the product is unlikely to be considered under the regulations for medicines. Most general claims related to use in common and minor complaints, such as 'refreshing' or 'calming' herbal teas and botanical drinks, or help with the symptoms of colds and coughs, are unlikely to be considered medicinal.

MANY HEALTH PRODUCTS SUSTAINABLY HARVESTED FROM ONE TREE SPECIES

NAME: Priestlands Birch

LOCATION: Somerset, UK

ACTIVITY: The birch (*Betula pendula*) tree is a fantastic source of products for healthy living, from soaps to teas. Lisette de Roche has built a whole business based on a range of quality handmade products from this one tree species! The source birch material is collected, with permission, from wild trees on Exmoor. Priestlands Birch sap is tapped from the trees for four weeks only in spring, resulting in a pure, delicate tasting drink. The sap is just one of many useful ingredients offered by birch trees. Priestlands Birch also uses the leaves, leaf buds, twigs and inner and outer bark to create tea, birch oil and birch tar, balms, moisturising soaps and moisturisers. This range of birch products has many health benefits. The business has been developed with considerable attention to marketing and locating good sales opportunities ranging from farmers markets in London to local food and gardening fairs.

KEY POINT: Through extensive networking and marketing, a demand can be established for a range of natural health products based on a sustainably harvested tree species.

INFO: www.priestlandsbirch.co.uk

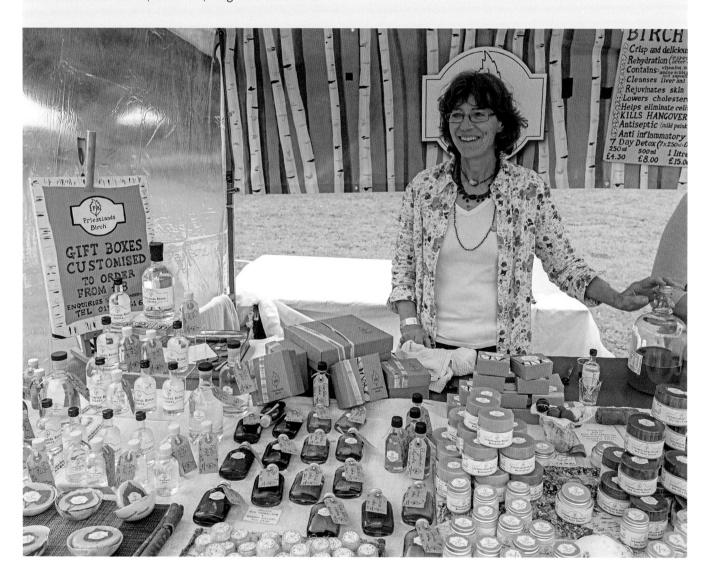

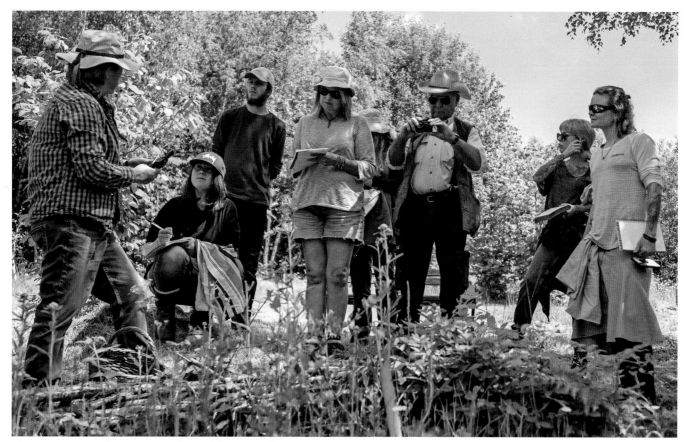
Courses are popular in the medicinal forest garden

(iii) Cosmetic sales

In recent years, regulation has been brought in by the European Union to govern the safety of cosmetics placed on the market, including general body care items such as bath products and skin care creams. Prior to public sale, cosmetic formulations have to be assessed by a recognised qualified person to determine whether they are safe. This safety assessment means that details such as plant constituents, shelf life and instructions for use are identified for labelling purposes and also registered online for each cosmetic product.[16] Cosmetic products sold in the European Union are also required to contain sufficient preservatives to limit the risk of growth of micro-organisms,[17] unless regarded as low risk, for example due to lack of water content. Some preservatives, such as phenoxyethanol and benzyl alcohol are vegetable derived and accepted in organic formulations. In the US such safety assessments are not currently required, although there are minimum requirements concerning labelling information on cosmetic products.[18] Like foods, herbal skin and body care products can be described in general beneficial terms such as 'preventative', 'toning' or 'restorative'. If you make such claims about these plant preparations then it is advisable to ensure that you have some evidence to justify them in case of queries. This could include herb monographs and research articles as well as the advertising claims of other reputable producers.

Generally speaking, healing plants and their products can be sold over the counter to the public so long as medicinal claims are avoided. Something to consider is how to encourage potential customers to be better informed about the herbal products they might want. Offering visits, open days, talks and courses to interested contacts and members of the public will help to broaden the range of interest in particular plants and their uses. Networking is a way forward, making connections with other growers, manufacturers, supportive advisers on health matters including local herbal practitioners, aromatherapists, nutritionists, wholefood suppliers, self-help groups and medical personnel.

Quality control and herbs

In addition to selling directly to the public or through retail outlets, growers could be supplying the trade with wholesale fresh or dried herbs. The buyers at manufacturing companies may be purchasing for varied uses in health foods, food supplements, herbal teas, cosmetic products etc. as well as herbal medicines. So they may have varying requirements in terms of quality standards. For pharmaceutical and food uses, testing is likely to be carried out on herbal material for microbiological quality, and contaminants such as pesticides and heavy metals.[19] Most companies will have testing using both macroscopic and microscopic techniques (see table below). Manufacturers of herbal medicines have to ensure that

Tests for quality of plant material

Nature of test	Details
Identity of species	Macroscopic observation of botanical features
Microbiological	Tests for specific organisms with limits for contamination
Foreign organic matter	Amounts of foreign organic matter permissable
Total ash	Maximum amount of ash permitted
Loss on drying	Permitted moisture loss
Pesticides	Maximum limits for pesticides
Other purity tests	Specific tests for extracted items and key constituents such as high performance liquid chromatography (HPLC)
Heavy metals	Analysis of heavy metal content and maximum limits
Radioactivity	Tests for radioactive residues
Chemical assay	Levels of key constituents required, assessed by spectrophotometry or HPLC

Details adapted from World Health Organization (2004) *WHO Monographs on Selected Medicinal Plants. Vol. 2*. Geneva: World Health Organization

their medicinal plant supplies are up to standard using published pharmacopoeia standards. If the plant material is not of sufficient quality then it is likely to be rejected.

Certification and premium prices

Growers and manufacturers have found that there is a premium to be gained from concerned consumers looking for certificated sources that indicate organic or fair trade provenance.[20] For growers of non-timber forest products, some form of certification could be very helpful in raising the value of medicinal plants and products. Certification of growers is usually based on a set of criteria and annual evidence has to be provided of having met those standards. Standards which might be relevant include those for organic and biodynamic cultivation as well as for forestry and wildcrafting, not to forget good agricultural and manufacturing practices. As yet there is no set of standards which readily applies to the harvest from a medicinal forest garden. The problem for growers is which form of certification to choose. While certification can provide recognition of sustainability and potential for premium value, cost is also an issue for the small-scale grower. The key characteristics of the different sets of standards are outlined below.

(i) Organic certification

Organic principles can be summarised under four headings – health of the soil and living beings, ecological sustainability, fairness of environment and life opportunities, and care for current and future generations and the environment. The certification process assesses whether detailed organic standards based on these principles are being met, and a conversion period of up to four years is involved for sites with permanent trees and shrubs. Ongoing certification involves an annual visit for visual inspection together with a review of business practice and accounts, and detailed record-keeping is fundamental.[21] Additional sets of organic criteria and standards are available for wild-harvesting and for manufacturers and processors.[22] The demand for organically certified medicinal plants continues to grow (see Organic Herb Trading in South West England, p.115, opposite).

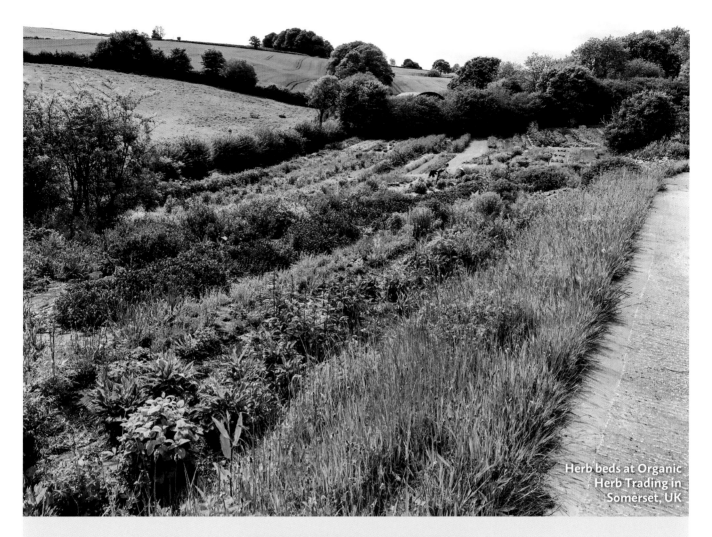

Herb beds at Organic Herb Trading in Somerset, UK

ORGANIC HERBS IN DEMAND

NAME: Organic Herb Trading

LOCATION: Somerset, UK

ACTIVITY: Organic Herb Trading has grown from a business set up by Mike Brook in the 1980s. Now it is probably the largest UK provider of organic herbs, supplying a wide range of premium dried herbs. Medicinal plant supplies are purchased from the company by manufacturers of teas, cosmetics and supplements, as well as herbal practitioners and pharmaceutical companies. Turnover annually is around £3 million and increasing. Some fresh field herbs are grown and harvested on site in Somerset, UK, with drying and processing facilities designed for specific requirements. However, many herb supplies have to be imported, and batch testing has shown that quality can be variable due to contamination and adulteration. The company builds relationships with growers to raise the quality of supplies. Wholesale quantities of herbs for a company of this size need to be substantial, from 50kg upwards. There is increasing interest amongst UK organic growers in meeting this kind of challenge and Organic Herb Trading is developing links with individual growers to foster trust and good practice.

KEY POINT: There is demand for organically grown herbs and potential for more home production of good quality.

INFO: www.organicherbtrading.com

(ii) Forest management standards

Forestry stewardship principles focus on yields of forest products (largely timber) which are sustainable, with soil and water resources being maintained and conserved, alongside social responsibility for the long-term social and economic wellbeing of the community.[23] These management standards have been widely adopted, and some certification bodies do include non-timber forest products. A plan is based on harvest rates at sustainable levels, and records of production are needed for effective monitoring. Organic standards and Forestry Stewardship Council certification might seem to be natural partners in promoting sustainable growing but, so far, studies suggest that the systems cannot be fully aligned, reflecting the often separate worlds of agriculture and forest management.[24]

(iii) Good agricultural practice

Good agricultural practice is based on a collection of principles relating to on-farm production and post-production processes. It is intended to provide best practices in farming situations to grow safe and healthy food without damage to the environment.[25] These guidelines have been adapted more specifically for medicinal plants and products, aiming for accurate identification, avoiding adulteration or contamination, and ensuring quality. World Health Organization guidelines were published in 2003 on good agricultural and collection practices for medicinal plants.[26] Similar guidelines are also available in the UK, Europe, Canada,[27] and in the US. Guidelines from the American Herbal Products Association are intended for use both with cultivated and wild-harvested medicinal plants.[28] The guidelines draw on principles of accurate identification, quality assurance, cleanliness, environmental stewardship, legal conformity and optimal harvest conditions.

(iv) FairWild certification

The FairWild standards concern wild-harvesting of plants and are based on principles of ecologically sound collection, social responsibility of the operation, economically viable business practices, respect of customary rights and fair trade relationships. In 2010, the standards were updated.[29]

Getting a head start in commerce

Existing farms or smallholdings are likely to have many of the resources needed for upscaling cultivation and harvest of medicinal trees and shrubs. To access further funding it is essential to draft a business plan which addresses the main purpose of your project and issues such as demand, feasibility and practical considerations, legislation, quality and marketing. This planning provides an opportunity to anticipate budgetary requirements, as additional initial investment may be needed for tools or machinery for cultivation, drying and processing, and storage facilities.[30] Running costs for the operation will need to be considered including labour costs, and additional costs for certification, advertising, packaging, repairs, sundries and transport. Aside from loans, grant aid might be sought in various ways, from direct approaches to charitable organisations keen on environmental benefits or business organisations wishing to support ethical and organic products. Crowdfunding through small contributions from many individuals has become one way in which some dedicated projects can get off the ground, by advertising rewards for variable contribution amounts within a fixed time frame. There may be government funding available to support planting of trees for various reasons from environmental improvement and water management to innovative agricultural techniques and community projects.[31] At the time of writing, further sources of funding for agroforestry and agroecology development were being discussed in Europe.[32] You could also join forces with other growers using sustainable methods and link up with initiatives to boost marketing and promote good practice.[33] Once you have a plan with specific aims and requirements, then you can tap into some of these developments and get going!

Looking Ahead

Plants offer incredible healing opportunities. In this book I have highlighted positive steps towards sustainable and regenerative uses of medicinal trees and shrubs, particularly through developing a medicinal forest garden. In this section I aim to identify further steps forward. I look forward to a time when healing plants, especially trees and shrubs, will be more widely recognised, valued and creatively integrated into many contexts, including gardens, parks, farms and woodland planting. Here I identify a fourfold approach to further development. First, growers of all kinds need advice and practical information on how to design with the inclusion of medicinal trees and shrubs. Second, greater awareness and more education is needed on sustainable harvesting and using medicinal trees and shrubs, whether for self-help or for wider use. Third, support is needed for research in order to gather and share evidence about the best ways of growing, managing, harvesting and using medicinal trees and shrubs in sustainable ways. Lastly, there is a need for more initiatives to promote collaboration and co-operative links between growers, manufacturers, clinical practitioners and consumers.

Advice on design with medicinal trees and shrubs

Practical information for growers and others interested in the inclusion of medicinal trees and shrubs is vital, and should be of interest to gardeners, smallholders, farmers and small woodland managers. Managers of larger scale forestry could also consider the longer-term benefits of including medicinal trees and shrubs in diversification and replanting schemes. But there remains a 'credibility problem' for farmers and other growers in relation to agroforestry and non-timber forest products, since the commercial possibilities are somewhat uncertain. Regarding the economics of using trees in agriculture, silvoarable and silvopastoral production examples in Australasia and North America have shown that favourable returns are possible. However, most studies have been inconclusive for European farmers so far, in comparison with mainstream agriculture which is well supported from the public purse.[1] There is increased interest in learning about forest gardening and growing networks of permaculture practitioners and designers.[2] In relation to small woodlands, more planning for medicinal products might be possible if non-timber forest products are better appreciated as having value.[3] Tree-planting schemes with public financial support could include consideration of the inclusion of medicinal trees and shrubs.

Awareness and education about sustainability of healing plants

Consumers are keen to hear more about sustainable sources. Within Europe, and elsewhere, there have been substantial steps in identifying sustainable wild-harvesting guidelines.[4] Education about the supply and use of healing plants is needed both for cultivated and wild-harvested sources. In the US, a new visitor centre for conservation of medicinal plants has been established at a botanical sanctuary in Ohio. Linking up with other sanctuaries, this development will be furthering the goal of United Plant Savers to promote more sustainable populations through cultivation of endangered woodland species.[5] Education about herbal medicine can also start young, and initiatives in forest schools can be a focus, such as the UK-based forest school where children learn about safe use of selected healing plants (see below).

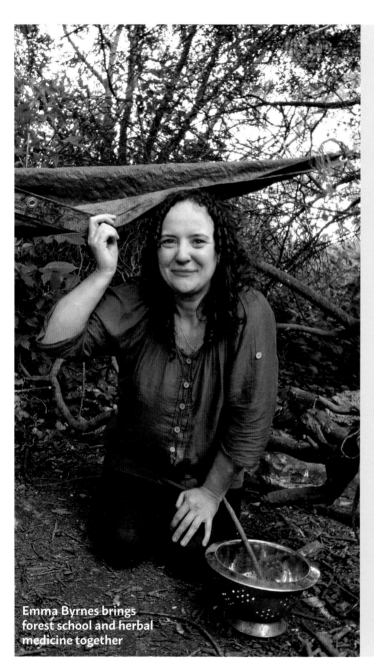

Emma Byrnes brings forest school and herbal medicine together

FOREST SCHOOL & HEALING PLANTS

NAME: Copplestone Primary School Forest Garden School

LOCATION: Devon, UK

ACTIVITY: One forest school now includes activities through which children are learning about healing plants. Emma Byrnes, Forest School leader, has been running the forest school at Copplestone Primary School since 2018, having previously been involved in 12 years of forest school activities. Emma came on a course about medicinal trees at Holt Wood in 2018. Since then Emma has been developing her new concept of Forest Garden School. Inspired by the course, Emma has recently focused on developing ways to help children learn safely about selected herbs. Activities are based on a small woodland area alongside the school. The forest school activities are based on ideas from the children and include games about plant identification and uses. The children also gain many social skills and develop resilience through their activities. As Emma describes, the children are excited to learn about healing plants. They particularly enjoy helping her to make creams and potions as well as using a capsule-maker.

KEY POINT: Educating the next generation about identification and uses of healing plants is fun and can be safely built in to forest school practice.

Gathering experience and research on cultivation and harvest

On a world scale, there have been research studies indicating the importance of forests for livelihoods, biodiversity, healthy ecosystems, and human health and wellbeing. The AGFORWARD project in Europe has brought together examples of research into existing practices in using trees in agriculture and their benefits, including cultivation of aromatic and medicinal plants.[6] Developments in the permaculture community have also brought research to the forefront, through networking between designers, growers and academics.[7] Dissemination of experience and research identifying good practices will encourage more growers to get involved and contribute to projects involving medicinal trees and shrubs.

Collaboration and co-operation between growers, practitioners and manufacturers

If herb growers and manufacturers collaborate then more sustainable and better quality supplies of medicinal plants can result. Socially responsible companies can show the way. For example, a US company, Traditional Medicinals, has worked with local people in the Upper Yangtze region in China to develop co-operative working around wild-harvested medicinal plants, sustaining a significant cash income for families.[8] In the UK, forest co-operatives have previously been mostly concerned with timber production,[9] but further development could help with marketing, research and training relating to new non-timber forest products.[10] A significant step has been the formation of a UK Organic Herb Growers Co-operative, which aims to encourage and support growers using organic and agroecological methods. Clinical herbal practitioners are also keen to access more sustainable supplies and to liaise with growers, and they can advise on plant provenance, herbal pharmacology and safety issues.

A future path

When I started out to write this book, it was a time of excitement and transformation embodied in creating a medicinal forest garden at Holt Wood out of a redundant conifer plantation. Our experience of growing and harvesting medicinal trees and shrubs has been hugely positive. Not only has the harvest benefitted human health but also the land has been rejuvenated with greater biodiversity of flora and fauna. This book is a means to share the experience of this bonanza of healing plants, and develop a future path.

For the future, I dream of replacing swathes of redundant conifer plantation with woodland plantings including native and introduced trees having uses for health and wellbeing. I foresee medicinal non-timber forest products as a sustainable spin-off. Such products could provide additional income to growers supported by co-operative networks. Most of all I want everyone to stop thinking of medicinal trees and shrubs as interesting but not a practical proposition. Many medicinal trees and shrubs are easily managed and can be productive

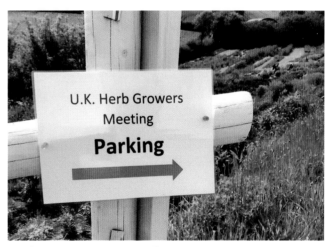

Herb growers getting together

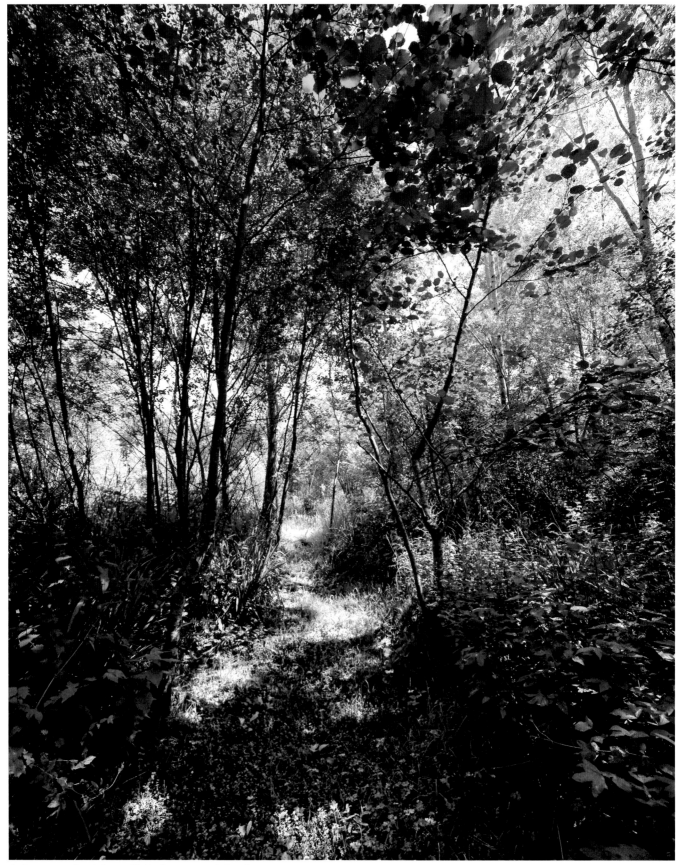

A future path with medicinal trees and shrubs

within a few years. There is no time better than the present to get started!

There is so much to gain from the growing of healing trees and shrubs, presenting considerably more opportunities for both earth care and people care. So, how would our landscapes look if we took up the opportunities for cultivating and harvesting medicinal trees and shrubs? Agroforestry projects and forest gardens are one way forward although medicinal trees and shrubs can be incorporated into many other contexts, large or small, from garden beds to hedges and windbreaks, as well as copses, parklands and farm woodlands. Where coppiced and pollarded, medicinal trees are not only ornamental and productive but encourage lower growing plants to flourish in newly opened up areas. Using a range of niche spaces at different levels for healing plants supports greater biodiversity, providing for sustainability and resilience in the face of climate change. Planting medicinal trees adds to the overall tree population and benefits the environment directly in many ways, including through soil regeneration, carbon sequestration and improved water management. As we become more independent from imported medicinal herb products, there will be further indirect environmental benefits of reduced packaging and transport costs.

And how will human health and wellbeing benefit? Whether helping or harvesting, working or walking in a medicinal forest garden, there is wellbeing and satisfaction for people in working with nature. By planting these amazing medicinal trees and shrubs, we can become more self-sufficient in herbal remedies, many of which are traditionally tried and tested, and some are backed up further by modern scientific research. As interest in herbal products continues to grow there will be more demand for domestically grown non-timber forest products that can be used as medicines, cosmetics and body care products. Not only can we become more self-sufficient but there are opportunities to develop sustainable businesses to supply the market for herbs used in food supplements, botanical drinks, herbal teas and more. These medicinal trees and shrubs integrate well with many other plants already offering human benefits from foods to fuel and floristry, as well as animal benefits in veterinary remedies. In the longer term, healing plants provide a reservoir of untapped potential, and conserving their many complex constituents means that we could develop resources not only for maintaining health but also for dealing with ageing, antibiotic-resistant infections and chronic disease.

PART 2

Directory of medicinal trees & shrubs

The 40 profiles listed here provide possibilities for the inclusion of medicinal trees and shrubs in a range of growing projects. The profiles are intended to provide sufficient information for you to make choices according to your situation and purpose. We have grown many of these healing plants at Holt Wood, and have enough experience of them to believe they are worth considering. This is not an exhaustive list as there are many more medicinal trees and shrubs which could be worthwhile growing in a temperate climate. In this Directory, the 40 medicinal trees and shrubs are listed alphabetically by their accepted Latin name. These healing plants have been selected for varied medicinal benefits and practicality in terms of cultivation and harvest; some are well known in the herbal medicine world while others deserve to be better known. For a quick access table showing the growing needs and medicinal uses of these medicinal trees and shrubs, see p.23 and p.24.

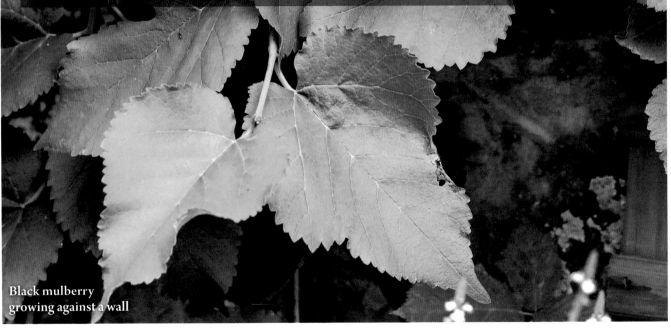

Black mulberry
growing against a wall

Each plant profile has the following sections:

- An overview summary section which gives a brief outline for quick reference and identifies scientific name, common name, plant family and parts used.

- The description section provides more detail on the size of tree and its appearance, the natural habitat in which it grows and related plants which might be considered as alternatives.

- The cultivation section gives information on hardiness and growing requirements, with details of significant pests or diseases, and suggested techniques of propagation. The hardiness of the plant is indicated by reference to the United States Department of Agriculture (USDA) or UK climate zone, and these zones are shown in Appendices 4 and 5. This section includes useful detail on harvesting practice.

- The therapeutic use section provides a brief overview of traditional uses and identifies the main medicinal actions and uses of the plant. Supporting evidence for clinical applications and research are outlined with references drawing on published research studies. While recent research articles are identified, this should not be taken as conclusive evidence but as a starting point for further reading. Note that preparations and doses given are examples only, they may need to be adjusted according to age, particularly for children or the elderly. Therapeutic use should always be based on professional clinical advice in chronic and serious complaints or where the person is taking other medications.

- The constituents and commerce section provides brief details of key constituents and an indication of how the plant might be commercially cultivated and used.

- The safety section provides important safety considerations and describes significant warnings, adverse events, interactions and contraindications.

- Finally, an other uses section is given for some plants to help plan use in an integrated growing project.

- There has not been space to include details of all sources used in compiling these profiles. If you wish to delve further, there are a number of online databases which are recommended for further investigation of cultivation, propagation and other details, and they are listed in Appendix 7: Resources and links.

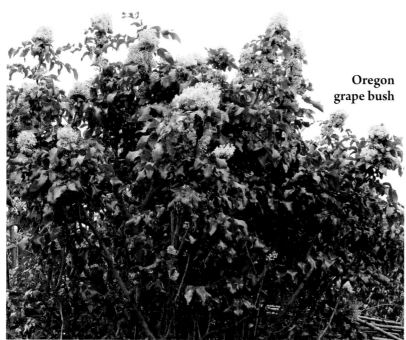

Oregon grape bush

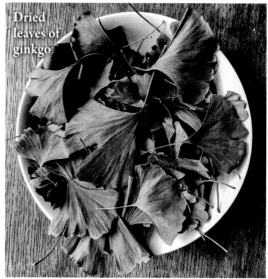

Dried leaves of ginkgo

Aesculus hippocastanum, Horse chestnut

An attractive large tree, native to western Asia, bearing large seeds or 'conkers', used to make an extract for complaints arising from venous congestion such as haemorrhoids and varicose veins.

SCIENTIFIC NAME *Aesculus hippocastanum*, L.

FAMILY Hippocastanaceae

PARTS USED Seed and bark

Description

A large deciduous tree growing rapidly to 30m by 15m. Showy whitish-pink flowers in erect panicles appear in May and are pollinated by bees and the spiny fruits with brown nut-like seeds ripen in September. Large sticky buds unfurl rapidly in spring and the palmate leaves are divided into five to seven leaflets with finely toothed margins. Characteristic tiny horseshoe marks are left on the twigs when the leaves fall.

Habitat

Indigenous to the mountain woods of western Asia, horse chestnut is widely cultivated, particularly in Europe, Russia and the US. Naturalised in the UK.

Related plants

Closely related are the Red and Yellow buckeye (*A. flava* and *A. pavia*) of North America.

Cultivation

The tree is hardy to USDA zone 4 (UK zone 3), and grows rapidly in shaded or sunny places. It can tolerate atmospheric pollution and poor soils. Grows best in eastern and southern parts of Britain. The tree can be pruned severely and coppices well. Seed bearing occurs in trees aged 20 years or more.

Pests and diseases

Horse chestnut trees suffer from a leaf miner (*Cameraria ohridella*), causing discolouration and defoliation of leaves, although not necessarily affecting tree health. Removal of fallen leaves in winter may help to reduce overwintering larvae.

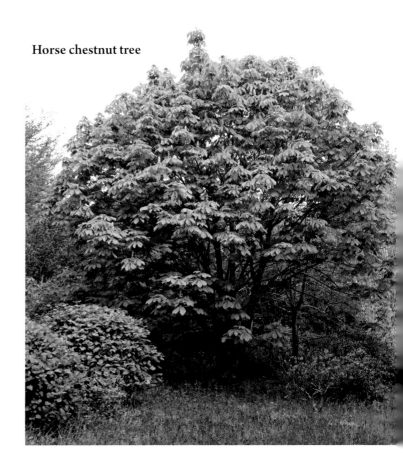

Horse chestnut tree

Propagation

Fresh ripe seed can be sown outdoors or in a cold frame with the scar downward. Stored seed should be soaked for 24 hours before sowing. This plant grows quickly and needs to be potted on in the first summer or planted out.

Harvesting

The seed is collected when ripe in the autumn; it is highest in flavonoids and aescin content 13-16 weeks after the start of flowering.[1] The seed is chopped for drying to avoid mould. The bark is stripped from younger branches in the autumn or spring and dried.

Therapeutic use

Historically, the horse chestnut was used for many ailments including rheumatism, bladder and gastrointestinal disorders, fever and leg cramps. The bark was used for its tonic, astringent, febrifuge and antiseptic properties,[2] and tea made from the bark was used for malaria and dysentery.

Medicinal actions and uses

Astringent, anti-inflammatory, anti-oxidant, venous tonic and circulatory stimulant. The horse chestnut seed extract strengthens the walls of small blood vessels, and is used in varicose veins and other complaints related to venous insufficiency.[3]

Clinical applications and research

Clinical data supports both internal and external use of a horse chestnut seed extract for symptoms of chronic venous insufficiency including varicose veins and haemorrhoids. A review of randomised controlled trials showed the superiority of horse chestnut seed extract over placebo and equivalence to use of compression stockings.[4] The research findings show that the extract increases venous tone and improves venous return, all of which lead to swelling reduction. Standardised extracts of internal dosage equivalent to 100-150mg aescin daily were found to improve swelling, pain and itching. This remedy can also be applied topically as a gel containing 2% aescin.[5] Other reports have suggested that horse chestnut leaf and bark extracts have considerable anti-oxidant and anti-inflammatory effects, although studies remain to be carried out.[6]

Sample preparations and dosage

A lotion or bath can be made using a decoction of the seed or bark, using 50g in 500ml water. Horse chestnut tincture can be made from the seed, and stirred into cream or gel for external application. Internal use of the seed tincture is based on a dose of 0.2-1ml three times a day but is best taken with professional advice.

Constituents and commerce

Constituents

The brown seeds contain a starchy inner rich in triterpene saponins (collectively known as aescin), also flavonoids, condensed tannins, sterols, fatty acids (including linolenic acid, palmitic acid and steric acid) and coumarins (including aesculetin, fraxin and scopolin).[7] The bark and leaves contain smaller amounts of aescin but are rich in flavonoids.

Commerce

Horse chestnut bark extract is in use in commercial skin care preparations. Horse chestnut seed extract preparations are widely sold in Europe for chronic venous insufficiency, sold as standardised products providing 50-75mg aescin every 12 hours.

Safety

Standardised horse chestnut seed extract is generally regarded as safe in adults at recommended doses for

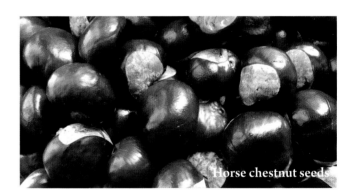

Horse chestnut seeds

short periods of time. The coumarin content may have anticoagulant effects, and toxicity to the renal system is suspected in very high doses of aescin, otherwise there are few adverse reports except for allergies and stomach upset.[8] Horse chestnut is not recommended in pregnancy due to insufficient data.

Other uses

Wood fuel. Dyeing. Saponins and tannins can be leached out of the crushed seed by steeping in water, and the water can then be used as a soapy substitute. Bach flower remedy.

Aronia melanocarpa, Black chokeberry

Black chokeberry is a North American shrub with tasty black berry fruits having astringent and anti-oxidant properties of use in treating colds with possibilities of use in cancer and diabetes.

SCIENTIFIC NAME   *Aronia melanocarpa* Michx. Elliott

FAMILY   Rosaceae

PARTS USED   Fruit, leaf, juice

Description

Black chokeberry is a woody shrub with glossy bright green leaves growing to 2m tall by 2m wide. Bunches of small white flowers are produced from late April. It is self-fertile and carries pendulous clusters of black fruit, ripening in September.

Habitat

From eastern North America, in swamps and low woodlands. Chokeberry is now widely cultivated in Europe and Russia and in drier soils.

Related plants

Closely related to the mountain ash (*Sorbus acuparia*) and hybrid cultivars have been developed for ornamental use ('Viking', 'Aron') and larger fruit production ('Nero'). The red chokeberry is *Aronia arbutifolia* and can be planted in wetter soils. This plant should not be confused with chokecherry (*Prunus virginiana*).

Cultivation and harvest

Cultivation

Black chokeberry will grow in full sun or light shade, fruiting best in open conditions. It will tolerate most soils whether wet or dry, and withstands salt and pollution. It is hardy to USDA zone 5a (UK zone 4). To encourage bushiness the stems can be pruned back in winter to a leaf node, 50cm from the ground. As the stems thicken the older ones can be removed to maintain vigour.

Pests and diseases

There are few problems, occasional leaf spot and rust. Twigs and fruit may become covered in powdery mould due to blight. Resistant to honey fungus.

Propagation

Sow seed fresh when ripe in a cold frame. Soak stored seed overnight and stratify in the cold for three months. Seedlings can be grown on in a cold frame for the first winter and planted out in the following late spring. Cuttings can be taken in July. Division of suckers when dormant, or branches can be layered.

Harvesting

Fruit is best harvested when fully ripe, and can stay on the plant for some weeks. It is estimated that three years after planting, up to 2kg of fruit is produced per bush, increasing further in subsequent years. Leaves can be harvested and dried for use in infusion.

Therapeutic use

Traditional

The fruits of chokeberry were primarily used by Native Americans for food.[9] Traditionally, fruits of both the black chokeberry and the red chokeberry were used by the Potawatomi tribe for treating colds.[10]

Medicinal actions and uses

Anti-oxidant and astringent. High concentrations of polyphenols and anthocyanins help to stimulate circulation and strengthen the heart as well as protect the urinary tract. High vitamin C content means the fruits are useful in treating colds and respiratory infections.

Clinical applications and research

The quality of clinical trials in recent years has been promising but more rigorous studies are needed of the indications of chokeberry extracts.[11] It has been suggested that this fruit could be used to prevent oxidative stress and vascular complications of diabetes, in addition to cancer therapy.[12]

Sample preparations and dosage

Infusion of leaves makes a tea based on 1 tsp per 1 cup of water. Preparations can be made such as fruit leather (see recipe p.92), or using the fruit juice.

Constituents and commerce

Key constituents

The fruit contains anti-oxidant polyphenols, phenolic acids (such as neochlorogenic and chlorogenic acids), and flavonoids (including anthocyanins, proantho-cyanidins, flavanols and flavonols).[13] A polyphenolic leaf extract has been shown to contain quercetin (11.70%), naringenin (9.01%) and gallocatechin gallate (10.02%).

Commerce

Chokeberry is grown as a commercial crop in Eastern Europe on a large scale for vitamin C content, and as a source of dietary anti-oxidants.[14]

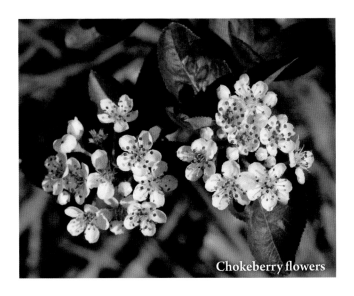

Chokeberry flowers

Safety   No known issues.

Other uses

Wildlife friendly. Commercial use for culinary extracts such as pectin.

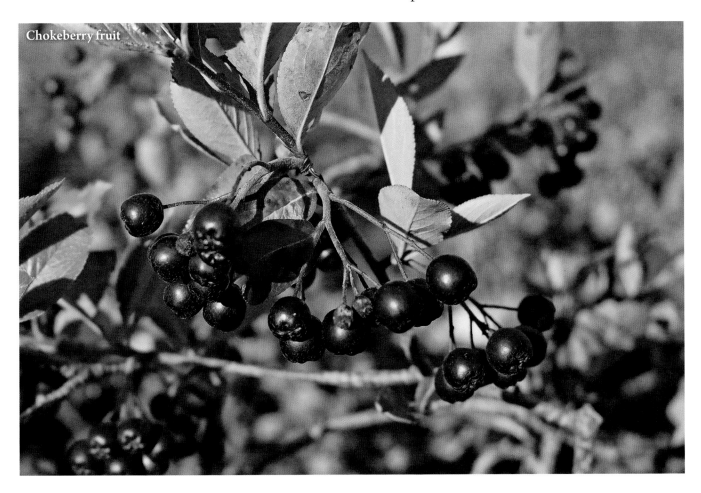

Chokeberry fruit

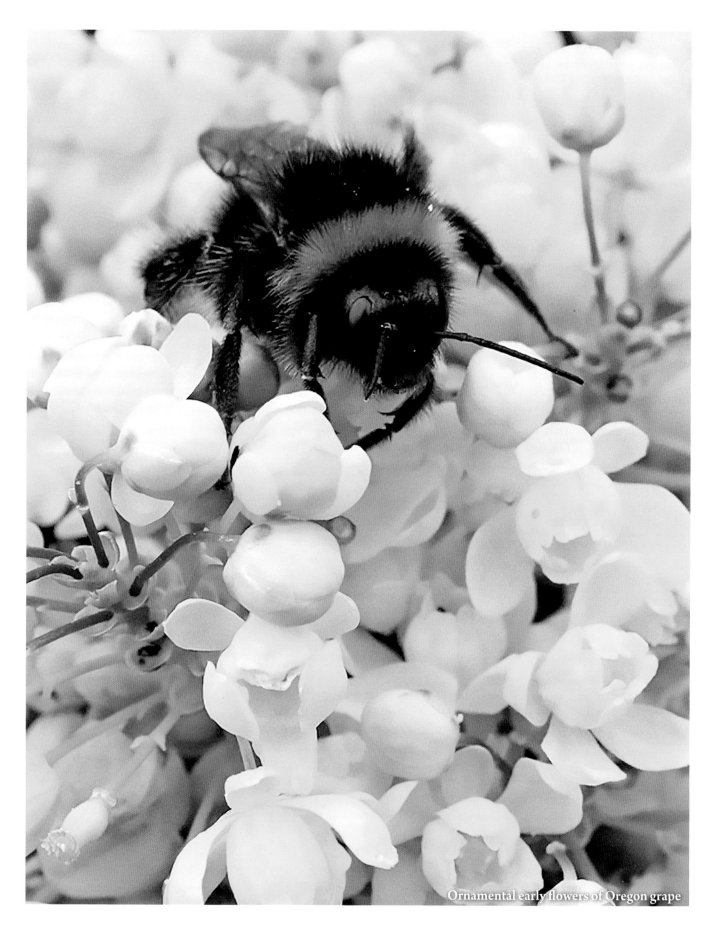
Ornamental early flowers of Oregon grape

Berberis aquifolium, Oregon grape

An ornamental evergreen shrub with early spring scented flowers that grows well in shade. The roots can be used in a range of digestive and skin complaints.

SCIENTIFIC NAME   *Berberis aquifolium* Pursh. (synonym *Mahonia aquifolium*)

FAMILY   Berberidaceae

ALTERNATE NAMES   Holly-leaved barberry, Oregon holly

PARTS USED   Roots and bark

Description

Oregon grape is an evergreen perennial growing up to 3-4m and spreading to 3m wide. It has leathery green pinnately compound leaves with sharp spiny teeth resembling holly. Early yellow flowers are produced in dense racemes from January onwards (p.123). The scented flowers are hermaphrodite and are pollinated by insects. The blue-black fruits ripen from August to September.

Habitat

Native to the western parts of North America especially in rich woods among rocks. Oregon grape has been widely grown in Europe for its ornamental value, and cultivated forms are regarded as invasive in some countries including Belgium and Germany. Oregon grape is considered a plant 'to watch' on the 'species-at-risk' in their native habitat.[15]

Related plants

The deciduous European barberry (*B. vulgaris*) is related and the bark, leaves and fruit can all be used for their berberine content.[16] The lower growing shrub, creeping Oregon grape (*B. nervosa*), is also collected in North America.[17] There are many varieties of Oregon grape developed for ornamental value of the flowers.

Cultivation and harvest

Cultivation

The plant is hardy to USDA zone 5 (UK zone 5). It can grow in full shade or semi-shade or no shade. Oregon grape will thrive in a wide range of soils provided they are well drained. It prefers cold dry winters but does not do well in a windy situation. Our initial plantings at Holt Wood suffered from wind rock and staking is recommended until plants are established. Oregon grape is tolerant of pruning in spring, and can be cut back, coppiced or pollarded to suit the space available.

Pests and diseases

Resistant to honey fungus.

Seed propagation

Blue-black berries are harvested when ripe in the autumn, cleaned and sown in a cold frame and kept moist with a mulch. Fresh seed can germinate within six weeks. Stored seed should be cold stratified for three months. Prick out the seedlings when they are large enough to handle and grow them on in a cold frame for at least their first winter. Plant them out in late spring or early summer. Leaf buds or stem cuttings can be taken in the late autumn, and placed in pots in a cold frame. Division of suckers in spring.

Harvesting

The root is harvested late autumn to early spring, washed and then dried. Roots can be removed from one side of a well-established plant, which is then allowed to recover for several years. Alternatively, plan to harvest the whole plant and replace with a new one. The rootstock and root are knotty, and hard, with a yellow tinged wood covering. After harvest, clean, chop and spread in a thin layer, turning daily for up to a week.

Therapeutic use

Traditional

Oregon grape has been traditionally used by Native Americans to treat various ailments, including digestive problems and inflammatory skin conditions. Early settlers to the Montana region of North America used the berries to make jam.

Medicinal actions and uses

The root and root bark is alterative, antibacterial, chola-gogue, diuretic, laxative and tonic. It is used to stimulate the kidney and gallbladder function and to treat catarrhal problems and skin disorders such as psoriasis. Internally, it can be used as a gargle for sore throats.

Clinical applications and research

Clinical trials have shown some effectiveness against atopic dermatitis and psoriasis.[18] The anticancer properties of berberine have been the subject of continued research. In animal and in vitro studies, berbamine, an alkaloid constituent of Oregon grape, has shown antiproliferative activity against leukaemia cells so may help to promote recovery from chemotherapy and radiation therapy for cancer.[19] Laboratory studies have indicated that Oregon grape may contain a specific multidrug resistance pump inhibitor named 5'-methoxyhydrocarpin which works to decrease bacterial resistance to antibiotics and antibacterial agents.[20]

Sample preparations and dosage

Used as a tincture 0.5-1ml three times daily.[21] Use as an infusion (5-15g of chopped roots boiled in 500ml of water for 15 minutes) strained and cooled, and taken in spoonfuls throughout the day.

Constituents and commerce

Key constituents

Active constituents of Oregon grape include bisbenzyli-soquinolines, protoberberines and aporphine alkaloids.

Commerce

The Oregon grape is used primarily in floristry and in the horticultural trade as a landscaping plant.

Safety

Should not be used in large doses or for more than a few weeks, and should not be taken during pregnancy or breastfeeding due to the alkaloid content.

Other uses

Ornamental floristry. The fruit is very acidic and has large seeds but can be eaten raw or cooked. Traditionally barberries were made into a tart jelly.

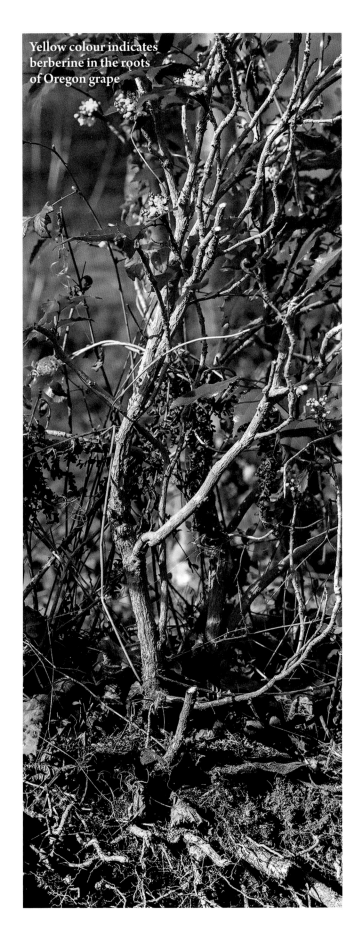

Yellow colour indicates berberine in the roots of Oregon grape

Betula pendula, Silver birch

A slender delicate tree with attractive white peeling bark that has many traditional medicinal uses from skin repair to rheumatic disease.

SCIENTIFIC NAME *Betula pendula* Roth.

FAMILY Betulaceae

ALTERNATE NAMES European birch, white birch, common birch

PARTS USED Bark, buds, leaves

Description

Silver birch is a graceful deciduous tree growing up to 25m tall by 10m wide within 30 years, limited to 6m on poorer sites.[22] It flowers in April and seeds ripen from July to August. Flowers are either male (10cm catkins) or female (initially upright and later drooping up to 4cm) and are monoecious. Diamond-shaped leaves are small with toothed margins, borne on slender warty twigs. Prolific seed is produced by trees aged 15 years or older.

Habitat

Silver birch is found throughout most of Europe, northern Africa and central Asia, and is widely distributed on open woodland and heathland. As a pioneer species, the birch is often first to colonise open or waste ground.

Related plants

Downy birch (*B. pubescens*) is another European birch that can be planted in moister areas, and can be coppiced. Black or sweet birch (*B. lenta*) and paper birch (*B. papyrifera*) are North American species.

Cultivation and harvest

Cultivation

Birch needs no special treatment if given plenty of light. Lower branches in shade will die back and the tree will not survive in full shade. It prefers a well-drained soil and though it grows best in rich soils it can grow in poor and very acid soils, growing in sites favoured by Scots pine. It is hardy to USDA zone 2 (UK zone 2). Birch is not suitable for very windy or maritime sites. It regenerates quickly from dormant basal buds after cutting;

coppice shoots are fast growing and produce a large leaf area. In forestry production, birch stands can include up to 1600 trees per hectare.

Pests and diseases

Birch is not a long-lived tree, usually lasting less than 70 years. The trunks of older trees may be more fissured and prone to colonisation by fungi such as the birch polypore fungus, *Fomitopsis betulinus*. Young plants may be damaged by voles and deer.

Propagation

Seed can be sown as soon as it is ripe in a sunny position. When seedlings are large enough to handle they can be pricked out into individual pots and grown on in a cold frame for the first winter. Plant out in late spring or early summer.

Harvesting

Leaf buds are harvested in early spring and leaves can be harvested in later spring, and these can be dried for later use. The bark can be harvested in late spring.

Therapeutic use

Traditional

The birch tree has longstanding medicinal use in Europe. Birch bark tar was used by the Yakut of Siberia for wounds and bandaging.[23] The Lapps chewed birch bark tar or pine pitch for toothache, and used it for coughs and rheumatism. The inner bark is bitter and astringent and was used in treating intermittent fevers. Tea using the bark has been used in Estonian traditional medicine for cancerous disease, as well as birch bud extracts for tumours.[24]

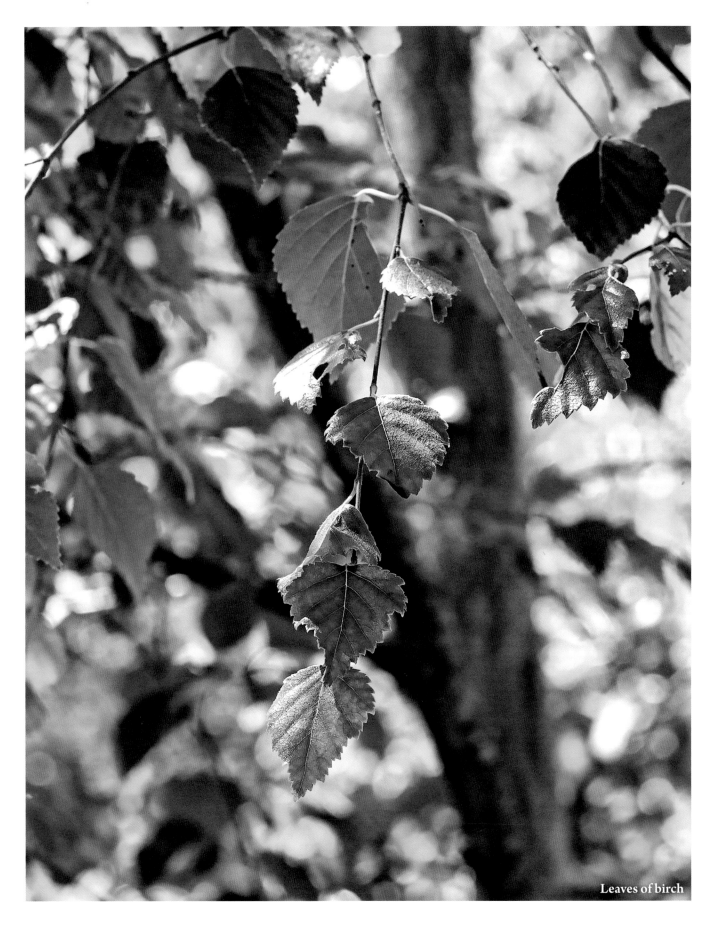
Leaves of birch

The leaves have been used in an infusion for gout, rheumatism and dropsy.

Medicinal actions and uses

Birch bark has constituents which are anti-inflammatory, antiseptic, anti-oxidant and cholagogue.[25] The leaves have diuretic and anti-inflammatory effects.[26] The leaves can be used in treating infections of the lower urinary tract.

Clinical applications and research

The wound healing effects of birch bark are likely due to triterpene constituents (betulin and others) which promote restoration of the skin barrier.[27] Research has suggested use of the bark for treating actinic keratosis, a precancerous skin condition.[28] Betulinic acid has been further researched for its role in causing cell death in certain kinds of cancer.[29] Betulin-rich extract from birch bark has assisted wound healing for patients with diabetic foot ulcers.[30] Birch leaves have been shown to inhibit enzyme xanthine oxidase, which is related to purine metabolism involved in gout and rheumatic disease,[31] and this supports the traditional uses in Central and Eastern Europe. The resinous leaf buds have anti-oxidant activity.

Sample preparations and dosage

Dried leaf infusion: pour a cup of boiling water over 2-3g of leaves, and strain after 10-15 minutes, up to three cups per day. Bark tincture: 2-5ml per dose up to three times a day. Birch bud glycerite up to 20 drops per dose.

Constituents and commerce

Key constituents

Birch bark contains proanthocyanidins and triterpenoid derivatives (including betulin, betulininc acid, oleanolic acid), tannins and saponins. The dry bark contains up to 30% betulin.[32] The tar oil (from destructive distillation of the bark) contains phenolics (including guaiacol, cresol and pyrogallol). The leaves contain flavonoids (about 3%), mainly hyperoside (up to 0.8%) with luteolin and quercetin glycosides, as well as sesquiterpene oxides, monoterpene glycosides, triterpene alcohols and esters. The leaf buds are rich in essential oils including a-copaene, germacrene D and d-cadinene.[33]

Commerce

The source of birch leaves in trade is mainly from China, Russia, Poland and other Eastern European countries. Distillation of the bark yields birch tar oil which is rich in methyl salicylate (like wintergreen oil) and has been used in treatments for eczema and psoriasis.

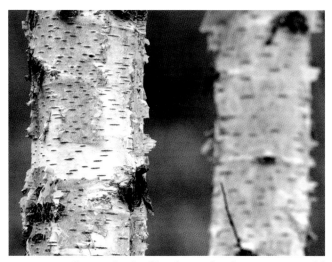

Shining bark of birch trunks about 12 years old

Safety

People sensitive to aspirin should not use birch as it contains aspirin-like compounds. There are reports of allergic reactions to the tree pollen which is produced in April/May from birch catkins. There are no known reports of interactions or contraindications in pregnancy although the use of birch is not recommended in pregnancy.

Other uses

Birch has many uses, the bark being traditionally applied in boatbuilding and roofing. Previously used in tanning. The sweet sap can be used to make wine or syrup.

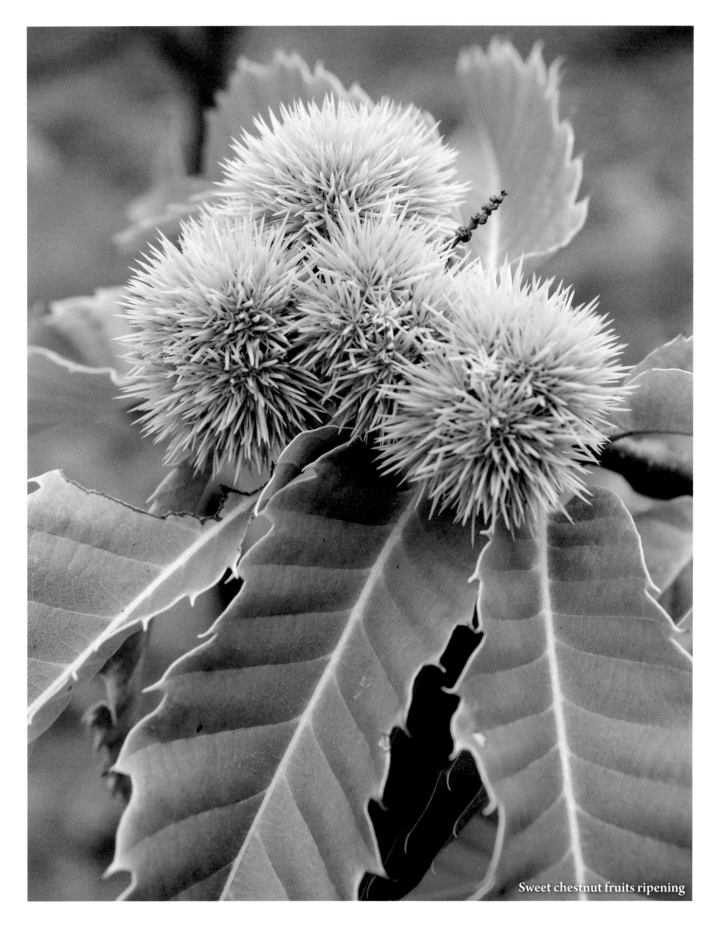

Sweet chestnut fruits ripening

Castanea sativa, Sweet chestnut

An attractive tree with edible nuts and glossy leaves; tea can be made from the leaves for coughs and colds.

SCIENTIFIC NAME   *Castanea sativa* Mill.

FAMILY   Fagaceae

ALTERNATE NAMES   European chestnut, Spanish chestnut

PARTS USED   Leaves, buds, fruits

Description

Sweet chestnut is a deciduous tree growing to 30m by 15m. It has large leathery leaves 15-20cm long with sharply toothed margins. It flowers in July and the fruits ripen in October. Flowers are monoecious and both sexes can be found on the same plant. The catkins hold both male and female flowers and are pollinated by bees. Chestnuts form inside spiny husks. Trees grown from seed may take 15 years to begin to produce edible nuts.

Habitat

This species may have originated in the eastern Mediterranean and was then deliberately cultivated in south Europe and Asia,[34] and it is now naturalised from north Africa to southern Scandinavia.

Related plants

Many edible sweet chestnut cultivars exist; over 100 are known. Both 'Marron de Lyon' and 'Paragon' produce fruits with a single large kernel (rather than 2-4 smaller kernels) and so are preferred for commercial production. The American sweet chestnut is *C. dentata*.

Cultivation and harvest

Cultivation

Sweet chestnut is hardy to USDA zone 5, and is naturalised in the UK where it is hardy to zone 5. Although the plant is hardy, the young growth in spring can be damaged by frost. The tree prefers well-drained soil and can grow in poor or acid soil. It is resistant to drought. It cannot grow in the shade. Warm dry summers are needed to ripen fruit in the UK. Sweet chestnut can be readily coppiced or pollarded; for timber poles this is done every 10 years. The trunk is cut at 30cm and the side shoots left to grow on; the shoots have a natural capacity to thin themselves, the base or stool becoming wider with repeated cropping. Planting density of 590 per acre is reported.[35] This plant will probably tolerate some rises in climate temperature.

Pests and diseases

Sweet chestnut is resistant to honey fungus. However, the Chinese chestnut has been affected by blight and introduction of this species into the US is the reason why American chestnuts are now almost extinct in the wild.

Propagation

Sow the seed as soon as it is ripe in a cold frame or in a seed bed outdoors, and protect from rodents. The seed can be stored in a cool place, such as the salad compartment of a fridge, for a few months if it is kept moist. The plants can be put out into their permanent positions in the summer or autumn, making sure to give them some protection from the cold in their first winter. Young shoots can be grown on as cuttings.

Harvesting

Leaves are picked in June and July and used fresh or dried. Buds may be a future source to note as they are rich in anti-oxidants.[36]

Therapeutic use

Traditional

The medicinal value of sweet chestnut has been appreciated since classical times for its astringent, stomachic

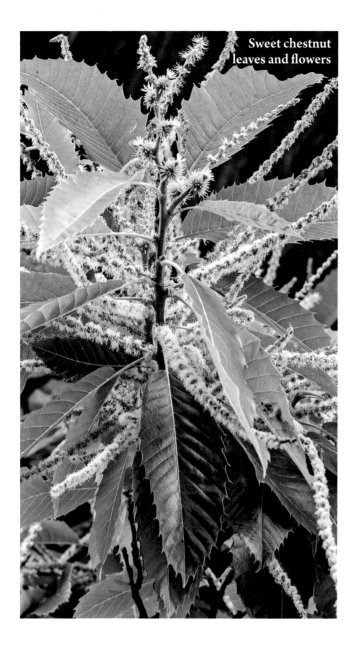
Sweet chestnut leaves and flowers

Clinical applications and research

Chestnut leaves contain polyphenolics which are anti-oxidant, and the flowers have considerable anti-oxidant activity.[38] The leaves are antimicrobial[39] and block the virulence of *Staphylococcus aureus*. Chestnut bark has anti-atherogenic, antithrombotic, anti-inflammatory and anti-oxidant activity.[40]

Sample preparations and dosage

The dried leaves can be infused as a tea for catarrh and coughs in the proportion of 25g to 500ml of water. The leaf or bark infusion can be used as a gargle.

Constituents and commerce

Key constituents

Sweet chestnut leaves contain tannins and are rich in pentacyclic terpenes, ursene and oleanene derivatives. The fruits contain starch, free sugars, proteins, vitamins and minerals, as well as polyphenolics, gallic and ellagic acids and ellagitannins (such as castalgin and vescalagin).

Commerce

Sweet chestnut is primarily grown in China and Korea for its edible nuts.

Safety

Extracts of sweet chestnut leaf have been shown to be safe for use on the skin. Chestnut pollen can cause hypersensitivity.

Other uses

Widely used as an edible crop. As a gluten-free source of carbohydrate, protein and other essential nutrients, the chestnut fruits can be eaten by people with coeliac disease. Useful timber and fuel crops. Bark and wood rich in tannins have been used in leather processing and wine making. A hair shampoo can be made from the infused leaves and fruit husks. Bach flower remedy.

and tonic characteristics. Chestnut flower honey was used for dressing wounds, burns and skin ulcers. Sweet chestnut bark was regarded as drying and binding and the powdered nuts were taken in an electuary with honey for cough and spitting blood. The leaves have been used in infusion against colds, whooping cough, diarrhoea, as well as for skin complaints and infections.

Medicinal actions and uses

The leaves are antitussive, expectorant, astringent and anti-inflammatory.[37] Chestnut fruits are a good source of dietary fibre, beneficial for digestive processes and colonic problems.

Ceanothus americanus, Red root

A low-growing shrub from North America that provides a refreshing tea for sore throats and lymphatic complaints.

SCIENTIFIC NAME *Ceanothus americanus* L.

FAMILY Rhamnaceae

ALTERNATE NAMES New Jersey tea, wild snowball, mountain lilac

PARTS USED Leaves and twigs, root

Description

Red root is a fairly fast-growing deciduous shrub growing to 1m tall by 1m wide. It has greyish finely toothed leaves, and clusters of small white flowers June to August. The flowers are hermaphrodite. The seeds ripen August to October, in a round capsule which dehisces (explodes) ejecting the seed away from the plant.

Habitat

From open woods and dry gravelly banks of eastern North America.

Related plants

Of comparable use is the snowbrush or sticky laurel (*C. velutinus*) which is evergreen, hardy to USDA zone 5 (UK zone 5) though may need protection in the UK, and is native in moister soils of western North America.

Cultivation and harvest

Cultivation

Red root is hardy to USDA zone 5 (UK zone 5) and it can grow in part shade or sun. It prefers well-drained soils and can grow in poor soil. It is recommended to plant out in permanent positions when young as the plant dislikes root disturbance since the roots are brittle. Avoid heavy pruning; ideally cut branches less than pencil thickness in spring. This plant can fix nitrogen and so acts as a soil improver.[41] It has high drought tolerance and is said to be quick to recover from fire. It will form suckers and spread so may be useful as ground cover.

Pests and diseases

Problems may include aphids, powdery mildew and leaf spot.

Propagation

Sowing ripe seed is best, though it can be difficult to collect as it dehisces. Stored seed has dormancy and needs to be placed in boiling water for five minutes and then soaked in warm water for 12 hours, followed by 2-3 months, cold stratification. Softwood cuttings root well in late summer but need protection under glass over winter.

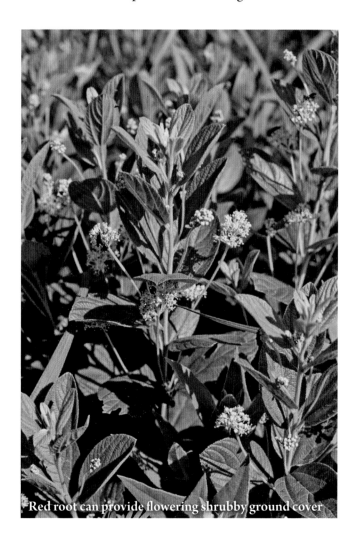
Red root can provide flowering shrubby ground cover

Mature wood cuttings with a heel can be placed in a cold frame over winter.

Harvesting

Leaves are harvested when the bush is flowering and dried for use as a tea. Caution as stems may be thorny. The roots are unearthed and partially harvested in the autumn or spring when their red colour is at its deepest. They need to be washed to remove gravel and other matter. Fresh roots should be split and cut up into small pieces before drying.

Therapeutic use

Traditional

The astringent roots of red root were used extensively by Native Americans to treat fevers and problems of the

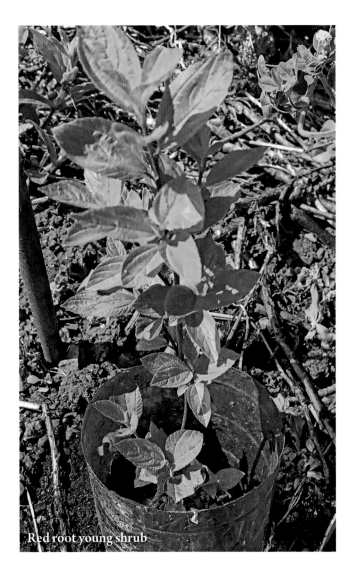

Red root young shrub

mucous membranes such as catarrh and sore throats. The powdered bark was used to dust sores, and a decoction of the bark used as a wash for skin complaints. The dried leaves were used as a tea for fevers by early settlers in the US.

Medicinal actions and uses

Astringent, lymphatic tonic, expectorant, antispasmodic, anti-inflammatory. As a stimulant for the lymphatic system, red root is used to relieve swollen glands, and to shrink fluid-filled cysts.[42]

Clinical applications and research

Red root has demonstrated inhibitory effects against *Streptococcus mutans*, *Actinomyces viscosus* and *Porphyromonas gingivalis*.[43] From the related *C. coeruleus* of Mexico, a methanol extract of the flowers has been found to inhibit *Staphylococcus aureus* and the leaf and root extracts were active as an anti-oxidant.[44]

Sample preparations and dosage

The root tincture can be taken, take 0.5-1.5ml in water, 3-4 times a day. Dried leaves are used to make a refreshing tea; steep 1 tsp of dried leaves in a cup of boiling water for 15 minutes. Can be cooled and also be used as a gargle.

Constituents and commerce

Key constituents

Red root contains triterpenes (ceanothic and ceanothetic acids), flavonoids, alkaloids and tannins (8% in the root).

Commerce

New Jersey or red root tea is not widely available in commerce, though it is sold as a drought-tolerant flowering shrub in North America.

Safety

Not for use during pregnancy or breastfeeding. Do not take alongside anticoagulant medications.

Other uses

Used as a dye for wool giving a cinnamon colour. Good source of nectar.

Chionanthus virginicus, Fringe tree

An ornamental North American small tree with dangling fragrant white flowers, having bark and roots used in liver and gallbladder disorders.

SCIENTIFIC NAME *Chionanthus virginicus* L.

FAMILY Oleaceae

ALTERNATE NAMES Snowdrop tree, old man's beard

PARTS USED Root and stem bark

Description

Fringe tree is a deciduous small tree or multi-stemmed large shrub growing to 5m tall by 3m wide, with large leathery leaves. The dangling pure white flowers appear in May-June on two-year-old wood when the plant is 5-8 years old. It is dioecious and seeds ripen to bluish fruits in October if both male and female plants are grown.

Habitat

From south-eastern North America and found in damp woods and scrub or by streams.

Cultivation and harvest

Cultivation

Hardy to USDA zone 5a (UK zone 4), and prefers a rich moist soil which is acidic to neutral. Can grow in sun or light shade, but is best in full sun. Fringe tree can be cut back to one main stem or can be pollarded. It is intolerant of wind but tolerant of air pollution and drought.

Pests and diseases

Related to the olive family and may be susceptible to ash die back.

Propagation

Sow ripe seed in autumn. Stored seed should be scarified and soaked in warm water for 24 hours and then given three months, warm and three months cold stratification – the seed may not germinate till second spring. Prick out the seedlings into individual pots when they are large enough to handle and grow them on in a greenhouse or cold frame. Plant them out into their permanent positions the following spring or early summer. Fringe tree is known to be difficult to grow from cuttings[45] and we agree (we have tried). Layering in spring or autumn takes 15 months.

Harvesting

Bark can be harvested at any time of year, then dried for later use.

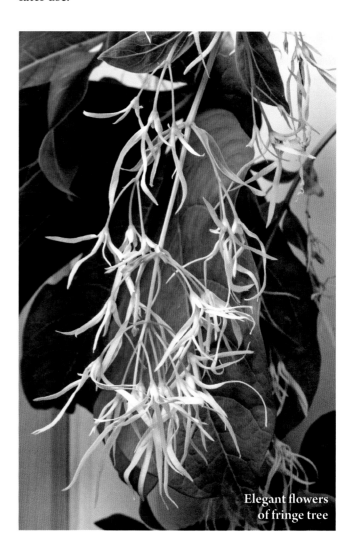

Elegant flowers of fringe tree

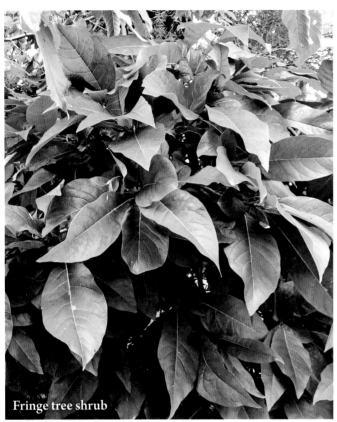

Fringe tree shrub

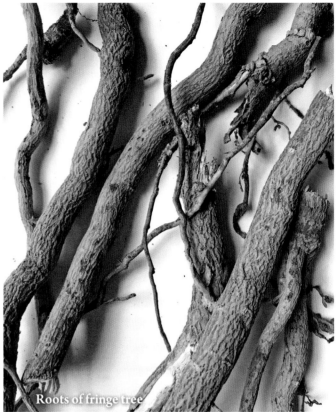

Roots of fringe tree

Therapeutic use

Traditional

Traditionally the root bark was used in fevers or externally for inflammations or wounds. The Choctaw tribe used the bark to treat cuts, bruises and wounds.[46] Use of the tincture and fluid extract for liver congestion was reported by a physician in the early twentieth century.[47]

Medicinal actions and uses

The root bark is bitter, alterative, cholagogue, digestive, diuretic, laxative and tonic. Used in present day herbal medicine for disorders of the digestive system, especially gallbladder inflammation. It has been shown that the active ingredients in the root bark are also present in the stem bark.[48]

Clinical applications and research

Little research has been carried out on the fringe tree. Polyphenolic lignans, phillyrin and pinoresinols in the root bark extracted with alcohol have been shown to have considerable anti-oxidant activity.[49]

Sample preparations and dosage

Tincture of the bark 1-2ml three times daily. This remedy is best used with professional supervision.

Constituents and commerce

Key constituents

The stem and root barks contain resin and lignan glycosides (including phillyrin), saponin glycosides and secoiridoids.[50]

Commerce

Fringetree bark and root is not widely sold as a herbal medicine but the tree is occasionally available in horticultural outlets as an ornamental flowering small tree.

Safety

Overdoses can cause vomiting, headache and a slow pulse. This plant should not be used if there is a possibility of impacted gallstones or growths obstructing the gall-bladder duct.

Crataegus monogyna, Hawthorn

A small European tree with early sprays of fragrant flowers followed by red berries, significant for wildlife and all parts can help to relieve anxiety and benefit the circulation.

SCIENTIFIC NAME *Crataegus monogyna* Jacq. (previously referred to as *C. oxyacantha*)
FAMILY Rosaceae
ALTERNATE NAMES English hawthorn, whitethorn, haw, oneseed hawthorn
PARTS USED Flowers, leaves and fruits (berries) are all used.

Description

A long-lived deciduous, thorny, large shrub or small tree growing up to 10m high and 6m wide. Small-toothed leaves with three to five acute lobes are borne on thorny branches. Pinkish-white flowers with five petals and 15-20 stamens are produced from May to June with the seeds ripening from September to November. The flowers are hermaphrodite and are pollinated by midges.

Habitat

Hawthorn is native to the northern wooded zones of Europe, parts of northern Africa and western Asia. It has become naturalised in parts of North America and other temperate locations as a garden escape. This plant is considered invasive in some parts of North America.

Related plants

There are some 280 species of hawthorns in the genus *Crataegus*, including some with attractive flowers and others with edible fruits. In the US, *C. monogyna* is an introduced species, and other native species could be used such as *C. douglasii*. All species are likely to have some medicinal effect, including the Midland hawthorn (*C. oxyacanthoides* or *C. laevigata*) which has less deeply lobed leaves.

Cultivation and harvest

Cultivation

Hawthorn suits most soils, and prefers moist soil although it tolerates drought, maritime exposure and atmospheric pollution. Will grow in light woodland or on woodland sunny edge, but not in heavy shade. The hawthorn is hardy to USDA zone 4 (UK zone 3).

Hawthorn can be repeatedly pruned and will form an impenetrable bush. In a woodland context it may need regular pruning to avoid people coming into contact with thorny branches. Suckers may need to be removed from the base. Pollarding is not recommended unless a young tree; at Holt Wood we found that pollarding a mature tree produced many dozens of spiny shoots. Seedlings take from 5-8 years before they start to bear fruit. A study of different methods of hedgerow management, predominantly hawthorn, found that the unmanaged areas were substantially more productive of berries, producing around 150g (dry weight so about half the fresh weight) per 2.5m^2 surface area of hedgerow.[51]

Pests and diseases

Hawthorn like other *Prunus* family plants is susceptible to apple scab, leaf blights and rusts.

Propagation

Fresh seed can be cleaned and planted immediately in a cold frame. Seed can be stored 2-3 years in a sealed container in a refrigerator. Stored seeds need 7-8 hours soaking, followed by three months, warm stratification and a further three months, cold stratification. Cuttings are rarely successful.

Harvesting

Flowers and leaves can be harvested in May; they may have a fishy smell (trimethylamine to attract insects) which disappears on drying. Berries are gathered in September/October when ripe and also dried. Take extra care, and wear thick gloves, to avoid the sharp thorns when harvesting.

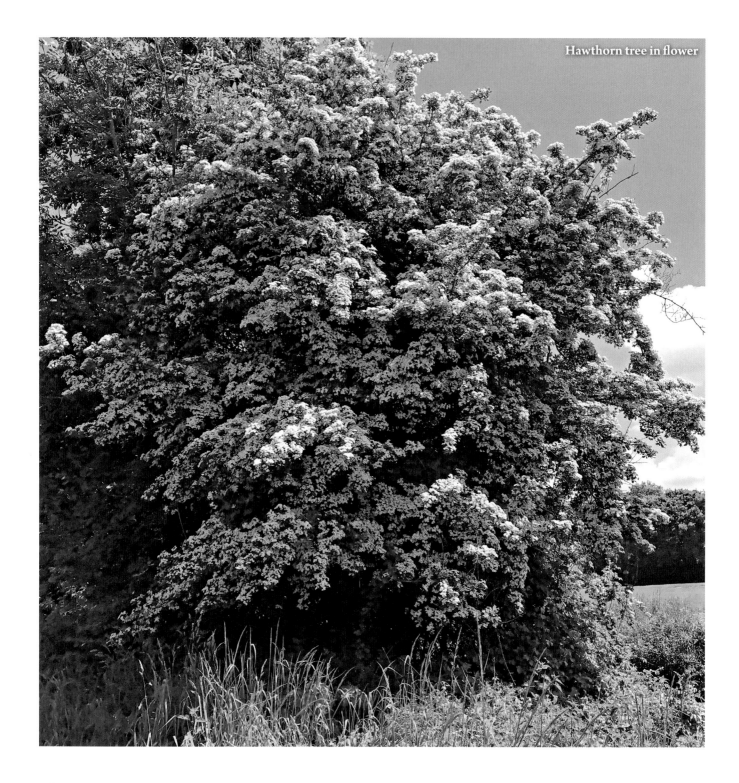
Hawthorn tree in flower

Therapeutic use

Traditional

Hawthorn has a considerable history of magical association and folklore. It was particularly associated with May Day festivities, and is also frequent in place names and boundary charters. Although used for decoration outside, there was a belief that it should not be brought into the house for fear of illness and death. The World Health Organization describes folk medicine use of the leaves and flowers as an antispasmodic for asthma, diarrhoea, gallbladder disease and uterine contractions, and sedative for insomnia.[52]

Medicinal actions and uses

Flower, leaf and fruit actions are anti-oxidant, coronary vasodilator, diuretic, astringent, anti-inflammatory and hypotensive.[53] Hawthorn leaf and flower can be used in heart palpitations and stress,[54] hypertension and hypercholesterolaemia. The World Health Organization includes hawthorn treatment in stage II chronic congestive heart failure.[55]

Clinical applications and research

Anxiety was shown to decrease in a trial using an extract of magnesium, hawthorn (*C. oxyacantha*) and Californian poppy (*Eschscholzia californica*) twice daily for three months: patients showed a significant decrease in anxiety measured by self-report and the Hamilton Anxiety Scale.[56] Hawthorn has a history of use and clinical evidence to support its cardiovascular benefits, especially cardiotonic activity. Hawthorn extract has been shown to lower blood pressure in a number of studies.[57] Research has shown that hawthorn preparations have been of benefit in ischaemic heart disease.[58] Hawthorn preparations contain bioflavonoids which are anti-oxidant and help to prevent degeneration of blood vessels; they relax and dilate the arteries so increasing blood flow to the heart muscle. However, the benefits of this herb are felt only after prolonged use, at least 4-6 weeks.

Sample preparations and dosage

Dried flowers and leaves, up to 6g per day, can be steeped in tea for 10-15 minutes. Dried berries, tincture 1:5, 1-5ml three times daily. A liqueur can be made with hawthorn berries steeped in brandy.

Constituents and commerce

Key constituents

Leaves and fruits of hawthorn species contain polyphenolic flavonoids (such as quercetin glycosides and flavone-C-glycosides), and oligomeric proanthocyanidins providing a high level of anti-oxidant activity in addition to strong antibacterial activity against gram-positive bacteria.[59] Other constituents include quercetin, quercetrin, triterpene saponins, vitamin C and cardio-active amines. Flowers revealed the highest tocopherol and ascorbic acid contents, and also the best essential

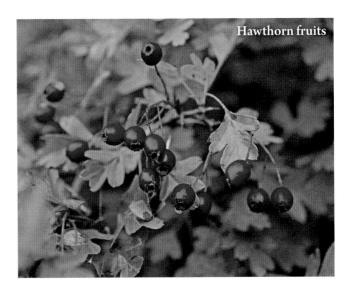

Hawthorn fruits

fatty acids ratio.[60]

Commerce

Commercial preparations are standardised to 5% or more oligomeric proanthocyanidins and 2% flavonoids, with doses ranging from 160-900mg of the dried extract. The material of commerce for the phytomedicine industry is obtained from European countries including Albania, Bulgaria, Romania, the former Yugoslavia and Poland.[61]

Safety

Use of hawthorn in heart complaints must be supervised by a clinical practitioner. Studies have found that hawthorn preparations are well tolerated with little evidence for anything other than infrequent mild adverse effects of headache, nausea and palpitations.[62] However, hawthorn preparations may potentiate the actions of digitalis, antihypertensives and lipid-lowering medications, so medical advice should be sought if taking prescription medications for circulatory complaints. Seeds in the hawthorn fruits (like apple seeds) contain amygdalin, a cyanogenic glycoside, and should not be eaten to excess as they can produce cyanide toxicity.

Other uses

Hedging. Fruit is edible, best cooked in preserves. Important wildlife plant providing haws for birds in winter.

Cytisus scoparius, Broom

An arching shrub with fragrant yellow flowers long used for fluid retention and arthritic complaints.

SCIENTIFIC NAME *Cytisus scoparius* (L.) Link. previously known as *Sarothamnus scoparius*

FAMILY Fabaceae

ALTERNATE NAMES Common broom, Scotch broom

PARTS USED Flowering shoots

Description

Broom is a deciduous shrub growing to 2m tall by 1.5m wide. It has alternate leaves and produces fragrant yellow pea-like flowers between May and June. The flowers are pollinated by bees and the fuzzy seed pods explode when ripe.

Habitat

Broom is found throughout Europe on sandy heaths and acidic soils.

Related plants

Spanish broom (*Spartium junceum*) has similar medicinal effects but is more active and toxic to the heart and likely to cause nausea, vomiting and purging. *C. villosus* or hairy broom from the southern Mediterranean may be worth considering in warmer areas.

Cultivation and harvest

Cultivation

Broom is hardy to USDA zone 5 (UK zone 5). It does best in acid soils and in sun but tolerates some shade and maritime or polluted conditions. The plant dislikes root disturbance and should be planted out in its final position as soon as possible. Once established, the plants are drought tolerant, and can be used to help stabilise soil in sand dunes. Broom can be cut back and regenerates quickly from the base. Broom is a nitrogen fixer. It is considered a weed in forestry especially in pine and eucalyptus plantations, and is classified as invasive in a number of states in North America.

Pests and diseases

Generally pest-free but may suffer from gall mites.

Propagation

Fresh ripe seed can be sown direct in a cold frame in the autumn. Soak stored seed in hot water for 24 hours, followed by four weeks cold stratification. Softwood cuttings taken in July-August can root in 4-5 weeks.[63] Cuttings of mature wood can be taken in October/November and placed in a cold frame. Layering can also be used.

Harvesting

The tips of flowering shoots are harvested in May and can be used fresh or dried for later use. The active ingredients break down in storage beyond 12 months.

Therapeutic use

Traditional

A decoction of twigs and tops was used traditionally for dropsy and arthritic complaints. 'Salts of Broom' (*Sal Genistae*) was made from the ashes of burnt tops infused in wine. Powdered seeds were also used to infuse a spirit which was taken for liver complaints and ague.

Medicinal actions and uses

Bitter, diuretic, emetic, hypertensive, peripheral vasoconstrictor, anti-oxidant, vermifuge, oxytocic.[64] Broom has been used for fluid retention, heart complaints and reducing blood loss after childbirth, but dosage is somewhat uncertain due to variation in active constituents.

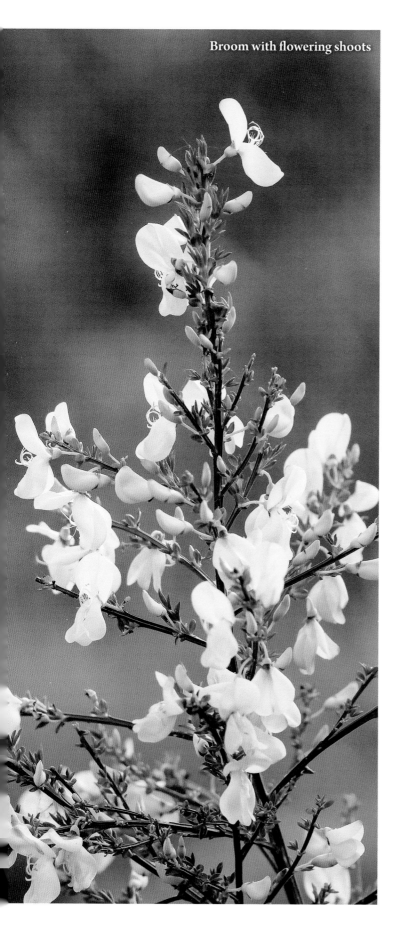

Broom with flowering shoots

Clinical applications and research

A number of studies have shown ways that broom species extracts might be used clinically. Flavonoid and carotenoid-rich extracts from broom could have application in topical extracts to protect against oxidative damage from UV light radiation.[65] Isoflavonoids in the leaf extract from a related broom species (*C. striatus*) have been shown to increase the effect of antibiotics against MRSA.[66] Another related broom species (*C. villosus*) has been researched for extracts with monoamine oxidase inhibition effects which could have value in neurological degenerative diseases such as Parkinson's and Alzheimer's diseases.[67]

Sample preparations and dosage

Dried flowering tops 1-2g in infusion. Used as a tincture 0.5-2ml three times daily. This plant is best used with professional advice. A decoction of young twigs and leaves can be used as an insecticide.

Constituents and commerce

Key constituents

Contains flavonoids and alkaloids (including sparteine, a heart stimulant), and the glycoside scoparin which has diuretic effects.[68]

Commerce

Other than uses in dyeing and paper making, broom is largely cultivated as an ornamental plant.

Safety

Not for use in high blood pressure. Do not take in pregnancy since sparteine can cause the uterus to contract.

Other uses

Can be used for fibre and paper making. Used to stabilise sand dunes. Used in dyeing and tanning. Thatching roofs in Spain.

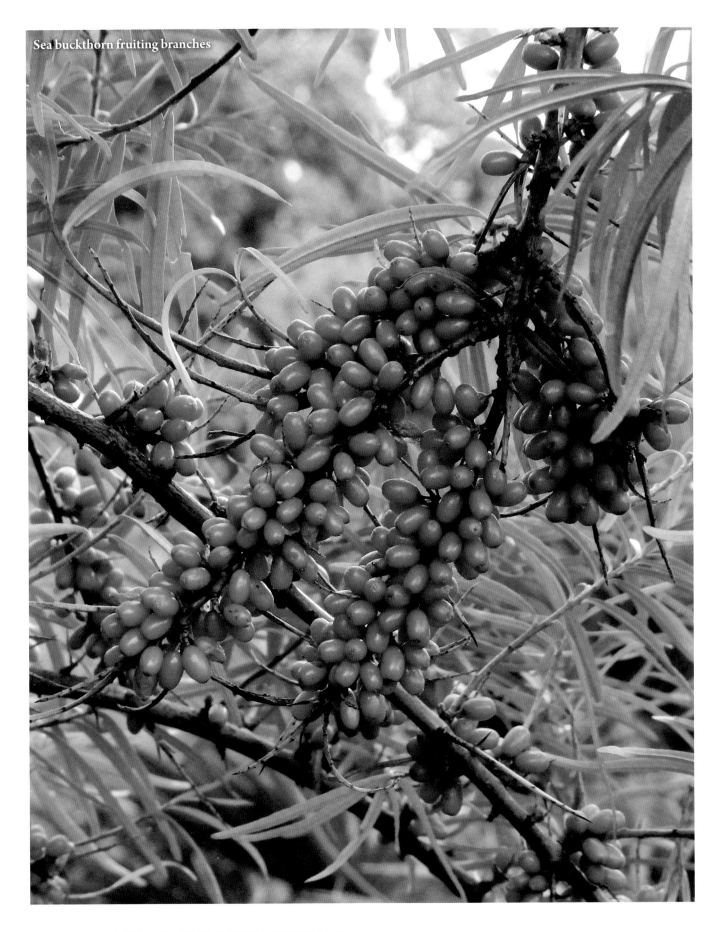

Sea buckthorn fruiting branches

Elaeagnus rhamnoides, Sea buckthorn

A tall shrub of coastal areas which can be hugely productive of bright orange fruits which are strongly anti-oxidant and promote the immune system.

SCIENTIFIC NAME   *Elaeagnus rhamnoides* (L.) A. Nelson, previously known as *Hippophaë rhamnoides*

FAMILY   Elaeagnaceae

ALTERNATE NAMES   Seaberry, sallow thorn

PARTS USED   Fruit and leaves

Description

Sea buckthorn is a tall deciduous shrub with spiny grey branches growing up to 6m tall and 3m wide at a medium rate. It is dioecious and wind-pollinated, flowers forming in May on wood from the previous year. The fruit ripens from 12-15 weeks after flowering, from late July until early October depending on the subspecies and location.

Habitat

Sea buckthorn is a native shrub of temperate zones of Europe and Asia. It can be found in thickets near the coast, and also grows in wet woods and scrubland.

Related plants

The Russian olive (*E. angustifolia*) is closely related and its fruits and flowers have been used traditionally in complaints such as nausea, cough, asthma, fever, jaundice and diarrhoea.[69]

Cultivation and harvest

Cultivation

Sea buckthorn can grow in a variety of soils from sand dunes to mountain slopes, preferring gravelly soils. It is hardy to USDA zone 3 (UK zone 3). It has extensive roots which seek out water, making it drought tolerant, and unsuitable for planting near buildings. It is a light-demanding species and cannot grow in shade. Sea buckthorn fixes atmospheric nitrogen in its root nodules and so is capable of improving soil fertility. Due to the suckering capability of sea buckthorn, it may be unsuitable as invasive in some locations. For the production of fruit, planting of males is necessary, estimated at one male per 7-10 females required as pollinators, and fruit is produced from the third year. Management like blackcurrants is advised for maximising fruit, cutting out one-third of stems at the base each year.[70]

Pests and diseases

Insect larval and moth pests in China damage crops in plantations. Aphids can damage shoot tips. Birds, deer and rodents will feed on sea buckthorn.

Seed propagation

Sow seeds in the autumn in a cold frame. Soak 12 hours before planting and scarify. Prick out seedlings when large enough to handle and grow on for their first winter. Plant out in late spring into their permanent positions. To distinguish male and female plants, male seedlings in spring have very prominent axillary buds whilst females are clear and smooth at this time. Rooting from cuttings is poor. Division of suckers can be done in the winter. Layering in autumn is also possible.

Harvesting

Fruit yield has been estimated from 5-7kg per plant up to as much as 15kg from a mature tree. Harvesting is carried out before the first frosts, has to be carried out by hand and is labour intensive and difficult due to the thorny stems and branches. The fruits are very juicy and one way is to remove twigs and small branches with secateurs, leaving a stump with several buds to sprout the following year, and then squeeze the juice direct into a pan (described as akin to milking a cow) and strain. Alternatively, freeze the branches and then the berries will shake off. In commercial plantations, the berries are

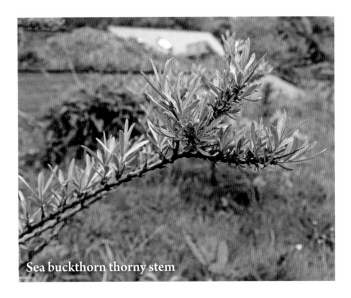
Sea buckthorn thorny stem

shaken off the branches every other year, allowing a year for recovery between crops.

Therapeutic use

Traditional

There are references to sea buckthorn in ancient Greek and classic Tibetan texts, particularly for diseases of skin and the digestive system. The leaves have also been used for treating diarrhoea and skin disorders. Sea buckthorn fruits have been used in Indian, Chinese and Tibetan traditions as medication for lung, heart, blood, stomach and other disorders including fever, tumours and abscesses.

Medicinal actions and uses

The fruit is anti-oxidant, anti-anaemic, anti-inflammatory. The leaves are antimicrobial, anti-inflammatory and antifungal.[71]

Clinical applications and research

Vitamin-rich freshly pressed juice of sea buckthorn fruit is used as a treatment for colds, fevers and exhaustion. Sea buckthorn oil has been used internally for heart and intestinal disorders,[72] and externally has been shown to promote skin cell and mucous membrane regeneration and so is used in treating burns.[73] Clinical research is continuing into the use of sea buckthorn preparations in cardiovascular disease and cancer.[74]

Sample preparations and dosage

A tea can be made from the leaves to help weight loss, and used as a wash. Sea buckthorn fruits can be infused in cider or wine vinegar. Fruits can be pressed for juice as a tonic and immune stimulant.

Constituents and commerce

Key constituents

The young leaves and fruits are rich in vitamin C and trace elements.[75] Mature seeds and fruit residue contain up to 20% oil, and are rich in essential fatty acids. Sea buckthorn berry oil is rich in flavonoids (such as carotene), and sea buckthorn seed oil is rich in essential fatty acids. Vitamin C content of sea buckthorn fruits is high, at 120mg per 100g, and the fruits also contain vitamins B1, B2, E and K as well as niacinamide, pantothenic acid, carotenoids in addition to oil (up to 9.2%), sugar, malic acid, amino acids and pectin.

Commerce

The whole fruits are stored frozen because of the high level of oil. Oil expressed from the fruit and oil from the seeds are both used in skin repair products. The oils and juice have been widely used in cosmetics and shampoos. Extensive plantations in northern China have been established with many processing plants, and there are commercial plantations elsewhere, such as in Canada. Weleda sources organic juice and seed oil from berries grown in Tuscany, Italy, and varieties are selected for either juice or seed oil production.

Safety

There are no documented adverse reactions. As sea buckthorn preparations may slow blood clotting, intake should be stopped two weeks prior to any surgery, and medical advice should be sought if taking anti-inflammatories and blood-thinning agents.

Other uses

Hedging, stabilising sand dunes. The acidic fruit is edible with a tart, bittersweet taste and is used in a wide range of food preparations.

Eleutherococcus senticosus, Siberian ginseng

An important bushy shrub from Asia with tonic and adaptogenic properties that help the body to deal with exhaustion and stress.

SCIENTIFIC NAME *Eleutherococcus senticosus* (Rupr. and Maxim.) Maxim. Previously *Acanthopanax senticosus* (Rupr. and Maxim.) Harms.

FAMILY Araliaceae

ALTERNATE NAMES Thorny ginseng, taiga root

PARTS USED Underground runners or rhizomes, stem bark and leaves

Description

Siberian ginseng is a deciduous shrub growing to around 3-4m tall. It flowers in July-August and berries ripen in September-October. The youngest stems may be covered in prickles while the older stems are unarmed. Palmate leaves on long reddish stalks are composed of five elliptical leaflets with toothed margins. Flowers are small, occurring toward the tips of stems in single or paired clusters that have long stalks. The fruit, a drupe, resembles that of ivy (*Hedera helix*).

Habitat

Siberian ginseng originates from southeast Asia, parts of China, Korea, Japan and the Russian Federation. An understorey shrub of mixed evergreen and deciduous forests, often forming dense thickets. Also cultivated in Siberia and Ukraine.

Related plants

The Araliaceae family includes American ginseng (*Panax quinqefolius*). Siberian ginseng is distantly related to ivy (*Hedera helix*), which is also in the Araliaceae family, and ivy leaf extract is used as a cough remedy.[76]

Cultivation and harvest

Cultivation

Siberian ginseng is hardy to USDA zone 3 (UK zone 3). It grows well in partial shade, is very hardy and prefers a cool climate. A moderately rich, moist and well-drained soil is ideal. Siberian ginseng can deplete soil nutrients[77] and so regular mulching similar to fruit trees is helpful.

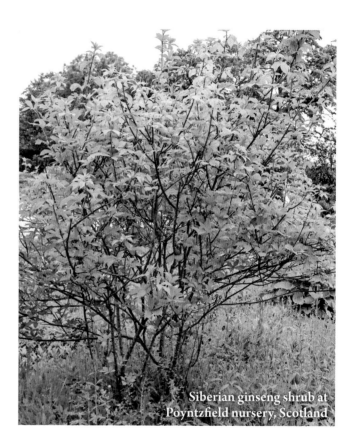

Siberian ginseng shrub at Poyntzfield nursery, Scotland

Flowers and seed are produced after 3-4 years of growth. Since Siberian ginseng grows competitively, forming thickets in its native habitat, care needs to be taken to ensure it does not spread invasively.

Pests and diseases

Few diseases and pests are reported, though we find that Devon slugs appear very partial to young Siberian ginseng leaves.

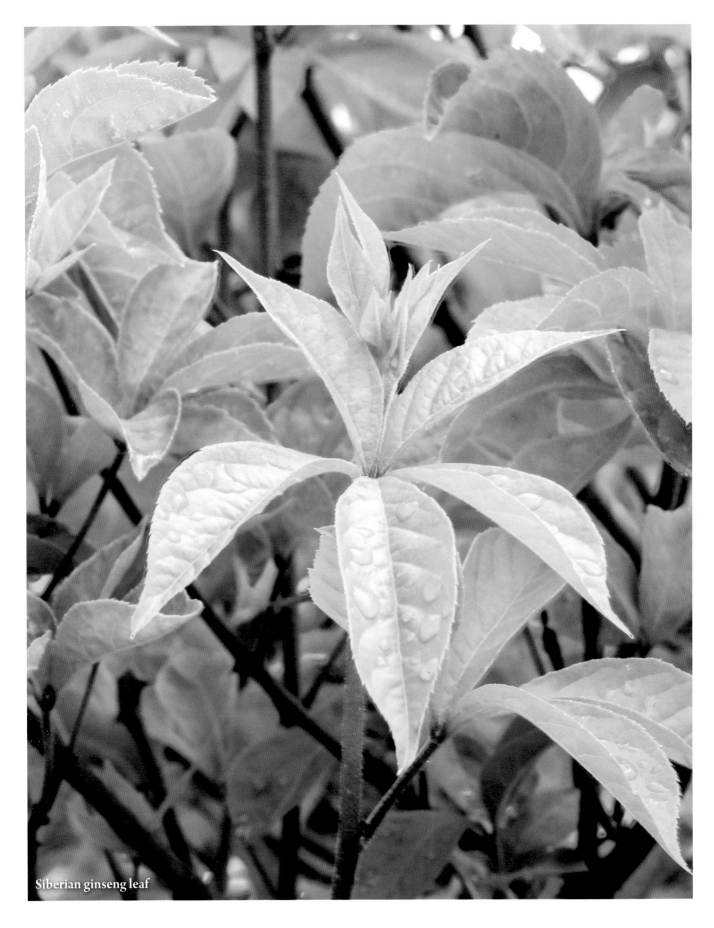

Siberian ginseng leaf

Propagation

Collect ripe seed in September/October and give six months warm stratification followed by three months, cold stratification, keeping an eye on the seed which may germinate earlier. Softwood cuttings about 15cm long, with two nodes, can be taken in the latter half of June, placed in free-draining compost, and kept moist, producing roots within four weeks.[78] Sections of the previous year's growth, 15-30cm, can be cut in August-September and placed obliquely in the soil to root within 2-3 weeks.[79] Suckers can be dug away from the parent plant in early spring and then replanted.

Harvesting

The root is best harvested when the plant is dormant, at least 4-5 years old. Lateral rootlets are cut off and the root thoroughly cleaned. Leaves are harvested when mature and can be dried for later use. The bark is harvested in late summer or autumn.

Therapeutic use

Traditional

Siberian ginseng has been used for centuries for increasing stamina and promoting overall health. In Chinese traditional medicine, Siberian ginseng root is used to invigorate qi (chi or energy), strengthen and nourish the spleen and kidney and balance vital energy.

Medicinal actions

The root and bark are adaptogenic, anti-oxidant, antiviral, antitumour, hepatoprotective, hypoglycaemic, diuretic, antifatigue, anti-inflammatory, antistress, anti-ulcer, immunoenhancing and antidepressive.[80] This plant offers a tonic for mental and physical capacities in cases of weakness, tiredness and during convalescence.[81]

Clinical applications and research

Used primarily for chronic fatigue, stress and compromised immunity, Siberian ginseng has additional uses including as a carminative in the treatment of acute and chronic gastritis, for impotence and blood pressure regulation. It has been claimed that Siberian ginseng has a role in cancer treatments.[82] The mechanism of the antistress or adaptogenic activities appears to be threefold: extracts of the roots produce a nonspecific increase in the body's defence against exogenous stress factors and noxious chemicals; they also stimulate the immune system, and they promote an overall improvement in physical and mental performance. In a randomised, double-blind, placebo-controlled study, Siberian ginseng was included with Malabar nut leaf (*Justicia adhatoda*) and purple coneflower (*Echinacea purpurea*) in the treatment of upper respiratory infection and significant cough relief was found.[83]

Sample preparations and dosage

Leaves can be eaten raw, fresh flowers and roots can be made into tea, the bark can be dried for later use. Dried bark can be taken as powder in capsules, up to 2-3g per day. A root tincture can be made by placing 50g chopped fresh root in 250ml vodka (40% proof) for 15 days in the dark; strain and take 1-2ml half an hour before meals.

Constituents and commerce

Key constituents

Active constituents include lignans, eleutherosides, coumarins, immunostimulant polysaccharides, glycans and sterols. Siberian ginseng root contains 0.6-0.9% of eleutherosides, and eleutheroside A has some similarities to ginsenosides found in Korean ginseng (*Panax ginseng*), though eleutheroside E is thought mainly responsible for increasing resistance to stress and fatigue.

Commerce

Siberian ginseng is harvested from its natural habitat in Russia and northeast China but overharvesting has resulted in this popular herb approaching endangered species status. Studies in Poland suggest considerable potential for European cultivation of *Eleutherococcus* species.[84] Commercial extracts are standardised to eleutheroside B and E at 300-400mg per day.

Safety

Siberian ginseng should not be used during pregnancy or breastfeeding, or by patients with high blood pressure. It should be taken for limited periods of 6-8 weeks or less.

Eucalyptus pauciflora, Snow gum

An evergreen from Australia with aromatic foliage, traditionally used for a wide range of inflammatory conditions and infections including coughs and colds.

SCIENTIFIC NAME   *Eucalyptus pauciflora* Siber. ex Spreng.

FAMILY   Myrtaceae

ALTERNATE NAMES   Cabbage gum

PARTS USED   Bark and leaves

Description

The snow gum is an evergreen shrub or small tree growing fast to 12m tall. The bark is smooth, somewhat mottled white or brown due to shedding of strips of bark, and grey-green lanceolate leaves up to 20cm long are borne in pairs.

Habitat

This is a variable species from eastern Australia, which grows in mountainous areas up to 1500m.

Related plants

A closely related variety *E. pauciflora* subsp. *niphophila*, also known as the snow gum, is found in higher mountain areas up to 2000m, reported as hardy to USDA zone 7 (UK zone 7). It grows to 6m high. The tall-growing blue gum (*E. globulus*) and the cider gum (*E. gunnii*) are the usual sources of aromatic leaves containing an antiseptic essential oil.[85] Other sources of essential oil include lemon eucalyptus (*E. citriodora*), *E. polybractea* and *E. camaldulensis*.[86]

Cultivation and harvest

Cultivation

The snow gum is one of the hardiest kinds of eucalyptus, hardy to USDA zone 8 (UK zone 8), though it is best to avoid frost pockets. A number of UK forestry trials have grown *Eucalyptus* species for biomass and energy crops, finding that the fastest growing varieties tended to be more susceptible to cold damage, although individuals of both *E. gunnii* and *E. pauciflora* varieties were able to survive on challenging sites.[87] Eucalyptus trees prefer well-drained soils and can grow in poor soil.

Choose the planting site carefully as *Eucalyptus* species are known for being unlikely to transplant well after several years. Snow gum cannot grow in the shade, and needs a sunny sheltered position. A deep mulch around the roots to prevent water loss and reduce the likelihood of freezing may be helpful. Avoid feeding in windy sites as too much top growth can increase wind rock. Most *Eucalyptus* species coppice readily, normally being cut in plantation forestry to a maximum height of 12cm with recommendations to be thinned after 9-18 months to three or fewer stems.

Pests and diseases

Snow gum is largely pest- and disease-free unless stressed when it can become subject to fungal attack. Eucalyptus gall wasp can disfigure the leaves according to the Woodland Trust.

Propagation

Seed is surface sown in February/March in a greenhouse. Species that come from high altitudes benefit from 6-8 weeks' cold stratification at 2°C (35°F). Pot up the seedlings into individual pots as soon as the second set of seed leaves has developed. Plant out into their permanent positions in early summer and give them some protection from the cold in their first winter. Cuttings of mature shoots with at least one leaf bud, about 10cm in length, can be taken in June/July and placed in a free-draining medium in a moist environment at 27-32°C (80-89°F).

Harvesting

Bark and leaf can be harvested at any time and used fresh or dried for later use.

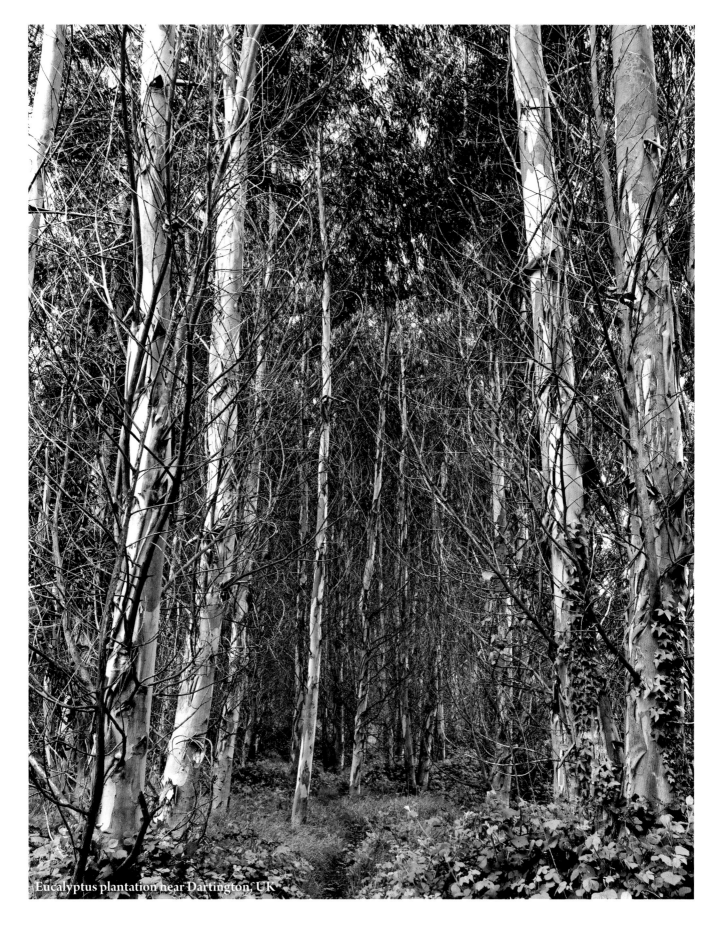

Eucalyptus plantation near Dartington, UK

Therapeutic use

Traditional

In traditional Aboriginal systems, the leaves of *Eucalyptus* species could be burned for inhalation, or used in a poultice, while the trees could also provide sap and gum for use in drinks and treating burns, cuts and sores.

Medicinal actions and uses

Eucalyptus essential oil is antiseptic, antibacterial, antispasmodic, expectorant, antiviral and antifungal, and has immune-stimulating and anti-inflammatory effects. Eucalyptus preparations can be used in a range of infectious complaints, particularly in coughs and colds.[88]

Clinical applications and research

The bark and leaves are rich in essential oils used for coughs and colds, with antiseptic effects exerted through direct application to the skin and through inhalation.[89] An Australian study showed 60% recovery in 50 patients with *Tinea* species fungal infections using an ointment formulated with essential oil from *E. pauciflora*.[90]

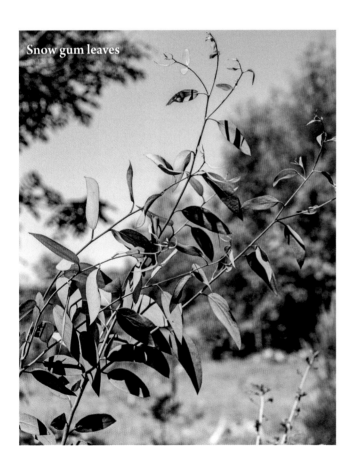
Snow gum leaves

Sample preparations and dosage

Distillation is the usual process to extract the essential oil. For inhalation use, 12 drops of the essential oil are dropped into boiling hot water in a basin. Alternatively, add 200ml of boiling water to a teaspoon of dried herb, then carefully inhale the steam placing a towel over your head. Dried leaves can be infused in a carrier oil; the oil can then be applied to the skin for treating fungal complaints.

Constituents and commerce

Key constituents

The leaves are rich in tannins, ellagitannins, triterpenes, sesquiterpenes and flavonoids. Essential oil constituents include the monoterpenes 1,8-cineole and α-pinene.[91] There is much variation in the constituents of essential oils of *Eucalyptus* species:[92] though the snow gum is reported to have higher levels of sesquiterpenes than other species.[93]

Commerce

In Australia, *E. polybractea* shrubs 1m high are harvested at between 18-24 months old. There are large plantations in China. Total world production in 1991 of medicinal eucalyptus essential oil was estimated at 3000 tons.[94] According to a market analysis in 2018, the global eucalyptus oil market will be worth over US$64 million by the end of 2025.[95] Eucalyptol or cineole content is the usual marker for medicinal eucalyptus essential oil.

Safety

Eucalyptus essential oil is not for internal use. For external use the essential oil should be diluted in case of skin irritation and use on the face should be avoided. Excessive use of the leaves can cause nausea, vomiting and diarrhoea.

Other uses

Biomass production of fast-growing trees. *E. gunnii* and *E. globulus* are cultivated in many subtropical areas including Portugal and Spain, for paper pulp manufacture.[96]

Ficus carica, Fig

A small spreading tree of Middle Eastern origin, long cultivated for its delicious fleshy fruits and having a range of further benefits in combatting high cholesterol and skin diseases.

SCIENTIFIC NAME *Ficus carica* L.

FAMILY Moraceae

ALTERNATE NAMES Edible fig, common fig

PARTS USED Fruit and leaves, latex

Description

The common fig is a fast-growing deciduous tree with many branches growing to 6m tall by 6m wide. Alternate leaves are large and deeply lobed. Both male and female flowers can be found on the plant. Unusually, the fig 'fruit' is actually a receptacle which encloses many flowers that have ripened their individual seeds.

Habitat

Fig is native to dry soils in southwest Asia, northern Africa and the Mediterranean region, and extensively cultivated worldwide.

Related plants

'Brown Turkey' is a common cold-hardy cultivar in the UK, self-fertile and with ripening fruit in August-September. Other cultivars reputed to be very hardy are 'Michurinska 10', 'Chicago' and 'Olympian'. 'White Ischia' is a dwarf cultivar up to 5m tall and wide.

Cultivation and harvest

Cultivation

The fig is hardy to USDA zone 8 (UK zone 7) and should be grown in a sheltered spot, such as against a southwest facing wall or fence. It does require light and cannot fruit readily in shade. Spacing depends on the varieties used, and in commercial plantings may be 3m × 4m. The fig has shallow roots and will tolerate a range of soils pH 6-8, appreciating a more chalky soil. Avoid waterlogging. If grown in a pot, it can be given a yearly mulch of compost (or tomato fertiliser feeds weekly in the growing season). The tree produces two

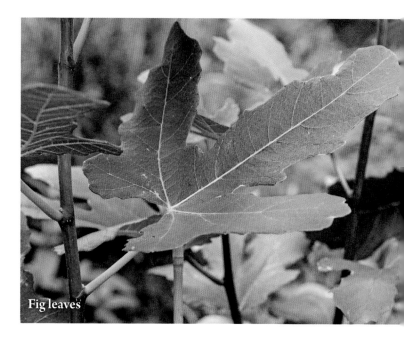
Fig leaves

to three crops per year but only one ripens in a cool temperate climate – the small pea-sized figs formed in the autumn overwinter to produce crops the following autumn; the other fruits produced in spring and early summer should be removed in August. Some winter chilling is helpful, and a dry period when flowering and fruiting avoids splitting of fruit. In cold winters, especially for younger trees, protection is needed. If a plant does die back it may sprout again the following year with many shoots. Fig roots can be very invasive. If planted in the ground then root restriction is advised to keep the tree compact and fruitful, by inserting concrete flags upright to full depth around the plant, allowing an area of one square metre.

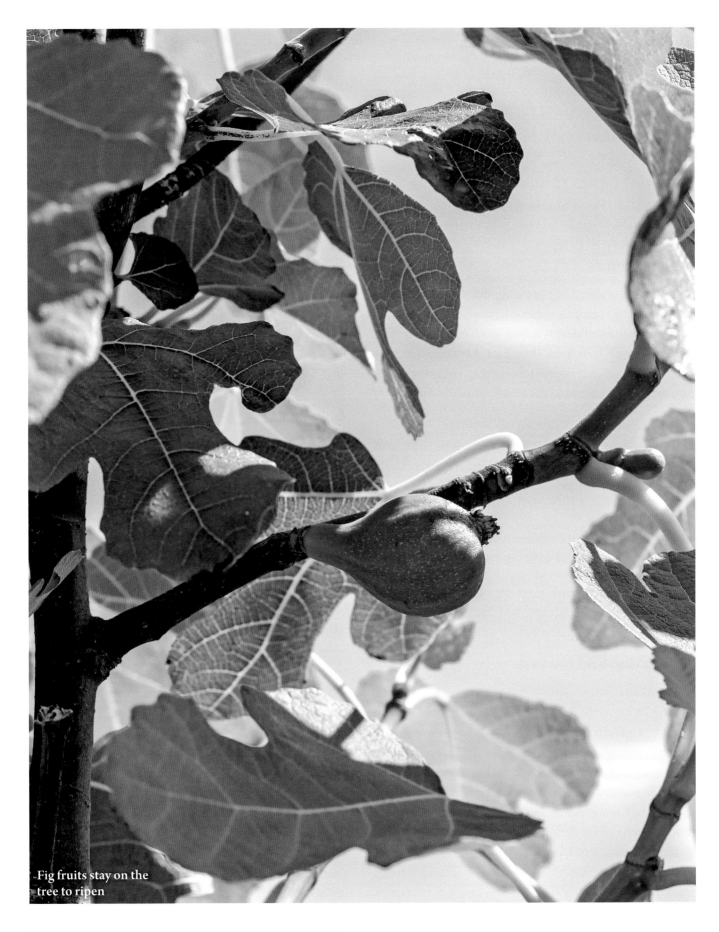

Fig fruits stay on the
tree to ripen

Pests and diseases

The fig is largely free of disease though it may suffer from coral spot fungus, pink pustules on dead twigs, or other moulds.

Propagation

The fig can be propagated by seed, but is very easy to grow from cuttings, 20-25cm long, taken in February or March. Remove any terminal bud and place the cutting into free-draining compost (half sand/half compost) and bring indoors until roots are forming. Then pot on and keep in a frost-free environment till well established. Fig branches can also be layered.

Harvesting

Fig leaves can be harvested and dried for later use. Fig fruits are ready to harvest when they darken and become soft and hang downwards. They should be picked once ripe and need to be dried if not used within 1-2 days. Dry the fruits by cutting in half and laying on a rack in the oven on the lowest possible setting. Turn occasionally for 8-12 hours until leathery. Take care when harvesting to avoid contact with drops of latex which can irritate skin.

Therapeutic use

Traditional

The fig has longstanding use in the traditional systems of Ayurveda, Unani and Siddha. It has been used in digestive, respiratory and cardiovascular disorders.

Medicinal actions and uses

Laxative, antispasmodic, anti-oxidant, cytotoxic, anti-inflammatory, astringent, carminative, galactagogue and hypolipidaemic. The leaves can be used as a vermifuge. Fig fruits are eaten as a mild laxative. The latex is used in treating warts and verrucas as it is corrosive on the skin, and further studies suggest there may be a use in treating skin melanoma and virus-related cervical cancer.[97]

Clinical applications and research

Leaf extracts have been shown to reduce triglycerides and moderate cholesterol secretion, and to provide natural antibacterial oral cavity care.[98] The ethanolic extract of the fruit is rich in polyphenols and flavonoids with potential as an antidiabetic agent.[99] Fig fruits are used as supplements in the treatment of constipation.[100]

Sample preparations and dosage

Dried fig leaves can be taken as an infusion to help lower blood fat and sugar levels. If used fresh then boil the fig leaves for 10-15 minutes. Fig fruits can be taken fresh or dried. Use the fig latex from the leaves or unripe fruits on warts direct.[101]

Constituents and commerce

Key constituents

Fig fruits contain numerous bioactive constituents including phytosterols, anthocyanins, amino acids, organic acids, fatty acids and phenolic components. Fig fruits are also a rich source of calcium and fibre. The leaves contain oxalic, citric, malic, quinic, shikimic and fumaric acids, and accumulate germacrene D[102] which acts as an antimicrobial. The main flavonoid in the leaf is luteolin with anti-inflammatory effects, also quercetin is an anti-oxidant, and biochanin-A is a phytoestrogen.

Commerce

The fig is an important crop worldwide for fresh and dry consumption of its sweet fruits. Some extracts of the fig are used in the production of sunscreen and colouring agents.

Safety

Avoid contact with the fig leaf latex which can be irritant and can cause a skin reaction.

Other uses

Edible fruits. Wrapping foods.

Forsythia suspensa, Forsythia

An arching ornamental shrub with abundant yellow spring flowers and seeds traditionally used in Chinese medicine, offering broad-spectrum antibacterial actions in respiratory and urinary infections.

SCIENTIFIC NAME *Forsythia suspensa* L.

FAMILY Oleaceae

ALTERNATE NAMES Weeping forsythia, golden bells

PARTS USED Flowers, young leaves and fruits

Description

A deciduous variable and somewhat straggly shrub with multiple stems and spreading branches growing to 3-4m tall by 4m wide. Copious yellow flowers are produced in March-April before the leaves, and they are pollinated by insects, mostly bees. The fruits are formed of narrow capsules with two chambers produced from July to September, though these are not always produced in European countries.

Habitat

From eastern Asia to China, a plant of hillsides and ravines and woodland margins, also cultivated in China and Japan. It was introduced in Holland in 1833 and then cultivated for sale in England from the 1850s.

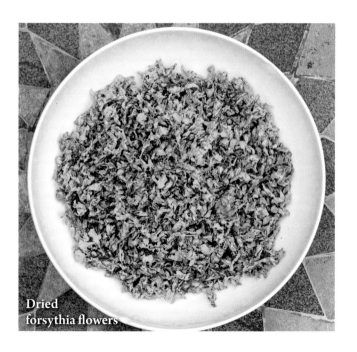

Dried forsythia flowers

Related plants

Forsythia × intermedia is the garden plant often used for ornamental value, a hybrid of *F. suspensa* and *F. viridissima*, and there are numerous cultivars. *F. viridissima* (with a low-growing habit) and *F. koreana* are used in Japanese and Korean traditional medicine.

Cultivation and harvest

Cultivation

Hardy to USDA zone 5 (UK zone 5). Forsythia prefers full sunlight, though it can grow in partial shade and is tolerant of urban pollution. Forsythia can grow in most soils, and is medium to fast growing. For the production of more flowers it should be pruned after flowering, as flowers are produced on wood more than one year old. This plant can form a thicket as the arching branches reach the soil and take root, and is considered invasive in some parts of the US.

Pests and diseases

Susceptible to honey fungus. As forsythia is a member of the olive family it may be susceptible to ash dieback.

Propagation

Seed can be sown in spring after 1-3 months' cold stratification. When large enough to handle, prick the seedlings out into individual pots and grow them on in the greenhouse for at least their first winter. Plant them out into their permanent positions in late spring or early summer, after the last expected frosts. Between May and September cuttings of half-ripe wood 10-15cm can be taken. Cuttings of mature wood

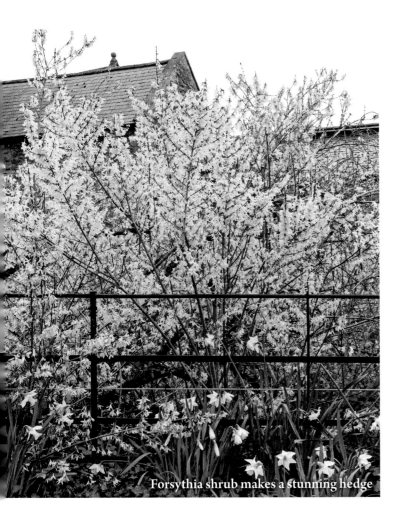
Forsythia shrub makes a stunning hedge

can be placed in a sheltered outdoor bed. Layering in spring or summer.[103]

Harvesting

The flowers, leaves and fruits can all be harvested and used raw or dried for later use.

Therapeutic use

Traditional use

Forsythia is a bitter tasting and pungent herb, one of the 50 fundamental herbs in Chinese traditional medicine, used for clearing heat and detoxification in childhood complaints. The fruits have been used to treat fever, inflammation and other conditions. The leaves and twigs have been used in decoction to treat breast cancer.

Medicinal actions and uses

Anti-inflammatory, bitter, astringent, anti-oxidant, antibacterial, antiviral, laxative, diuretic and tonic. The flowers have broad-spectrum antibacterial action, and can be used in the treatment of acute infectious diseases such as tonsillitis and urinary tract infections. The leaves can be used as an anti-inflammatory poultice for ulcerated glands or haemorrhoids.

Clinical applications and research

Research into the applications of forsythia is limited. Anti-inflammatory and anti-oxidant properties of the seed contribute to the anticancer and neuroprotective properties attributed to the fruits.[104] Research into the more widely grown garden plant *Forsythia × intermedia* has identified that the flowers and leaves are a potentially valuable source of active lignans of use in inflammatory diseases where there is excessive production of cytokines.[105]

Sample preparations and dosage

The flowers can be made into syrup or jelly. Flower or leaf infusion may be helpful as a gargle for a sore throat, and taken short term in colds and flu. A decoction of the fruit can be used for skin infections and acne. An infusion of flowers is used for a face wash.

Constituents and commerce

Key constituents

Lignans and phenylethanoid glycosides are active constituents of this herb, including forsythiaside, phillyrin, rutin and phillygenin. Levels of phillyrin are highest in the leaves.

Commerce

In Chinese traditional medicine the fruit is harvested in two forms, when green and starting to ripen (Qing Qiao) and when yellow and fully ripe (Lao Qiao).[106]

Safety

Avoid in breastfeeding or pregnancy. It is recommended that forsythia preparations should be avoided alongside anticoagulants or before surgery.

Other uses

Ornamental hedge. Flowers can be eaten as a bitter garnish in salads.

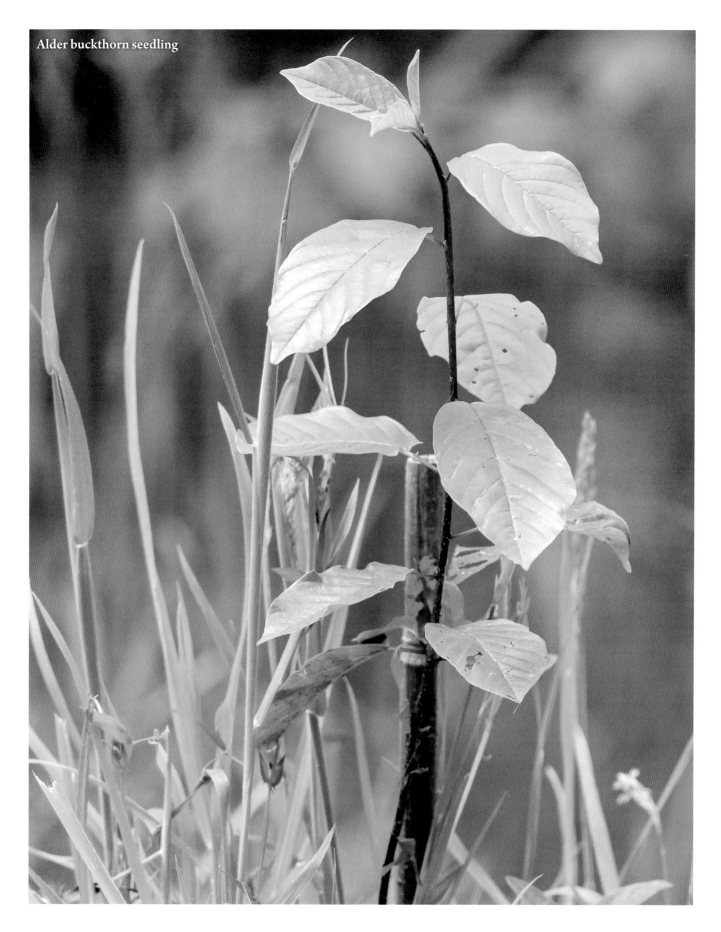
Alder buckthorn seedling

Frangula alnus, Alder buckthorn

An attractive small European tree that buzzes with bees and other insects, having traditional use of the bark as a laxative and new possibilities in viral and degenerative diseases.

SCIENTIFIC NAME   *Frangula alnus* Mill. previously known as *Rhamnus frangula*

FAMILY   Rhamnaceae

ALTERNATE NAMES   Alder dogwood, black alder, glossy buckthorn

PARTS USED   Bark

Description

Alder buckthorn is a deciduous shrub or small tree, erect and slender, growing to 5m by 4m at a slow rate. Leaves are alternate and have smooth wavy edges. Flowers are produced from May to June and are hermaphrodite and pollinated by insects. Small black fruits containing seeds ripen September to November.

Habitat

Native to Europe from southern Scandinavia to north Africa, the Urals and Siberia.

Related plants

Purging buckthorn (*Rhamnus cathartica*) is another European buckthorn, has spiny branches, and is more likely to be found in calcareous soils. *R. californica*, coffeeberry, is evergreen growing to 5m in western North America, with a dwarf shrubby habit. The bark of *R. purshiana* of western North America is the source of Cascara sagrada, a worldwide commodity promoted for use in constipation. Alder buckthorn provides an alternative to the use of *R. purshiana* which is on the UPS 'Species-at-risk to watch' list.[107] Alder buckthorn is not related to alders (*Alnus* species).

Cultivation and harvest

Cultivation

Alder buckthorn is hardy to USDA zone 3 (UK zone 3) and will grow on any reasonably good soil, though it does well on an acid soil. It can grow in semi-shade or no shade, and prefers a moist soil. It dislikes drought, exposure to high winds and a waterlogged soil. Alder buckthorn can be coppiced and regenerates well. A close relative, *R. purshiana*, can be readily coppiced if cut down to within 30cm of the ground, producing new shoots and flowering and fruiting within 3-4 years.[108]

Pests and diseases

The alder buckthorn is associated with crown rust which can affect grasses and cereal crops. It is considered invasive in north-eastern US states and eastern Canada and some states restrict it as a noxious weed.[109]

Propagation

Harvest the ripe black berries in autumn, if necessary taking these several weeks early to prevent losses to birds. Place the berries in dry sand in a box and allow to ripen. Rub the berries in sand to release the seeds and spread the mixture direct onto a seedbed in a cold frame. Stored seed requires 1-2 months' cold stratification at about 5°C (41°F) and should be sown as early in the year as possible in a cold frame or outdoor seedbed. Prick out the seedlings into individual pots when they are large enough to handle, and grow them on in the greenhouse or cold frame for their first winter. Plant them out in late spring or early summer of the following year. Softwood cuttings can be taken in early August and placed in a frame. Layering in early spring.

Harvesting

Young bark of alder buckthorn is collected in early summer from branches and dried. It must be stored for at least one year before use to remove harsh constituents.

Therapeutic use

Traditional

Both alder buckthorn and purging buckthorn have long been used for the cathartic and laxative effects of their bark and berries. The berries of purging buckthorn were once used to provide a nauseous bitter juice prepared as Syrup of Buckthorn. A pamphlet of the 1740s published by John Juxton explains that the 'Syrup of the Berries of Buckthorn are [*sic*] much in use and prepared at many Gentlemens Houses, and good Housekeepers, and likewise sold in the Apothecaries Shops', although he was advertising his own product as he claimed that his pills were stronger and cheaper than the 'bitter, heavy syrup'.[110] Alder buckthorn provides a milder action than purging buckthorn. The bark used to be boiled in ale by country people for jaundice, and it was also used as a tonic for the intestines and for relieving haemorrhoids. The alder buckthorn bark has been used in the UK as a substitute for Cascara sagrada.[111]

Medicinal uses

The bark is laxative, cholagogue and tonic and is mainly used for chronic constipation.[112] The bark contains anthraquinones which are inactive in the gastrointestinal tract until they reach the colon, where they are degraded by bacterial enzymes; within about six to eight hours this causes vigorous peristalsis.[113] Other actions of alder buckthorn include antimicrobial, antifungal, antiviral and insecticidal.[114]

Alder buckthorn young bark

Clinical applications and research

Alder buckthorn leaves and bark have shown promise for their therapeutic effects.[115] The high levels of hydroxybenzoic acids and flavanols in alder buckthorn bark have been considered for use against staphylococcal local infections.[116] The constituent emodin, an anthraquinone derivative, has been shown to inhibit replication of the herpes simplex virus, an effect comparable to acyclovir.[117] Furthermore, anthraquinones can inhibit the abnormal aggregation of tau proteins in paired helical filaments which is a hallmark of Alzheimer's disease.[118] In a study of a related species of buckthorn, *R. alaternus*, a methanolic extract proved cytotoxic to human monocytic leukaemia cells.[119]

Sample preparations and dosage

For constipation, 0.5-2.5g of alder buckthorn dried bark is taken directly in capsules or in decoction at night. Tincture 0.5-2.5ml administered at bedtime for constipation.[120]

Constituents and commerce

Key constituents

Contains anthraquinone derivatives, flavanoids, tannins and peptide alkaloids.[121]

The main active constituents are hydroxyanthraquinone glycosides (emodin, frangulin, iso-emodin, aloe-emodin, and chrysophanol). The bark contains a minimum of 7% glucofrangulins.

Commerce

Commercial preparations of alder buckthorn are standardised to contain 20-30mg hydroxyanthracene derivatives (glucofrangulin A) to be taken at bedtime or in two divided doses in the evening and morning.

Safety

Do not use fresh bark which contains anthrones and can cause severe vomiting. Avoid use in people with nausea or vomiting, inflammatory bowel disease, appendicitis, intestinal obstruction or acute intestinal inflammation. Not recommended for use in children under 12 years of age. Use of this remedy may colour the urine orange. Long-term use as a laxative is not advised as dependence may result. Due to insufficient data, this remedy should not be used during pregnancy or breastfeeding.

Other uses

Alder buckthorn is the source food for caterpillars of the yellow brimstone butterfly (*Gonepteryx rhamni*), and it is attractive to bees and other insects. Dye plant. Charcoal making.

Fraxinus excelsior, Ash

A widespread tall and elegant tree with bitter leaves and bark once used to treat fevers, with potential for wider use in arthritis and viral complaints.

SCIENTIFIC NAME   *Fraxinus excelsior* L.

FAMILY   Oleaceae

ALTERNATE NAMES   Common ash, European ash

PARTS USED   Leaves and bark

Description

Ash is a tall deciduous tree growing fast to 30m tall by 20m wide with greenish-grey twigs, and firm ridged bark. Flowers in bunches in April-May are small and lacking petals. The ash is wind-pollinated. Large compound leaves are divided into 9-13 leaflets of lanceolate shape with serrated margins. Characteristic identification in winter is by the large opposite black buds. The fruits are slightly twisted ellipsoid samaras (keys) with wide wings to aid wind dispersal, maturing from September onwards. The trees are dioecious so that both male and female trees are needed if seed is wanted.

Habitat

Ash is native throughout Europe and into western Asia. It grows in moist areas in deep soil, as well as meadows and hedges.

Related plants

In North America, the American white ash (*F. americana*) has similar uses. The manna ash (*F. orna*) is a smaller tree of southern Europe known for a sweet exudate from its trunk which is regarded as a gentle laxative and tonic. *F. pennsylvanica* of Canadian origin has been shown to have bark extract providing significant antibacterial activity.[122] *F. rhynchophylla* is the Chinese ash (Qin Pi) and the bark is used in traditional Chinese formulae for infections and inflammations.

Cultivation and harvest

Cultivation

The ash forms part of the woodland canopy and cannot tolerate shade. It needs moisture, and it will survive on a variety of soils. The ash can be used as a windbreak although it is one of the last trees to come into leaf, and is also known for its role in erosion control through protecting the soil. Although hardy to USDA zone 4 (UK zone 4), the ash is sensitive to late spring frosts which can cause forking of the main stem and branches. The ash coppices well.

Pests and diseases

As a fast-growing tree, the ash has not usually been prone to disease or pest damage. However, more recently it has suffered from ash dieback caused by the fungus *Hymenoscyphus fraxineus* (previously known as *Chalara fraxinea*), which causes branches and leaves to blacken and wither. No cure is known, and since infected trees can survive for some years, the general advice is to take no action unless a tree poses a safety risk. Leaves and logs should be composted and burnt on site and not taken off the site.

Propagation

Ash seeds have multiple dormancy and need both warm and cold stratification, germinating in the second spring following sowing. To speed up the process put fresh seed in a moist mixture of 50/50 organic compost and sand or perlite and provide warmth at 15°C (59°F) for up to 16 weeks and then chill in the refrigerator at 5-10°C (41-50°F) for 20 weeks. If seeds are germinating they can then be potted up. Harden off the seedlings over a three week period and plant out once the seedlings are 30-40cm tall. Cuttings of mature wood can be placed in a sheltered outdoor bed in the winter.

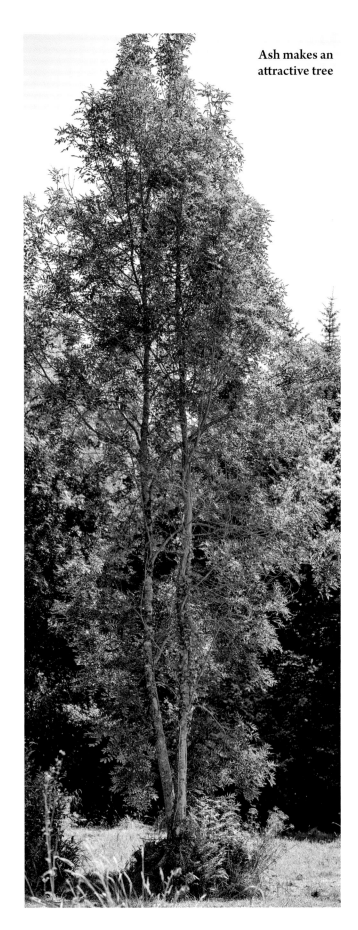

Ash makes an attractive tree

Harvesting

The leaves are gathered in June and dried for powdering and later use. The bark is collected from young branches which are 2-3 years old.

Therapeutic use

Traditional

The ash has considerable traditional use in Europe. The seeds have long been considered an aphrodisiac, and used to control flatulence. Ash bark has been used as a bitter tonic and astringent, and was used extensively as a substitute for imported Peruvian bark (*Cinchona* species) for ague and fever. Ash leaf has been used internally for fever, rheumatism, gout, oedema, stones, constipation, stomach symptoms and worm infestation; and externally for lower leg ulcers and wounds. The leaves in a distilled water were considered good for dropsy and obesity. Amongst other uses described by John Evelyn in 1670:

> There is extracted an Oyl from the Ash, by the processes on other Woods, which is excellent to recover the Hearing; some drops of it being distill'd warm into the Ears, and for the Caries or rot of the Bones, Tooth-ach, pains in the Kidneys, and Spleen, the anointing therewith is most soveraign.[123]

Medicinal actions and uses

Ash bark is anti-inflammatory and febrifuge with application in arthritis and rheumatism.[124] Ash leaves are diuretic, diaphoretic and laxative. Further research into the potential of ash in terms of anticancer, antioxidant and anti-inflammatory properties has been recommended.[125]

Clinical applications and research

Little clinical research data is available on ash despite a long tradition of use of the bark and leaves in Europe.[126] Extracts of the leaves have been found to suppress fungi and to have antiviral properties.[127] Recent trials have shown a use for an extract from ash keys in control of blood sugar levels in obesity.[128]

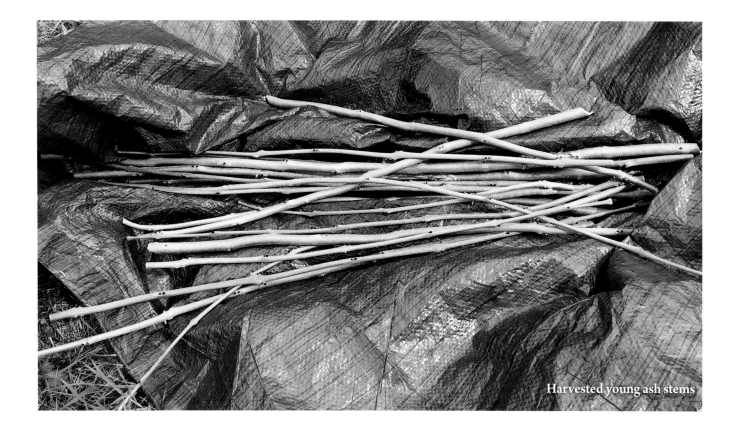

Harvested young ash stems

Sample preparations and dosage

Leaf can be juiced as a poultice for insect bites. Tea of 25g of leaf infused in 500ml water, divided into 2-3 cups per day. Powdered bark or leaf in capsules for arthritis and diuretic effects, 300-600mg three times daily. Tincture of ash bark can be taken, up to 20 drops before meals (see recipe p.88).

Constituents and commerce

Key constituents

Coumarin derivatives including aesculin, fraxin, fraxetin and fraxinol. Flavonoids based on aesculetin (including aescin) and others such as rutin and quercetin. Also iridoids and secoiridoids.

Commerce

A combination product of poplar (*Populus tremula*), goldenrod (*Solidago virgaurea*) and ash (*Fraxinus excelsior*) for use in rheumatism was reported on in the

1990s with favourable results comparable to the average dose of nonsteroidal anti-inflammatory drugs but with half the adverse effects.[129]

Safety

Toxicity data is lacking, and although no health hazards are recorded, use in pregnancy and breastfeeding should be avoided.

Other uses

Timber. Fuel. The fruits can be used as food, pickled in salt and vinegar like capers.

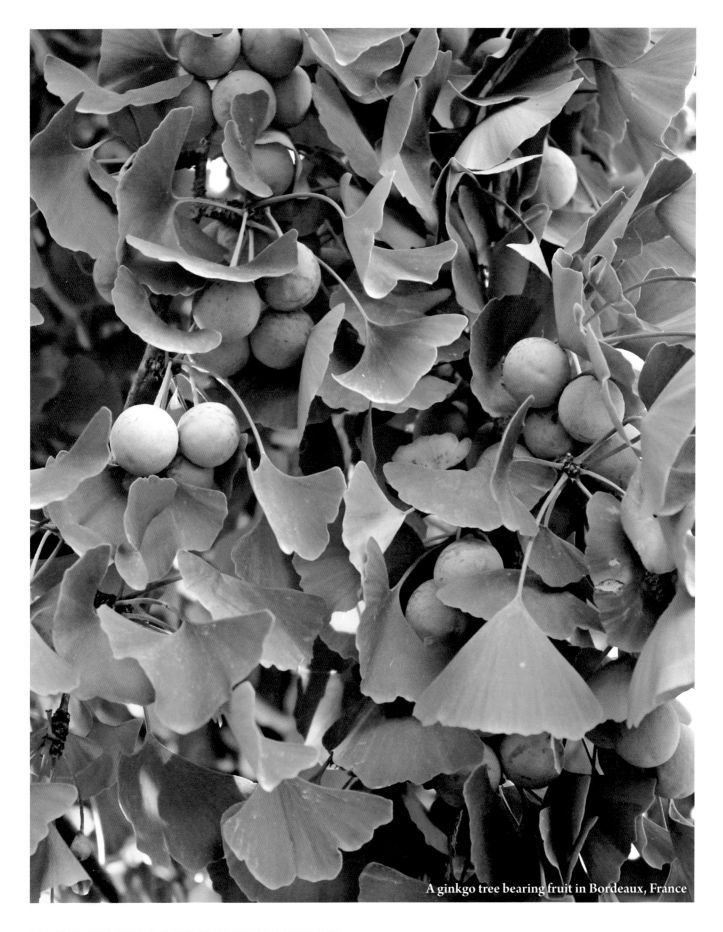

A ginkgo tree bearing fruit in Bordeaux, France

Ginkgo biloba, Ginkgo

A beautiful coniferous tree with fan-shaped leaves and a lengthy tradition of use in Asia, now recognised for its help to treat anxiety, poor circulation and dementia.

SCIENTIFIC NAME *Ginkgo biloba* L.

FAMILY Ginkgoaceae

ALTERNATE NAMES Maidenhair tree

PARTS USED Leaves

Description

A deciduous conifer tree growing up to 30m tall and 9m wide, having glossy green fan-shaped leaves with irregularly toothed upper margins. The ginkgo is regarded as a living fossil, related to tree ferns and cycads. Trees are dioecious and may be male or female; male specimens are said to be upright and irregular while females are lower and spreading. Flowers are inconspicuous and appear after 20-35 years. Yellow/orange plum-like seeds about 2cm long are edible and can be roasted but the fleshy coat does deteriorate and smell similar to rancid butter due to its butyric acid content.

Habitat

The ginkgo is a native of China, growing in silty soils along stream banks, but is endangered in the wild. It is widely grown in Europe and America, introduced in the UK in 1754.[130]

Related plants

The ginkgo is the sole survivor of an ancient tree family. 'Fastigiata' is a columnar form; 'Pendula' has spreading or weeping branches.

Cultivation and harvest

The ginkgo tree can grow in a wide range of soils, preferring deep fairly rich soil with a neutral pH[131] and full sun. It can tolerate drought and pollution, but does best in moist and well-drained soil. It is hardy to USDA zone 5a (UK zone 4) and does not need frost protection. Ginkgo is a relatively slow-growing tree, averaging less than 30cm per year, reaching 10m in 30 years. It can be readily coppiced or pruned, and this is best done while dormant in January or February. Ginkgo can be pot grown, in a well-drained container, using good quality multipurpose compost with 10% grit added. Keep moist and a little mulch can be added to the surface of the soil in spring.

Pests and diseases

Ginkgo has few pests or diseases.

Propagation

Collect ginkgo fruits in October and remove the pulp. The fresh seed is warm stratified for 1-2 months and then cold stratified for 1-2 months. The seed can be sown outside for spring germination in a moist seedbed. Cuttings taken in July root well.

Harvesting

The leaves are harvested in late summer not long before they start to turn yellow, and can be dried for later use (see p.123). Whole branches can be removed for stripping of leaves. Drying should be done in a single layer or with regular turning to avoid the leaves sticking together.

Therapeutic use

Traditional

Ginkgo has longstanding use in Asia, particularly for the seeds, which have been used as an aid to digestion and to reduce alcohol intoxication. The leaves were recorded for external use in a text of 1436 during the Ming dynasty, and then for internal use for diarrhoea in 1505. In traditional Chinese medicine, ginkgo is used for respiratory problems (asthma and bronchitis), brain disorders and urinary conditions.

Medicinal actions

Antihypoxic (increases peripheral and cerebral blood flow), anti-oxidant, cardiovascular tonic, anticoagulant and vasodilator. Uses of ginkgo are primarily indicated in poor circulation and in age-related cognitive impairment.[132]

Clinical applications and research

Almost all research on ginkgo has been performed with a German standardised extract known as EGb 761 or GBE, which is analytically controlled to 6% terpene lactones and 24% flavone glycosides. Studies have found evidence of improvements in circulation to the eye and brain[133] and decreases in intermittent claudication (poor circulation in legs). A double-blind placebo-controlled trial using doses of 240mg and 480mg of the standardised extract over four weeks found a significant decrease in anxiety in patients with anxiety disorders.[134] Studies have also considered possible benefits in dementia, memory and tinnitus.[135] The broad spectrum of medicinal activities of gingko make it useful for an extremely wide range of chronic degenerative conditions.[136]

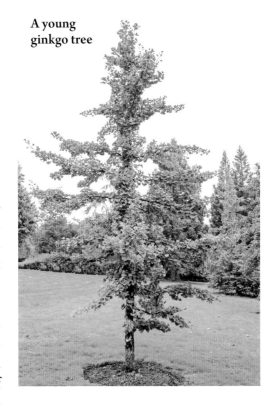

A young ginkgo tree

Sample preparations and dosage

Leaf tincture 2-5ml three times daily. Dried leaf infusion or powder in capsules, 6-12g per day.

Constituents and commerce

Key constituents

The leaves contain flavonoids including flavonol glycosides (including quercitin, kaempferol), biflavones, diterpenes (including terpene lactones), triactonic diterpenes (including ginkgolides A, B, C, J, M), the sesquiterpene bilobalide, and other organic acids and tannins.[137] The maximum active terpenoid ingredients are found in late summer and early autumn, then declining until leaf fall.

Commerce

For medicinal use, leaves are harvested from trees of 2m or higher planted at a spacing of 3-6m. The leaves are dried in drum dryers and yields are 2-4 tons of dried leaves per hectare depending on site.[138] World supplies of ginkgo come from plantations in the US, Japan, Korea, France and China. Ginkgo is commercially cultivated in plantations of up to 25,000 plants per hectare, where a row cultivation technique is used keeping the plants cut to 30cm in autumn, harvesting the leaves in late summer. Intensive growing can attain leaf yields of 20 tons per hectare after three years.[139] Ginkgo leaf extract is now a widely sold supplement throughout the world, particularly for circulatory and cognitive disorders. Manufacturers' preparations may vary, but most are standardised. However, there is concern about adulteration of ginkgo products with cheaper substitutes such as buckwheat or pea family ingredients as one study showed that 33 out of 35 products did not have the recommended levels of key ingredients.[140]

Safety

Tolerance of ginkgo extract is excellent and side effects minimal. The commonest problems are gastrointestinal upset, dizziness and headache. There have been isolated reports of adverse effects of bleeding when used alongside antiplatelet drugs so caution is needed in using ginkgo alongside anticoagulant medication.[141] For safety, ginkgo should be discontinued at least two weeks before having dental or surgical treatment.

Hamamelis virginiana, Witch hazel

A small tree from North America that produces spidery fragrant flowers in autumn, providing a distilled water that is widely used in skin care and common ailments.

SCIENTIFIC NAME   *Hamamelis virginiana* L.

FAMILY   Hamamelidaceae

ALTERNATE NAMES   Spotted or striped alder, snapping hazel, Virginian witch hazel

PARTS USED   Bark, leaves, twigs

Description

A deciduous shrub or small tree growing up to 5m tall and 3m wide, often multitrunked and with arching branches. The alternate leaves are simple and hazel-like. Spidery yellow fragrant flowers are produced in the autumn. The flowers are hermaphrodite with both male and female organs. Woody seed capsules are produced which stay on the branch until the following year and then burst open to project the small shiny black seeds over 3m. Witch hazel is highly ornamental as leaves turn golden in the autumn.

Habitat

Witch hazel comes from the eastern half of North America. It grows wild in dry to moist woods, often on the banks of streams on stony ground.

Related plants

Four related species of witch hazel exist, two in North America, and two in Asia. Most plants available from garden centres for ornamental use are Chinese or Japanese cultivars with showy flowers in early spring that are grafted on to Virgininan witch hazel rootstock.

Cultivation and harvest

Cultivation

Witch hazel is a hardy tree to USDA zones 5 (UK zone 5) and does not need frost protection. It can readily grow in partial shade, and is ideal for the woodland edge. It prefers a rich moist soil which must be on the acidic side (less than pH 6.5) and well drained. Witch hazel can be thinned or pruned, and this is best done while dormant in January or February.

Pests and diseases

Witch hazel appears to have few pests and diseases.

Propagation

Fresh seed harvested 'green' around the end of August can be sown immediately in a cold frame. Stored seed needs two months' warm stratification then one month cold followed by another two weeks' warm and then a further four months' cold stratification. Germination may take up to 18 months. Scarification may improve germination of stored seed. Prick out the seedlings into individual pots and overwinter them in a greenhouse, planting out in the following spring. Softwood cuttings can be taken in summer, though we have had limited success with cuttings at Holt Wood, preferring seed propagation. Layering can be carried out in early spring or autumn, taking 12 months for new roots to form.

Harvesting

Fresh young leaves and twigs can be harvested in the spring (at Holt Wood we give the bushes a yearly 'haircut' in spring). Leaves can be harvested in the summer and dried for later use.

Therapeutic use

Traditional

Historically, the leaves of witch hazel were used by Native Americans as a poultice for painful swellings, bruises and inflammations as well as a treatment for insect bites and burns. The traditional method of preparation was to boil chopped twigs in water for eight or more hours.[142] The leaves were used internally as a tea for their astringent properties, to relieve diarrhoea,

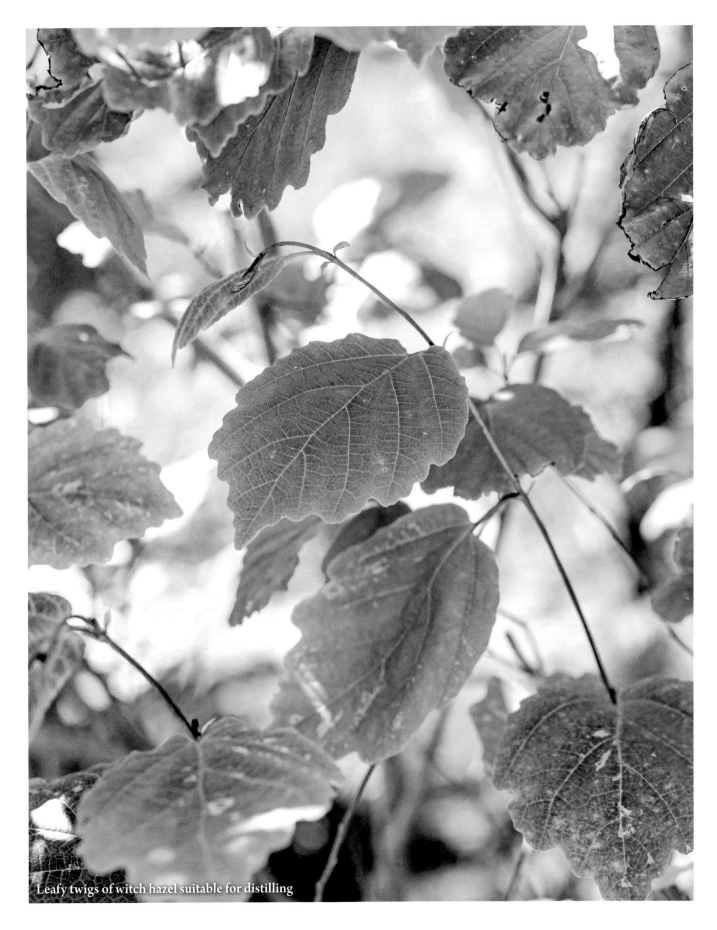

Leafy twigs of witch hazel suitable for distilling

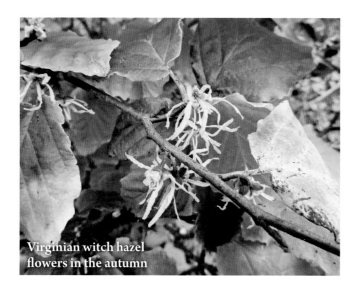

Virginian witch hazel
flowers in the autumn

metrorrhagia, haemorrhoids, vaginal discharge and digestive haemorrhage, and externally for nosebleeds and eye inflammation. A bark decoction was also used for these purposes, as well as for inflammation of the gums and mouth mucosa (as mouthwash or gargles). Witch hazel distillate was first developed in the 1840s in central New York by Theron T. Pond in collaboration with a medicine man from the Oneida tribe.[143] Alice Henkel described in 1909 how the farmers in New England states brought in cartloads of witch hazel brush to the distilleries, typically receiving 1-4 cents per pound of bark.[144]

Medicinal actions and uses

The leaves and bark have similar properties, being astringent and anti-inflammatory. Used externally in skin complaints. The leaves can be used as a gargle for sore throat.[145]

Clinical applications and research

Clinical data support use for topical relief of minor skin lesions, bruises and sprains, skin and mucous membrane inflammation, haemorrhoids and varicose veins.[146] An aftersun formulation with 10% distilled witch hazel showed significant anti-inflammatory effects compared to other lotions.[147] A study reported in 2014 on the antiviral effects of tannin-rich witch hazel, suggesting that the high molecular weight of condensed tannins in the bark caused a more pronounced antiviral effect. However, this was not the only active principle, as other

antiviral mechanisms were identified.[148] An antiproliferative effect on colon cancer cells has also been noted.[149]

Sample preparations and dosage

For topical use only. A distilled extract of the leafy twigs can be preserved with 14-15% alcohol. The distillate can be used on acne and eczema direct or diluted 1:3 with water. Otherwise 5-10g of dried leaf or bark can be decocted in 250ml water for poultices and wound irrigation. Used also to reduce inflammation in sprains.

Constituents and commerce

Key constituents

The plant contains 3-10% tannins (both hydrolysable and condensed), phenolic acids, flavonoids and other constituents. Volatile compounds are also obtained from the bark and leaves of witch hazel.[150] The bark has been shown to be high in phenylpropanoids and sesquiterpenoids, while the leaves are high in monoterpenoids.

Commerce

Witch hazel is a common ingredient in numerous over-the-counter topical preparations as well as eyewash preparations. According to pharmacopoeia standards, the steam distillate of Virginian witch hazel twigs is a clear colourless liquid prepared from partially dormant twigs to which 14-15% alcohol is added. Some forms of the distilled witch hazel water are sold with other preservatives such as benzoic acid, phenoxyethanol or parabens. The main supplier of distilled witch hazel is American Distilling, a company producing some 10 million litres per year based on continuous production with 10 stills, although there are some smaller artisan businesses offering organic supplies. In the UK, attempts were made to cultivate witch hazel in the earlier half of the twentieth century. The company Optrex had a plantation in Hampshire which operated on a five-year coppice cycle producing 133,000 litres per 2.8 hectares.[151]

Safety

Witch hazel extracts are regarded as safe and well tolerated on the skin, but are not for internal use due to the tannin content which can cause stomach irritation.

Juglans regia, Walnut

A large spreading tree, long cultivated in Europe for delicious large nuts, having aromatic bark and leaves that can be used for treating constipation and skin complaints.

SCIENTIFIC NAME   *Juglans regia* L.

FAMILY   Juglandaceae

ALTERNATE NAMES   English or Persian walnut

PARTS USED   Bark, leaves, fruit husks

Description

Common walnut is a large deciduous tree from Asia growing to 30m tall by 20m wide at a fast rate, having aromatic pinnate leaves. Flowers of both sexes are borne on the same tree and appear in early spring before the leaves. The fruit ripens with a husk containing the edible seed (walnut). The mature tree has deeply furrowed bark.

Habitat

The walnut is considered to originate from central Asia, with dispersion to Europe and other areas for early cultivation.

Related plants

There are similar uses for black walnut (*J. nigra*) which is a large deciduous tree of northern America, introduced as an ornamental tree into Europe since the seventeenth century. The leaves of black and common walnut differ in proportions of essential oils, such as eugenol and methyl salicylate and traditionally used to treat tooth-ache, rheumatism and fungal infection.[152] Butternut (*J. cinerea*) grows up to 12-18m and is another North American nut-bearing tree with root bark used as a mild cathartic and tonic.[153] There are many varied nut-bearing cultivars of walnut.

Cultivation and harvest

Cultivation

The walnut is hardy to USDA zone 5 (UK zone 5). It does best in a deep well-drained soil in a sunny position with shelter from winds. It can grow in slightly acid to slightly alkaline soil but will not succeed in poorly drained soil (we have repeatedly lost trees due to wet conditions at Holt Wood). Winter protection may be needed in the first few years of establishment, and frosts can damage the young shoots and flowers in spring. An annual mulch of cardboard and compost helps to suppress weeds around the tree and can provide additional fertility. Pruning should only be carried out when the tree is fully dormant in late autumn and winter as wounds bleed profusely. The roots of walnut trees produce substances which are toxic to many plants, and heavy shade is also cast by this tree, though many plants appear to be immune.[154]

Pests and diseases

Walnut is little troubled by insects, though slugs at Holt Wood seem to like the young leaves. Walnut is susceptible to fungal diseases so keep the stem clear of any mulch to reduce chances of any rot.

Propagation

Ripe fresh seed is sown in individual pots in autumn, 25-50mm deep, and placed in a cold frame with protection from rodents. Germination may be fast or occur the following spring. Plant out the seedlings into their permanent positions in early summer and give some protection from the cold for their first winter or two. The seed can also be stored in cool, moist conditions in a refrigerator over the winter and sown in early spring though it requires a period of cold stratification before it will germinate, 90-120 days at 0-3°C.

Harvesting

Leaves are harvested from the tree in June and July in fine weather, and are dried in a single layer. Young bark can

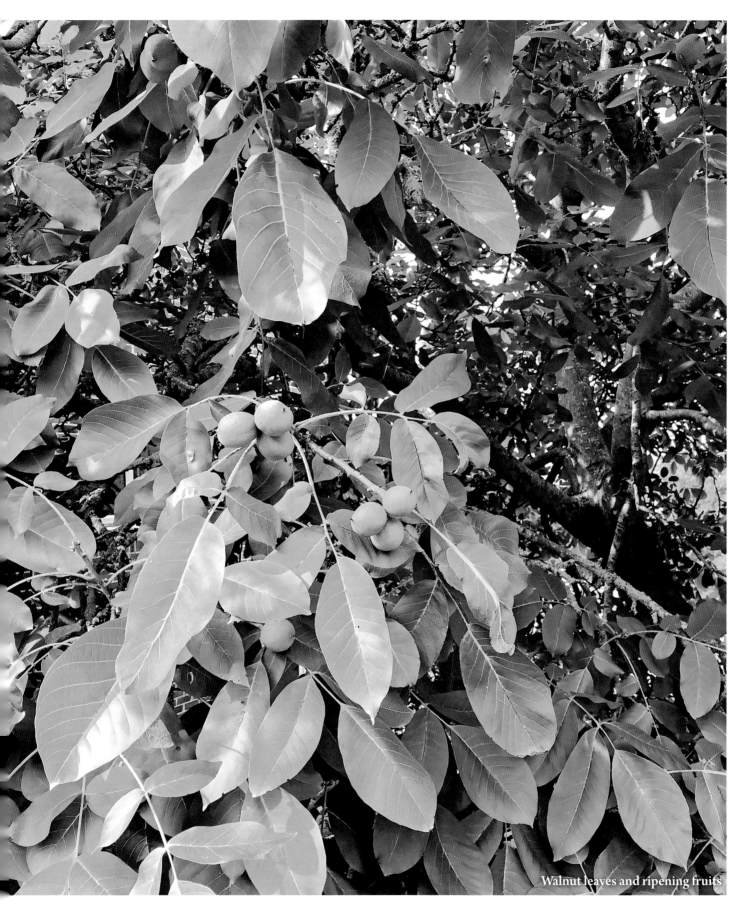

Walnut leaves and ripening fruits

be peeled from pruned branches and dried. The green husks of the walnut can be dried for later powdering.

Therapeutic use

Traditional

The walnut tree was introduced from eastern Asia into the Mediterranean area in classical times. In addition to providing a food, the walnut tree has provided a remedy for many skin problems and other infectious complaints. The distilled water of the husks was used as an application for wounds and internally as a cooling drink for agues. John Evelyn wrote in 1670 that 'The water of the Husks is soveraign against all pestilential infections, and that of the leaves to mundifie, and heal inveterate Ulcers'.[155] Walnut bark has been chewed to allay toothache.

Medicinal actions and uses

The bark and leaves are antifungal, antibacterial, laxative, astringent, anti-oxidant and alterative. The bark infusion acts as a purgative. A tea of the leaves is astringent and used in skin inflammations.[156]

Clinical applications and research

Walnut bark tincture has been shown to have antibacterial effects in oral hygiene against *Staphylococci* and *Streptococci* bacteria.[157] In addition to astringent and laxative effects, research on the uses of walnut leaves suggests a role in controlling high blood fat and sugar levels.[158] A water/alcohol extract of walnut leaves was used in a randomised double-blind placebo-controlled trial of 50 diabetic patients. Although the blood glucose level of patients was not significantly affected, the study found that body weight and blood pressure were significantly reduced after eight weeks.[159] Walnuts are also beneficial for improving levels of blood fats and sugar, as shown in a randomised trial providing metabolic syndrome patients (at risk of heart disease and diabetes) with 45g of walnuts per day for a period of 16 weeks.[160] Overall, walnut preparations contain highly active constituents of continuing interest in cancer prevention and treatment.[161]

Sample preparations and dosage

Tincture of bark or leaves 0.5-1ml three times daily can be used for laxative and alterative effects. Infusion of bark, at 25g to 500ml of boiling water and allowed to stand for six hours, can be used as a wash against dandruff, athlete's foot, ringworm and eczema. An infusion of the leaves can also be used on the skin, 5g in 200ml of boiling water.

Constituents and commerce

Key constituents

Active ingredients of all parts of the walnut are tannins and napthaquinones (including juglone). Juglone is an antifungal, antiparasitic and antimicrobial toxin, considered as having antitumour potential. The leaves also contain flavonoids, essential oils (including E-caryophyllene, germacrene and delta-cadinene). The phenolic content of the leaves is reported as higher in July and early September, lower in August.[162] The husks contain many polyphenols (including chlorogenic, caffeic, ferulic, sinapic and gallic acids).

Commerce

The top five countries for walnuts grown commercially are China, the US, Iran, Turkey and Mexico.

Safety

May cause skin discolouration and dermatitis if used externally and should be washed off. Short-term use is recommended, up to one week. Not for use internally in chronic conditions of the gastrointestinal tract, and not advised in pregnancy or breastfeeding.

Other uses

The nuts provide a nutrient-dense food and can be pressed for oil. Excellent timber. Dye plant using leaves and husks.

Juniperus communis, Juniper

An evergreen European shrub with aromatic spiky foliage and berries with powerful antimicrobial and diuretic effects, giving a range of uses from insect repellent to treating cystitis.

SCIENTIFIC NAME *Juniperus communis* L.

FAMILY Cupressaceae

ALTERNATE NAMES Savin, common juniper

PARTS USED Fruit, leaf

Description

Juniper is an evergreen shrub or small tree with aromatic prickly needle-like leaves and fruits. It can grow to 9m by 4m at a slow rate. The flowers are dioecious and only one sex is found on a plant, so both male and female plants are needed for fruit to be produced. Pollinated by wind, the fruits take 2-3 years to ripen on the branches, turning from green to blue-black. This is a coniferous

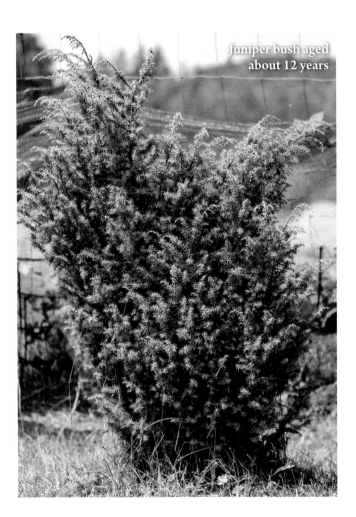

Juniper bush aged about 12 years

plant and the berries are actually composed of the fused fleshy scales of a cone.

Habitat

Juniperus is a native shrub of the northern temperate zone, ranging from Europe to Asia and North America. In southern England it is often found as a low-growing shrub on chalk downs and rocky areas, as well as in pine and birch woods in Scotland. According to the Woodland Trust, juniper populations in the UK are shrinking, and the species is a priority under the UK Biodiversity Action Plan.

Related plants

A dwarf form of juniper is *J. communis* subsp. *nana* mostly found in mountainous and coastal areas. There are many cultivated garden varieties of *Juniper communis* including spreading, creeping and dwarf forms. Eastern red cedar (*J. virginiana*), growing to 20m, is found in open woods of northern America and the fruit and leaves have similar properties.

Cultivation and harvest

Cultivation

Juniper is hardy to USDA zone 4 (UK zone 3). It prefers a slightly alkaline and well-drained soil but can grow in most soils including dry, poor soil or heavy, clay soil. The juniper shrub grows slowly but steadily in slightly acid and poorly drained soil at Holt Wood. It can grow in light shade or no shade. Juniper is tolerant of drought. Young growth can be damaged by late frosts. Prune in spring, removing dead or dying branches and thin out interior or crossing branches to enable more light to reach the plant.

Pests and diseases

Protection is needed for newly planted juniper which is very palatable to deer, rabbits, rodents and birds, ideally mesh covers which also insert 5cm into the soil. Mature juniper is more resistant to heavy grazing. Juniper resists honey fungus but may be infected by rust, and by *Phytophthora* root rot.

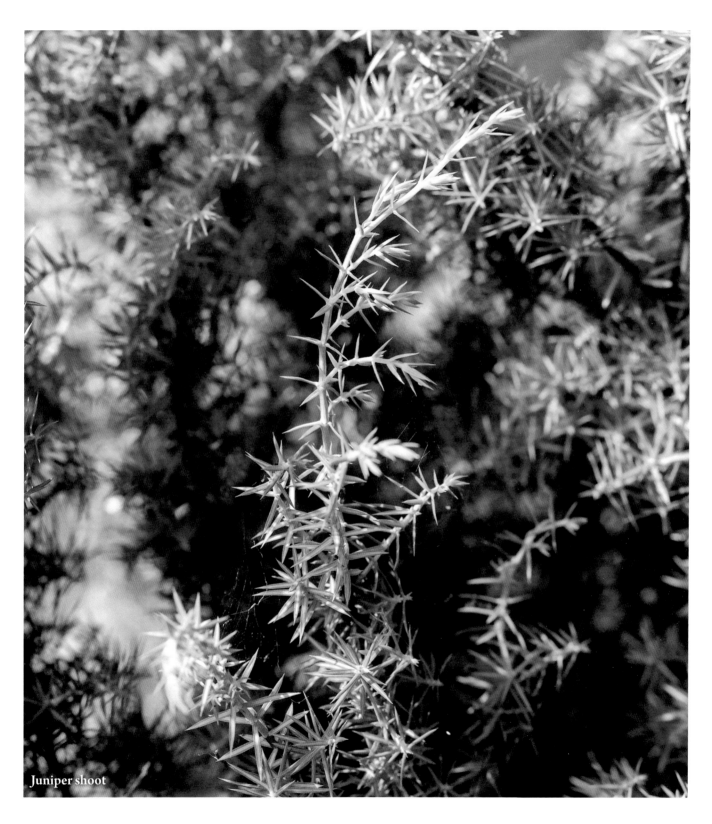

Juniper shoot

Propagation

The seed is slow to mature and only black berries should be picked.[163] It is best sown as soon as it is ripe in a cold frame. Some might germinate in the following spring, though this can take up to four years. Stored seed requires a cold period followed by a warm period and then another cold spell, each of 2-3 months duration. Soaking the hard seed for 3-6 seconds in boiling water, or scarification, may help. The seedlings can be potted up into individual pots when they are large enough to handle. Grow on in pots until large enough, then plant out in early summer. Studies for the Forestry Commission suggest that cuttings are faster than seed; 10cm long hardwood cuttings should be taken in February or March from the tips of branches and inserted into a well-drained medium, misting for 12 weeks. Rooting should commence after 6-8 weeks, and misting can be gradually reduced so that at 16 weeks the plants can survive in a greenhouse and potted on.[164]

Harvesting

The fruits are usually harvested in the autumn when ripe. Leaves can be harvested at any time but are very prickly so wear thick gloves.

Therapeutic use

Traditional

Juniper has a long tradition of use in Europe and the berries are recognised as a traditional herbal product for minor urinary complaints, stomach upsets and flatulence.[165] In northern America, juniper infusions were used as a tonic and for treating tuberculosis.[166]

Medicinal actions and uses

Diuretic, anti-inflammatory, antifungal, antimicrobial, anti-oxidant. The essential oil of juniper is strongly antibacterial,[167] being rich in monoterpenes, although there can be variation between wild and cultivated species in the levels of different constituents.[168]

Clinical applications and research

Little clinical research has been carried out in relation to juniper leaves and berries although a study of the phenolic components indicates that the leaves have anti-oxidant and hepatoprotective potential.[169] Another study argues that an extract of juniper berries has the potential for anticancer activity through suppressing cell growth.[170] The effects of essential oils of juniper and other cypress family members against ticks and mosquitoes have been researched. It was found that all of the oils were repellent to ticks, and juniper leaf essential oil was the most repellent against the mosquito.[171]

Sample preparations and dosage

Pour 150-250ml of boiling water over 1-2g of dried berries. Infuse for 20 minutes in a covered container, and take 2-3 times daily. Tincture of leaves: 1-3ml three times daily. Although juniper can be taken internally for its diuretic effects, it is probably more useful externally as an antiseptic and insect repellent, as a wash or lotion. An infusion in oil can be made using the leaves and/or berries and this can be applied to the skin as an insect repellent.

Constituents and commerce

Key constituents

The leaves contain flavonoids. The essential oil of juniper berries contains monoterpenes (mostly α-pinene, also β-pinene, apigenin, sabinene, β-sitosterol, campesterol and limonene).

Commerce

Studies have shown that waste products of forestry activity in Poland, leaves and twigs of *Juniperus* species can contain significant amounts of podophyllotoxinins which could be used in cancer treatments.[172]

Safety

Safety during pregnancy and breastfeeding has not been established and use then is not recommended. Use with under 18-year-olds not recommended. Juniper is contraindicated in conditions where reduced fluid intake is recommended or in severe renal disease. Consult a professional clinical practitioner if used internally for more than two weeks.

Other uses

Culinary spice. Flavouring for gin. Making incense sticks. Antiseptic shampoo.

Laurus nobilis, Sweet bay

An evergreen tree with glossy green spicy leaves and berries, used for supporting digestion since classical times and effective against respiratory infections.

SCIENTIFIC NAME   *Laurus nobilis* L.

FAMILY   Lauraceae

ALTERNATE NAMES   Bay tree, common bay

PARTS USED   Berries and leaves

Description

Sweet bay is a small to medium evergreen tree slowly growing to 10m tall (up to 20m in warmer climates) by 10m wide. It has dark green leathery leaves with pointed tips and a spicy aroma. Clusters of small yellow flowers are produced in April-May and pollination is by bees. Since male and female flowers grow on separate plants, both sexes are required for production of berries.

Habitat

Sweet bay originates from southern Europe and grows amongst damp rocks and ravines.

Related plants

L. nobilis angustifolia has narrower leaves and may be more hardy. Caution in confusing the sweet bay with other plants named as cherry laurels, which are in a different family and are potentially toxic.[173]

Cultivation and harvest

Cultivation

Sweet bay is hardy to USDA zone 7 (UK zone 7), and needs a sheltered position in most areas. It can grow in sun or dappled shade, and tolerates a range of soils so long as they are well drained. It may be best grown in a container to form a small shrub which can be brought indoors in temperatures below -5°C (23°F), or protected with fleece. In the ground the sweet bay tree can tolerate lower temperatures, especially if not pruned back to a bare stem. Sweet bay can be planted

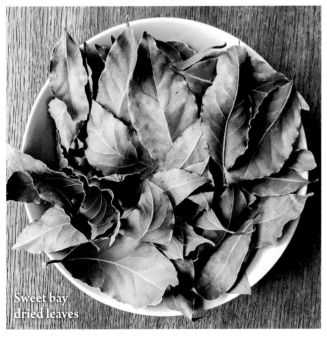

Sweet bay dried leaves

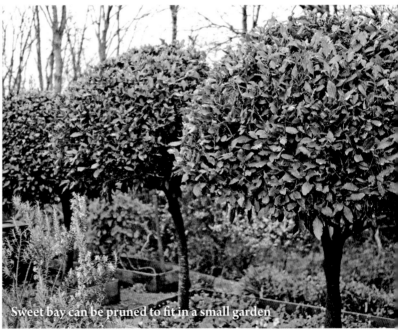

Sweet bay can be pruned to fit in a small garden

out at a spacing of 3m by 3m and is readily pruned for a harvest of leaves in spring or summer.

Pests and diseases

It is resistant to honey fungus, insects and rodents but can be susceptible to root rot and leaf spot fungus or infested with sap suckers or scale insects.

Propagation

Remove the fleshy berry outer casing from ripe fruits and sow seed as soon as possible in the autumn as seeds lose viability rapidly. Soak the seeds in warm water for 24 hours and sow in a shady mulched seed bed. Prick out the seedlings when large enough to handle and grow on in the first year. Plant out in the second summer and protect in the first winter. Softwood cuttings can be taken in early summer, though are not always successful. Hardwood cuttings with a heel can be taken in November-December. Layering is possible.

Harvesting

The leaves are harvested in spring and dried in a single layer for several weeks. Drying reduces bitterness in the leaves. The berries are harvested in the autumn and can be dried for later use.

Therapeutic use

Traditional

Sweet bay leaves have been used since classical times as an infusion for digestive, respiratory and urinary complaints and the berries used to promote appetite.[174] The leaves and berries have also traditionally been used for ague, arthritis and rheumatism, skin rashes and boils. Sweet bay has a longstanding reputation as an emmenagogue, and the berries have been used to promote expelling of the afterbirth in livestock.

Medicinal actions and uses

Sweet bay leaves are anti-inflammatory, anti-oxidant, antimicrobial, astringent, carminative, diaphoretic, diuretic, stimulant and emmenagogue. The essential oil is analgesic, antispasmodic, antibacterial and antifungal.[175] It can be used as an insect repellent.

Clinical applications and research

There have been few clinical studies of sweet bay, apart from the effects of the essential oil of bay. Extract of sweet bay leaves has been shown to be anti-inflammatory[176] and anti-oxidant,[177] and it is suggested that sweet bay extracts could help to prevent oxidative stress and the production of free radicals in diabetes.

Sample preparations and dosage

The leaves can be steam distilled to produce an essential oil. Infusion of the leaves or a few drops of essential oil in hot water can be used as an inhalation for respiratory complaints. Use a leaf-infused oil, or mix five drops of essential oil per 5ml of carrier oil (such as almond or olive oil), as an application for swollen or painful joints.

Constituents and commerce

Key constituents

The leaves contain flavonoids (especially epicatechin). The essential oil of sweet bay contains 1,8-cineole, pinene, sabinene, 1-linalool, eugenol, eugenol acetate, and other esters and terpenols.[178]

Commerce

Sweet bay berries and leaves are collected in Mediterranean countries especially Turkey, and also cultivated in the Canary Islands, Morocco, south-eastern US and Mexico. Grown commercially in southern Europe on a coppice system, especially if irrigated, the annual yield of leaves is 5-12 tons/acre.[179]

Safety

Not for internal use except under the advice of a professional clinical practitioner. Although used as a culinary spice, the leaves are emetic in large doses. The essential oil should not be used undiluted on the skin as it can cause dermatitis. Not for use with children or in pregnancy or breastfeeding.

Other uses

Food flavouring. Hedging. Seed oil is used for making soap. Veterinary uses. Insect repellent in storage of foods.

Liquidambar styraciflua, Sweet gum

A highly ornamental large tree from North America with aromatic leaves and bark, long used as a medicinal remedy for skin complaints and infectious diseases.

SCIENTIFIC NAME   *Liquidambar styraciflua* L.
FAMILY   Hamamelidaceae
ALTERNATE NAMES   Satin walnut, American storax
PARTS USED   Stem bark, leaves, sap/resin

Description

A medium to large deciduous tree, the sweet gum can grow at a moderate to fast rate up to more than 30m tall and 15m wide. The bark on the main trunk is furrowed and greyish and may be over 1cm thick on old trees, while younger branches are red-brown, often with corky ridges or spines. Glossy green and aromatic 3-5 lobed leaves make a star shape with a toothed margin. Autumn foliage is colourful, turning purple and red. This is a monoecious species with male and female flowers and pollination by wind. Fruits are produced after 20-25 years. The fruit is a globular, horny, woody ball, 2.5cm in diameter, hanging on a long stem and persisting through to the spring.

Habitat

Sweet gum is native to Central and North America, found in low, rich, moist woods and coastal plains. It exists in a range of climates from temperate to tropical, losing its leaves for a short period of one month in warmer areas.

Related plants

A number of ornamental cultivars are sold, and the cold-hardy cultivar 'Moraine' is said to be somewhat slower growing and reaches 20m. Another species of oriental sweet gum (*L. orientalis*) is of Asian origin and is somewhat frost tender to USDA zone 8 (UK zone 8) – though we have both kinds of sweet gum growing in sheltered positions in Devon.

Cultivation and harvest

Cultivation

Sweet gum is hardy through USDA zone 5 (UK zone 5). It prefers a sheltered site with rich moist soil which is well drained and acidic. It can grow in full sun or part shade. Frost tolerance is variable, and so provenance may be important for use in temperate areas where frost occurs regularly. The sweet gum dislikes root disturbance and needs to be planted in its permanent place. It coppices readily and will resprout and rapidly grow from a cut stump,[180] and we have found it pollards well. The roots are fairly aggressive and so take care to ensure the tree is planted away from buildings and water courses. Sweet gum is regarded as a competitor for resources in pine forests and plantations in the US.

Pests and diseases

Sweet gum appears to have few pests and diseases – in the native range in the US during summer a leaf spot fungus has been seen.

Seed propagation

Collect mature fruiting heads before they have completely dried. Spread out the heads at room temperature until they release the seeds after 5-10 days. Stratify 1-2 months at 5°C (41°F). Propagation by cuttings is said to be difficult, and root cuttings based on suckers may be better. Place in a well-drained medium in early autumn and keep the air moist until rooting occurs.

Harvesting

Sweet gum bark can be harvested in spring or autumn, leaves and twigs in the growing season.[181] When the tree is wounded in early summer, the inner bark produces an oily resin which is soaked up by the bark and this can be harvested in autumn. Pressing the bark in cold water, alternating with boiling in hot water, releases this resin to make the balsam known as storax.[182]

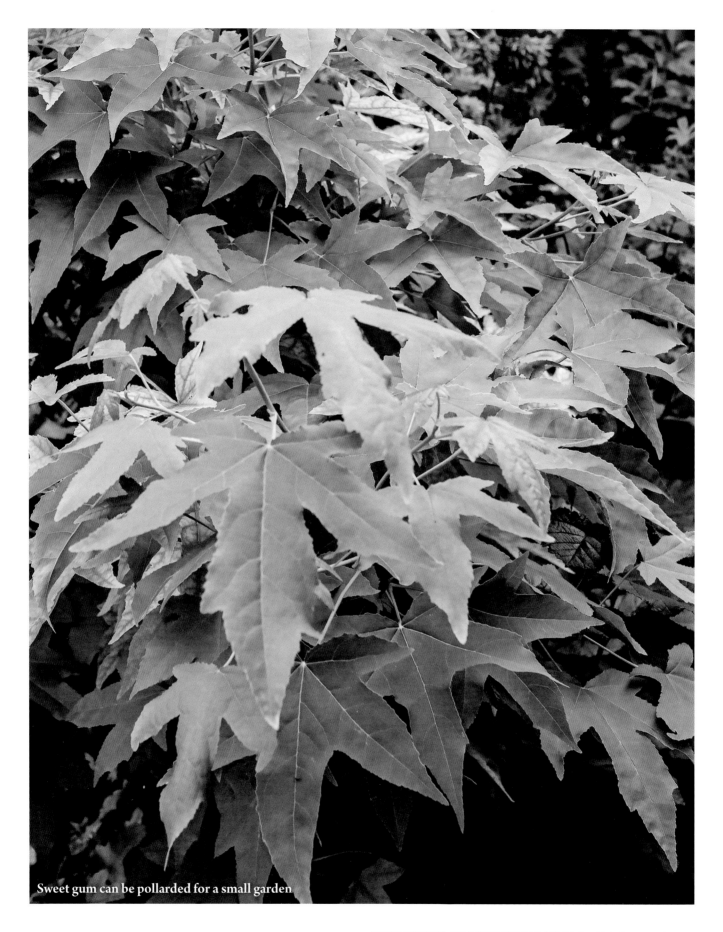

Sweet gum can be pollarded for a small garden

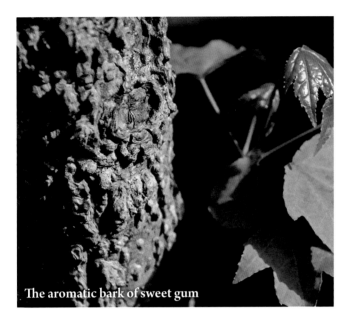
The aromatic bark of sweet gum

Therapeutic use

Traditional
The extract of sweet gum species, known as storax, has been used for centuries to treat common ailments such as skin problems, coughs and ulcers, and for treating acute stroke in Chinese traditional medicine.[183] The Aztecs collected storax for treating skin infections and other ailments. Native Americans used storax and the bark for coughs, dysentery and wounds.[184] Tea made from leaves was used to wash wounds.

Medicinal uses
Sweet gum provides stimulating expectorant, diuretic, vulnerary, astringent, antimicrobial and anti-oxidant actions. In 1898, *King's American Dispensatory* listed the syrup of sweet gum as 'a pleasant medicine … useful in bowel complaints of children's diarrhoea, chronic cough, and chronic mucous affections generally'.[185] Storax is the name given to the balsamic oleoresin extracted from the inner bark.

Clinical applications and research
Storax has proven to be a strong antimicrobial agent against multidrug resistant bacteria such as methicillin-resistant *Staphylococcus aureus* (MRSA).[186] Other extracts derived from sweet gum trees have shown potential as

anti-oxidants, anti-inflammatory, antihypertensive and antispasmodic agents. Hepatoprotective effects are shown by the phenolic compounds in leaf extracts.[187]

Sample preparations and dosage
An infusion of the leaves or bark (1 tsp in 1 cup) can be taken a mouthful at a time in flu and colds. A syrup of the bark can be made, based on powdered bark infused with water for 24 hours, then filtered and sugar added, the dose for an adult being 30ml up to 3-4 times per day. A decoction of the bark can be boiled down to make a balsam for external use on skin complaints.

Constituents and commerce

Key constituents
Essential oil from the leaves contains terpinen-4-ol and 1,8-cineole (similar to the Australian tea tree).[188] Other constituents include tyrene, cinnamic acid, cinnamyl alcohol, 2-phenylpropyl alcohol, 3-phenylpropyl cinnamate, cinnamyl cinnamate and vanillin. Cinnamic acid has known antimicrobial and anti-oxidant properties.

Commerce
Commercial storax, a fragrant resin used in perfumes and medicines, is derived from the oriental sweet gum (*L. orientalis*) of western Asia. It is an ingredient in Friar's balsam used for colds and skin problems. Shikimic acid is found in sweet gum, particularly in infertile seeds, and yields of 1.7mg/g have been reported, making it a possible alternative source for manufacturers of antiviral oseltamivir (Tamiflu).[189]

Safety

Information on contraindications and adverse events is lacking, though allergic rhinitis and kidney injury from excessive use on the skin have been suggested. In the absence of data, use in moderation and for short-term periods only. Not for use in pregnancy or breastfeeding.

Other uses

An important timber tree providing veneer and furniture. Chewing gum. Incense. Use in perfumery with some fixative effects.

Magnolia liliiflora, Lily magnolia

A small tree with fragrant pink flowers, long used in Chinese traditional medicine for sinus congestion.

SCIENTIFIC NAME   *Magnolia liliiflora* Desr.

FAMILY   Magnoliaceae

ALTERNATE NAMES   Mulan magnolia, tulip magnolia

PARTS USED   Bark and flower buds

Description

The lily magnolia is a large deciduous shrub or small tree growing to 4m and spreading to 3-4m wide. Large pink fragrant flowers are produced in April-May before the leaf buds open. The flowers are bisexual and pollinated by beetles. The fruit is cone-shaped and purple or brown, ripening August to October.

Habitat

Native to southwest China and also cultivated in Japan, and now widespread as an ornamental plant in North America and Europe.

Related plants

An ornamental variety of the lily magnolia is the cultivar 'Nigra' with deeper coloured flowers which is widely available and slightly more hardy (this is what we are growing at Holt Wood). The Yulan magnolia (*M. denudata*) is an alternative to consider, growing to 12m by 10m with large white tulip-shaped, fragrant flowers. *M. denudata* and *M. lilliflora* are the parents of the hybrid form *Magnolia × soulangeana* which is widely grown as an ornamental in the UK and US. Other medicinal magnolias include *M. officinalis*, a fast-growing deciduous tree reaching 20m high by 12m wide with large obovate leaves and fragrant white flowers and *M. acuminata* or the cucumber magnolia, a deciduous tree growing to 20m by 10m in the southern US. Species such as *M. officinalis* are at risk of extinction in the wild.[190]

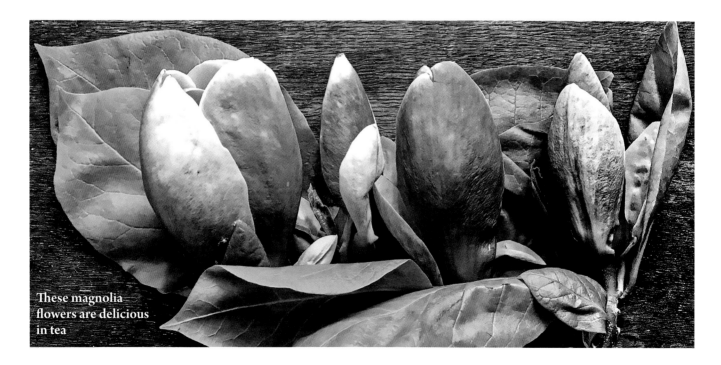

These magnolia flowers are delicious in tea

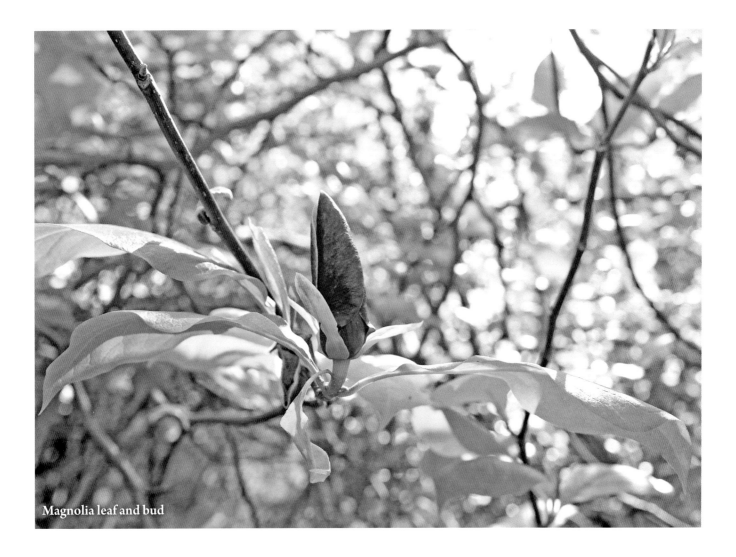
Magnolia leaf and bud

Cultivation and harvest

Cultivation

The lily magnolia is hardy to USDA zone 7 (UK zone 6). It prefers slightly acid soil which is organically rich, moist but well drained. The lily magnolia can grow in sun or light shade. A sheltered position is needed, particularly as the branches are brittle and vulnerable to wind. Once established, the lily magnolia is moderately drought tolerant. Pruning can be carried out after flowering though severe pruning is not recommended.

Pests and diseases

There are few problems though scale insects may suck the sap, and black sooty mould may form on the honeydew produced by scale insects. Mould and fungus can be discouraged by ensuring good air circulation through pruning out crowded branches.

Propagation

Seed can be sown in a cold frame and usually germinates in the spring but can take 18 months. Prick out the seedlings into individual pots when they are large enough to handle and grow them on in light shade in a cold frame or greenhouse for at least their first winter. They can be planted out into their permanent positions when they are more than 15cm tall, though should be well mulched and given some protection from winter cold for their first winter or two outdoors. Take softwood cuttings in early summer, or semi-ripe cuttings in autumn. Layering in early spring.

Harvesting

The flower buds are harvested in spring before the petals begin to show and are dried for later use. The bark can be harvested when pruning in summer and dried for later use though it does not store well so stocks should be renewed annually.

Therapeutic use

Traditional

A number of magnolia species have had longstanding use in traditional Chinese medicine for thousands of years. The aromatic pungent and warming bark has been used in formulae for various disorders of the digestive system, and many other complaints ranging from anxiety and depression to muscular pain and fever.[191]

Medicinal actions and uses

The general effects of the bark and flowers are bitter, anti-oxidant, anti-inflammatory, antibacterial, emmenagogue and antispasmodic. The aromatic and spicy flowers of the lily magnolia are used primarily for treating sinus congestion. The bitter bark may be used for flatulence, nausea, lack of appetite, shortness of breath and dysentery.

Clinical applications and research

Clinical studies are lacking despite the longstanding use of magnolia species and the pharmacological evidence on constituents. For example, the bark constituents honokiol and magnolol have cortisol-like effects supporting use in preparations for asthma. One pilot study involving lily magnolia investigated the effect on chronic rhinosinusitis in 55 volunteers of use of a herbal tea with the flowers in a formula with eucalyptus, fennel and liquorice. After six weeks, the self-reported health status of participants with sinusitis improved, including being able to sleep better.[192] Further uses of the bark of *M. officinalis* have been identified for anti-anxiety and antidepressant effects, and in cardiovascular and cerebrovascular diseases such as Alzheimer's disease.[193] The cytotoxic activity of lignan constituents of magnolia bark is viewed as a basis for anticancer drug development, and further therapeutic uses in diabetes have been suggested.[194]

Sample preparations and dosage

An infusion of the dried flower buds can be used as a tea for sinus congestion and headache. The infusion can also be used as an inhalation. Dried bark as a decoction may be of use in digestive disturbances with bloating and nausea, up to 9g per day.

Constituents and commerce

Key constituents

Lily magnolia flowers contain lignans and terpenoids, including monoterpenes and sesquiterpenes.[195] Major phenolic constituents in magnolia bark are magnolol and honokiol, and there are also alkaloids (magnoflorine and magnocurarine). A study of the phenolic compounds in the violet flowers of *M. liliiflora* and white flowers of *M. denudata* found that the violet flowers contained higher levels of anti-oxidant and anti-inflammatory constituents.[196] A study of *M. officinalis* from different provenances showed that the bark of seven-year-old trees varied considerably in magnolol and honokiol, so that the original area of growth may be important, as taught in traditional Chinese medicine.[197]

Commerce

M. officinalis bark extract is a constituent of many dietary supplements and cosmetic products. In China, harvesters cut down 20-year-old trees in spring and strip the bark from the roots, trunks and branches. The bark is dried and then it is decocted in boiling water and steamed, finally rolled into tubes and dried again. Commercially available magnolia bark extracts are marketed based on their high phenolic content, with magnolol and honokiol ranging from 40-90% of total polyphenols.

Safety

Magnolia has low toxicity and very few adverse effects, although large doses should be avoided. Due to emmenagogic effects this plant should not be used in pregnancy or breastfeeding.

Other uses

Flowers are edible; it is worth trying different varieties as some are delicious in tea.

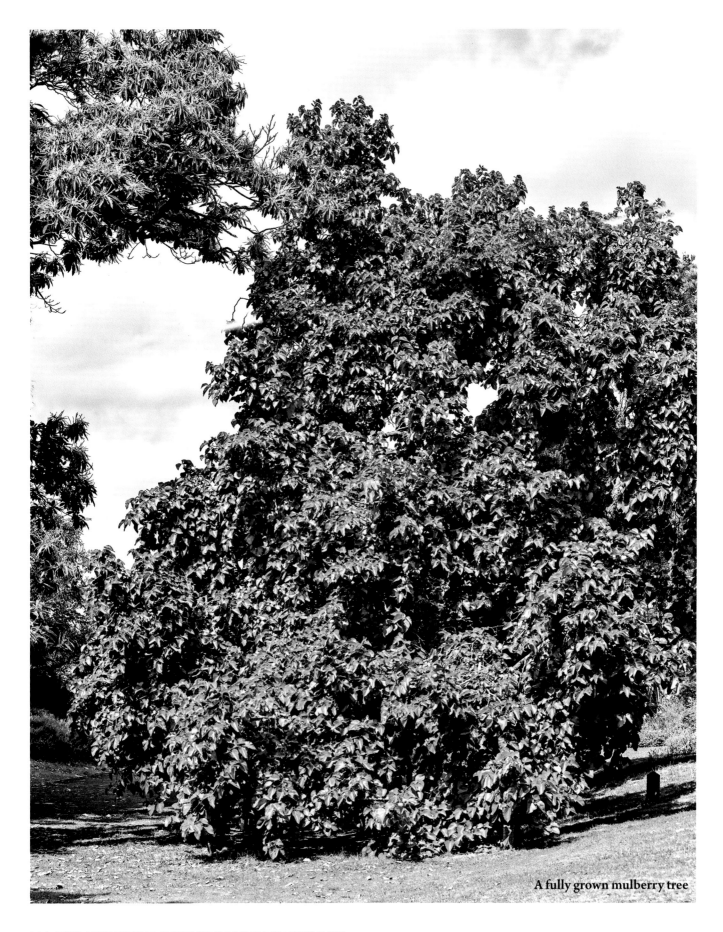

A fully grown mulberry tree

Morus nigra, Black mulberry

A spreading deciduous tree with juicy black fruits and leaves which can be used to lower blood sugars and with potential in anti-ageing disorders.

SCIENTIFIC NAME   *Morus nigra* Mill.

FAMILY   Moraceae

PARTS USED   Leaves and fruits

Description

A deciduous tree with numerous branches eventually growing to 10m tall by 10m wide. Leaves have rough surfaces, often varying in shape; some are multilobed and others not. Flowers appear in May-June as small scaly clusters and ripen into blackberry sized edible fruits from August to September. Trees are either monoecious or dioecious and can change from one to the other. Flowers are wind-pollinated and fruiting generally begins after 15 years of age.

Habitat

Black mulberry is a native shrub of southwest Asia, now widely planted in Europe, Africa and India.

Related plants

There are a number of black mulberry cultivars; the variety 'Chelsea', also known as 'King James', produces well-flavoured fruit. The red mulberry (*M. rubra*) is a native of eastern North America, growing up to 20m, and the white mulberry (*M. alba*) originates in northern, eastern and central Asia. Some mulberry cultivars do not produce fruit but have large leaves.

Cultivation and harvest

Cultivation

Black mulberry is hardy in USDA zone 5 (UK zone 5). After rapid growth when young, it is fairly slow growing. It likes a moist but well-drained soil and appreciates neutral to acid soil. It is resistant to cold but grows best in full sun, can grow in dappled shade, fruiting well in southwestern UK, and can be grown with protection further north. The tree can be grown in various forms as it tolerates pruning well: coppiced, pollarded as a tall standard, as a bush or fan-trained against a wall, or cultivated in a pot. It is not advisable to prune the tree heavily due to an inclination to bleed, so prune while it is dormant.

Pests and diseases

Black mulberry is generally free of pests and diseases, although cankers and dieback can occur. A white powdery coating on the lower leaf surface is a symptom of mildew spread by the pathogens *Phyllactinia corylea* and *Uncinula geniculata*.

Seed propagation

Seed-grown trees are said to be stronger. Sow the ripe seed in a cold frame. The seed usually germinates in the first spring, though it sometimes takes another 12 months. Prick out the seedlings into individual pots when they are large enough to handle and grow them on in the cold frame for their first winter. Plant them out in late spring or early summer after the last expected frosts. Cuttings of half-ripe wood, 7-10cm with a heel, can be taken in July/August. Cuttings of mature wood of the current season's growth, 25-30cm with a heel of two-year-old wood, taken in autumn or early spring are placed in a cold frame. Bury the cuttings to three-quarters of their depth. Older cuttings may also strike. Layering in autumn.

Harvesting

The leaves can be used fresh or dried. Fruits drop as soon as they are ripe and so a grass or protective layer on the ground helps when they are harvested, and they can be frozen.

Therapeutic use

Traditional

The black mulberry has similar properties to the white mulberry which has a long history of use in China as a medicine and traditional uses include preventing liver and kidney diseases, joint damage and degenerative diseases of ageing.

Medicinal actions and uses

The leaves are antimicrobial, anti-inflammatory, anti-oxidant, astringent, diaphoretic and hypoglycaemic.[198] The leaves are taken internally for colds and influenza. A tincture of the bark is used for toothache, is anthelmintic and purgative. The fruit has laxative and fever-reducing properties. It is used in urinary incontinence, tinnitus, premature greying of hair and constipation in the elderly.

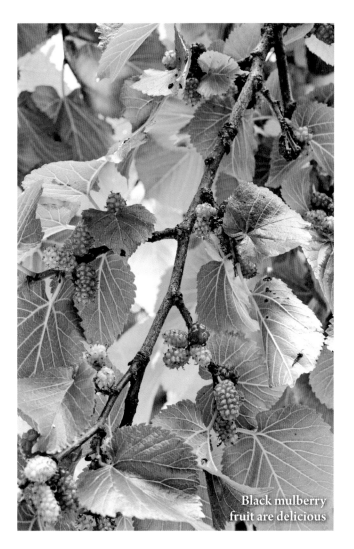

Black mulberry fruit are delicious

A leaf, flower or root decoction can be gargled for sore throat and swollen vocal chords.

Clinical applications and research

Black mulberry has attracted support for use in chronic disease as a nutraceutical especially due to anti-oxidant activity – both fruit and leaf.[199] The anti-oxidant effects are relevant to preventing diseases related to ageing. Flavonoids are hepatoprotective and use of the tincture extract of black mulberry leaves may be appropriate where the liver is affected by drugs, however so far most studies have been carried out on animals. Mulberry leaves provide a possible treatment in diabetes due to their hypoglycaemic effects, and the leaves may have fewer side effects than drugs such as metformin which can affect the liver and cardiovascular system.[200] Blood sugar reductions have been found in a trial with women with impaired glucose tolerance.[201]

Sample preparations and dosage

Tincture of mulberry leaf, 1-1.5ml three times daily. Mulberry leaf tea, 1 tsp in a cup of hot water, steep for 10 minutes and drink up to three times per day.

Constituents and commerce

Key constituents

The fruit of black mulberry contains anthocyanins and phenolic acids. The leaves contain sugar-mimicking alkaloids with hypoglycaemic properties that can affect the metabolism and transport of sugars in the body.

Commerce

The main use of mulberry in modern medicine has been for the preparation of a syrup obtained from the ripe fruit used to flavour or colour other medicines.

Safety

Male plants can produce copious pollen.

Other uses

Edible fruit. Animal forage. The leaves are repeat harvested in tropical areas for biomass and silkworm rearing.

Myrtus communis, Myrtle

A delightful, fragrant evergreen shrub with white flowers and glossy green foliage, having considerable antibiotic and anti-inflammatory uses including treating infections and dyspepsia.

SCIENTIFIC NAME *Myrtus communis* L.

FAMILY Myrtaceae

ALTERNATE NAMES Common myrtle, sweet myrtle

PARTS USED Leaves and berries

Description

Myrtle is an evergreen shrub growing to 4.5m tall by 3m wide, with aromatic small shiny green oval leaves. The attractive star-like white flowers from July to August are hermaphrodite and pollinated by bees. Seeds ripen in October-November as purple-black fruits.

Habitat

Southern Europe to western Asia and North Africa along coasts and on islands on scrubby acidic soils.

Related plants

There are a number of named myrtle varieties; the dwarf variety 'Tarentina' with narrow small leaves is reputed hardier and especially wind-resistant, growing slowly to 1.5m by 1.5m.

Cultivation and harvest

Cultivation

Myrtle is hardy to USDA zone 8 (UK zone 8) and is frost tender so needs a sheltered position, though it is fairly hardy when dormant. It can grow in most soils but prefers well drained soil. It can tolerate dry soil and maritime exposure. The plant readily tolerates clipping, and can be grown as a hedge in milder areas.

Pests and diseases

Myrtle is resistant to honey fungus.

Propagation

Clean the fruits by rubbing and washing off the fleshy coating and sow fresh seed into pots of well-drained sand/compost under glass. Pre-soak stored seed for 24 hours in warm water and then sow in late winter. Prick out the seedlings into individual pots as soon as they are large enough to handle and grow them on in a greenhouse for at least their first winter. Plant them out into their permanent positions in late spring or early summer, after the last frost. Cuttings of half-ripe wood, 7-10cm

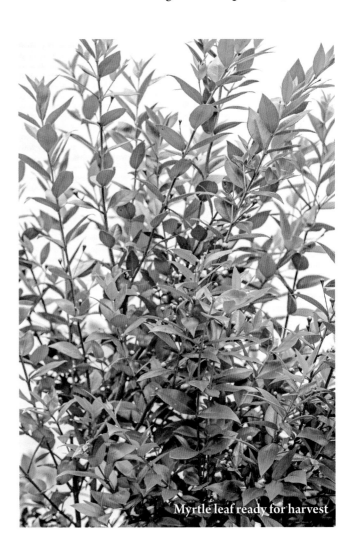
Myrtle leaf ready for harvest

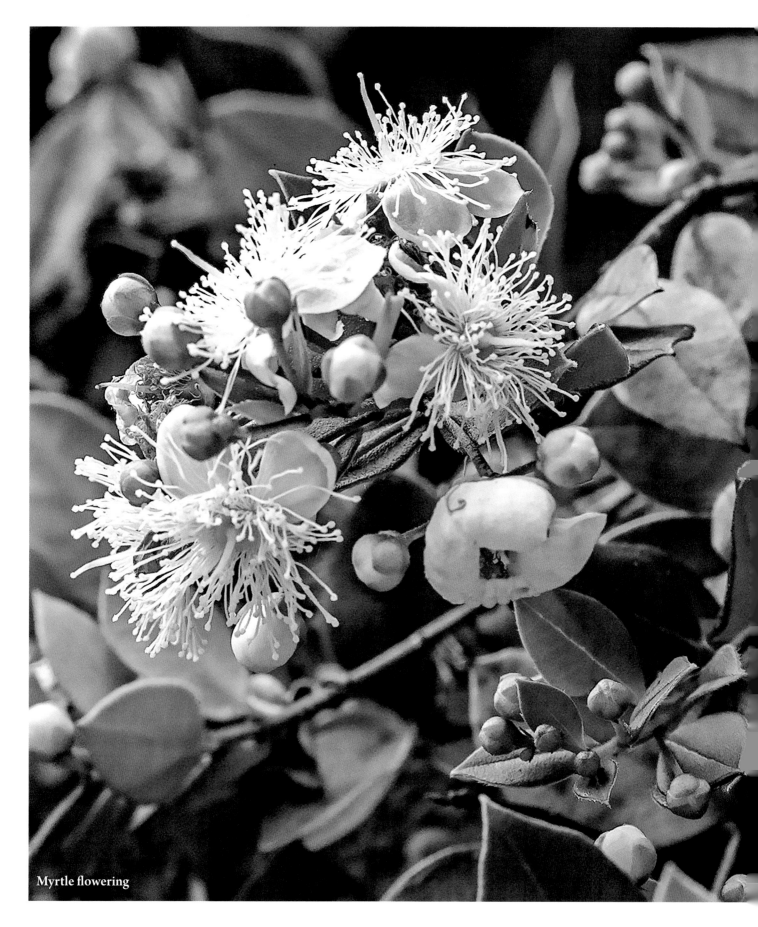

Myrtle flowering

with a heel, can be taken in July/August or cuttings of mature wood in November in a shaded and frost-free location. Plant out in late spring or early autumn. Layering is also possible.

Harvesting

Leaves can be picked in spring or summer and used fresh or dried. Fruiting may only occur in more sheltered areas, and the berries are harvested in late autumn for use fresh or for drying.

Therapeutic use

Traditional

Myrtle is an important plant in the Unani system of medicine,[202] and has been used traditionally for the treatment of many disorders such as diarrhoea, dysentery, peptic ulcer, haemorrhoids, inflammation, pulmonary and skin diseases. Externally, the essential oil has been used on wounds, gum infections and haemorrhoids.

Medicinal actions and uses

The leaves are anti-oxidant, anti-inflammatory, antimicrobial, astringent, haemostatic and tonic. The berries are carminative. The leaves have significant anti-oxidant activity, greater than the berries.[203] The plant can be taken internally in the treatment of urinary infections, digestive problems, bronchial congestion, sinusitis and dry coughs, and used as a wash or in a gel for vaginal discharge. The active ingredients in myrtle are rapidly absorbed and give a violet-like scent to the urine within 15 minutes.

Clinical applications and research

Clinical and experimental studies suggest that myrtle possesses a broad spectrum of pharmacological effects including anti-oxidant, anticancer, antidiabetic, antiviral, antibacterial, antifungal, hepatoprotective and neuroprotective activity.[204] A methanolic extract of myrtle has been shown to inhibit both gram-negative and gram-positive bacteria including *Staphylococcus aureus*.[205] In a double-blind randomised controlled trial, patients with digestive reflux were given myrtle berry extract 1000mg per day for six weeks to compare with omeprazole. A significant comparable reduction in reflux and dyspepsia was found, suggesting that myrtle berries

might have a use in treating gastrointestinal reflux disease.[206] The antifungal effects of myrtle leaves have been confirmed in randomised trials of women using a gel for bacterial vaginosis which also contained barberry (*Berberis vulgaris*) fruit extract, showing less recurrence of the infection compared to standard treatment with metronidazole.[207]

Sample preparations and dosage

Tincture of the berries can be used as a digestive aid, adding 1-2ml to half a cup of warm water before meals. An infusion of dried leaves can be used as a tea for digestion and also for diarrhoea, up to 10-15g daily. The infusion of the leaf can be used as an inhalation for coughs and sinusitis and a gargle for gingivitis. A hydrosol can be distilled from the leaves, for use as a skin toner (see p.102).

Constituents and commerce

Key constituents

Constituents of the leaves include terpenoids, flavonoids, flavonols, coumarins and benzoic acids. The berries also contain anthocyanins. Specific constituents include myrtucommulone, semimyrtucommulone, 1,8-cineole, α-pinene, myrtenyl acetate, limonene, linalool and α-terpinolene.

Commerce

Commercial sources are grown in the Middle East and North Africa. An essential oil can be made from the plant which is used in cosmetics and perfumery. Further uses of leaf extracts are as an organic insecticide and as an anti-oxidant in lipid-rich foods such as olive oil and sardines.

Safety

The essential oil is not for internal use. No other warnings have been reported but myrtle is best avoided in pregnancy and breastfeeding.

Other uses

Berries are used in food flavouring and as a pepper substitute. In floristry, myrtle has traditional use as a symbol of love and peace. Berries are macerated in alcohol to produce a myrtle liqueur.

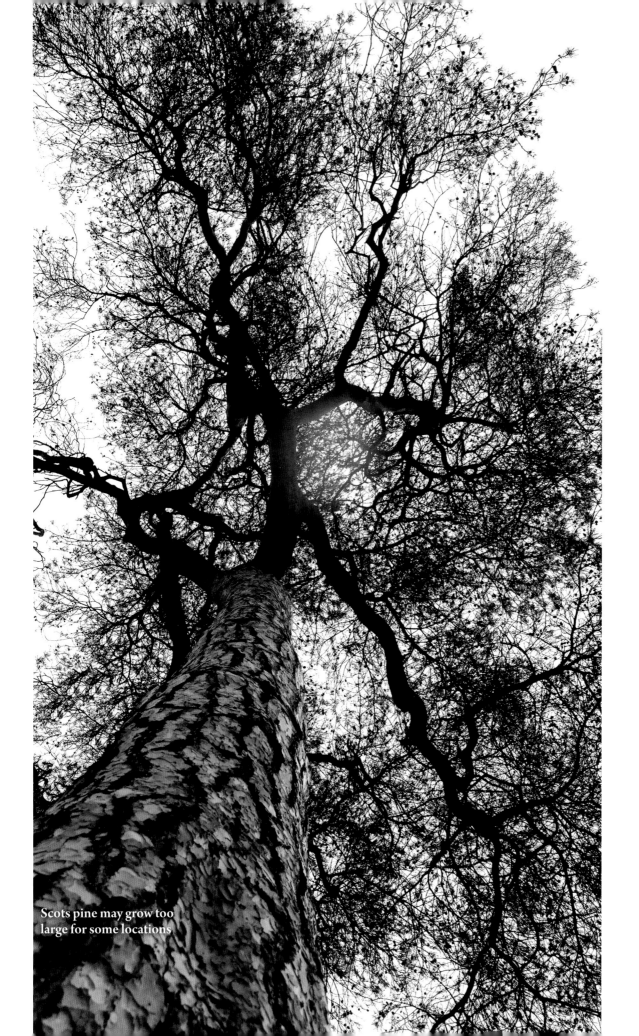

Scots pine may grow too
large for some locations

Pinus sylvestris, Scots pine

A stately conifer tree with aromatic needles and bark providing antiseptic and anticatarrhal effects.

SCIENTIFIC NAME   *Pinus sylvestris* L.

FAMILY   Pinaceae

ALTERNATE NAMES   Norway pine

PARTS USED   Needles, bark and resin

Description

Scots pine is a large evergreen pine growing fast up to 35m tall by 10m wide. It is monoecious with both sexes of flowers on the same plant. The flowers appear in May and are wind-pollinated. Cones develop the following season and ripen in March to June.

Habitat

European woods from temperate Asia to southern Scandinavia.

Related plants

Most pines and related conifers produce aromatic bark and needles and some resin. Smaller growing pines to consider include *P. parviflora*, the Japanese white pine, growing to 15m by 6m and hardy to USDA zone 5b (UK zone 5), or *P. mugo*, the dwarf mountain pine up to 4.5m by 3m. A pine that is tolerant of alkaline conditions is the Italian stone pine (*P. pinea*) growing to 10m.[208]

Cultivation and harvest

Cultivation

Scots pine is hardy to USDA zone 2 (UK zone 2) and tolerates drought and pollution. It grows best on light and acid soils and is short-lived on a shallow soil over chalk. Fairly shade tolerant, the pine soon overtakes other trees. Like most conifers, the pine does not readily coppice or pollard, since woody growth ceases if the leading stem is removed. However, the fresh shoot tips on branches (known as candles) can be pinched out in spring to produce a bushier plant. If a whole branch is removed then it is best to cut back close to the trunk, taking care not to damage the trunk itself.

Pests and diseases

Pines are liable to honey fungus as well as a number of blights and rusts.

Propagation

Sow ripe seed in individual pots in a cold frame. Cold stratification of six weeks at 4°C (39°F) can improve the germination of stored seed. Plant seedlings out into their permanent positions as soon as possible and protect them for their first winter or two. Plants have a very sparse root system and the sooner they are planted into their permanent positions the better they will grow. Cuttings can be taken only from very young trees less than 10 years old.

Harvesting

Pine needles can be harvested any time of year; ideally young needles are gathered in spring from pruned branches. Sap is harvested in the spring from v-shaped notches in the trunk bark. Pine sap exudes from the trunk of pine trees where they have suffered damage, and this stiffens to resin as it dries. The resin can be pried off with an old knife, aiming not to remove resin directly from the damaged area. Hard resin (it can be frozen) can be smashed into smaller bits with a hammer.

Therapeutic use

Traditional

All pines have some medicinal effect, and the bark, needles and resin have been used for centuries across the continents. Sap was tapped from pine trees to produce turpentine, and pitch tars and resin were also obtained from the wood. The resin was used for an antiseptic

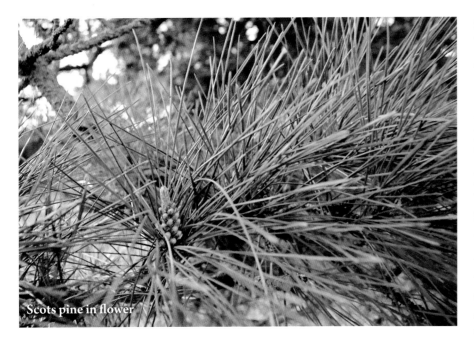
Scots pine in flower

improvements for blood circulation, blood pressure, platelet function and venous insufficiency.[213]

Sample preparations and dosage

For pine needle tea, pour a cup of boiling hot water over 1-2 tsp of fresh pine needles and stand for 15 minutes; take up to three times/day. The infusion can also be used as an inhalant, or use a few drops of essential oil added to boiling hot water, taking care with the steam. Pine tincture should be made with dried leaves and 40% alcohol to extract essential oils. Take up to 3ml twice a day. Pine resin is heated in a double boiler with twice as much oil till dissolved, then about 25% beeswax added to make a salve. Pine needles can be added to a bath for easing sore muscles.

ointment as well as cough cures, and a pine pillow can be made full of the needles or wood shavings.

Medicinal actions and uses

Pine needles are antiseptic, antifungal, tonic, decongestant, anticatarrhal, diuretic and stimulant, especially useful in bronchitis or sinusitis as an inhalant.

Clinical applications and research

Pine essential oil is used internally for a range of respiratory complaints including catarrh, and externally for rheumatic complaints.[209] Pine essential oils including that from Scots pine have antimicrobial effects, particularly against *Clostridium* species of bacteria.[210] An investigation of the effects of Scots pine needles on breast cancer cell lines found the greatest effects on cells responsible for tumours unresponsive to endocrine treatment[211] and pine bark extract has been shown to have a high total phenolic content with toxicity against tumour cells.[212] Considerable research has been carried out on extracts of the bark of the French maritime pine (*Pinus pinaster* subsp. *atlantica*) known as Pycnogenol. The fresh bark is extracted and then purified to a water-soluble powder with dosages of 20mg up to 200mg orally per day depending on complaint. Controlled clinical trials have shown evidence of

Constituents and commerce

Key constituents

The leaves and essential oil contain monoterpenes (particularly a-pinene, carene and limonene), and oleoresins. The needles are also rich in vitamin C.

Commerce

Pycnogenol is marketed for sustained relief in osteoarthritis.[214] Pine oil is widely used as a disinfectant ingredient in cleaning products.

Safety

Pine essential oil should not be used in pregnancy or breastfeeding. The essential oil is not for internal use and avoid use around the face and eyes. Since pine preparations may intensify bronchial spasm, use is not recommended in bronchial asthma or whooping cough.

Other uses

Scots pine is an important timber tree and is also grown for wood pulp. Can be grown as a windbreak. Pine resin can be burnt as incense, leaves made into smudge sticks.

Prunus padus, Bird cherry

A deciduous medium-sized tree with early spring flowers and attractive ringed bark which is used to alleviate respiratory and urinary complaints.

SCIENTIFIC NAME   *Prunus padus* L.

FAMILY   Rosaceae

PARTS USED   Bark, fruits, leaves and sap

Description

Bird cherry is a small to medium-sized deciduous tree growing to 16m tall by 7m wide. It has clusters of almond-scented white flowers in May and bitter black fruits ripen from July to August. The tree is hermaphrodite, and flowers are pollinated by bees. The fruit is eaten by birds and the seed is distributed through their droppings. The bark is shiny with characteristic rings and an almond-like scent.

Habitat

Bird cherry is native to northern Europe and Asia, and is found widely in woods and hedgerows, especially on alkaline soils by streams.

Related plants

Most cherries can be exploited for their bark as well as fruit. Wild cherry or gean (*P. avium*) is the ancestor of cultivated cherries. Black cherry (*P. serotina*) is the North American counterpart, native to central and eastern parts, a large tree growing to 30m.

Cultivation and harvest

Cultivation

Bird cherry is fully hardy to USDA zone 3 (UK zone 3), and flowers April to May. The flowers are hermaphrodite and pollinated by insects. This tree can grow in light shade. It will grow in most soils, preferring moist soils. The trees are shallow rooting and produce suckers, so they can form a thicket. Bird cherry is fairly vigorous and suitable for coppicing or pollarding in winter to produce young stems for the shiny bark. Otherwise, if pruning is required then it is done in late summer after new growth has matured, to avoid excessive bleeding and susceptibility to fungal or bacterial disease.

Pests and diseases

Susceptible to blossom wilt, silver leaf and bacterial canker.

Propagation

Ripe seeds need 2-3 months' cold stratification in a cold frame. Germination of the seed can be rather slow, sometimes taking 18 months. Prick out the seedlings into individual pots when they are large enough to handle. Grow them on in a greenhouse or cold frame for their first winter and plant them out in late spring

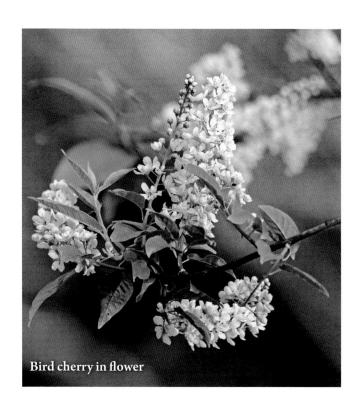

Bird cherry in flower

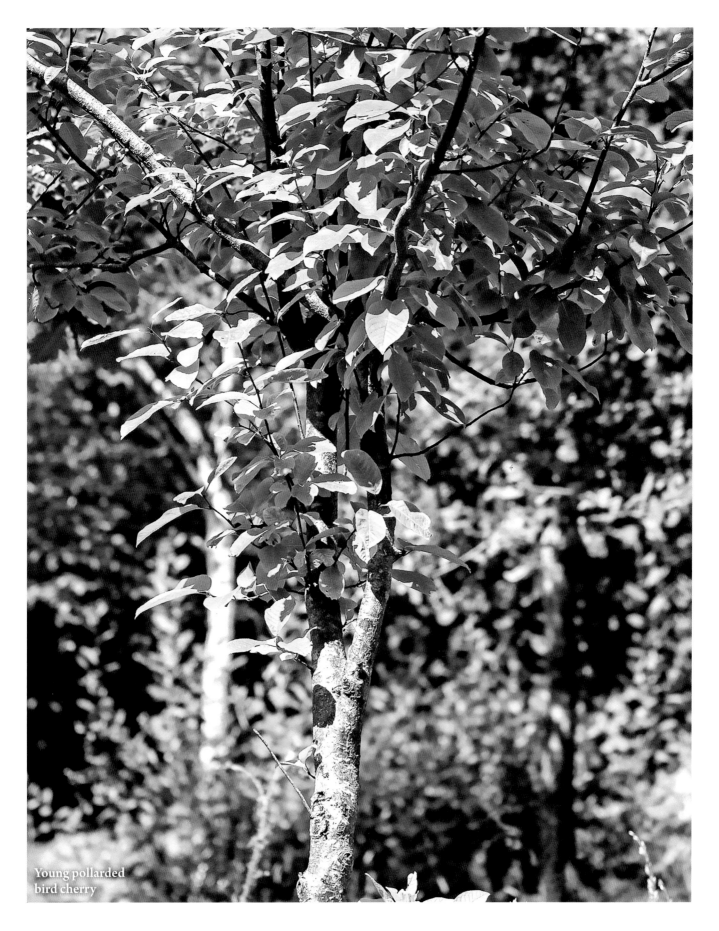
Young pollarded
bird cherry

or early summer of the following year. Cuttings of half-ripe wood with a heel can be taken in July/August and placed in a frame. Division of suckers should be done in the dormant season or layering in spring.

Harvesting

The aromatic resin can be obtained by making small incisions in the trunk in early spring to collect sap, then allowing the sap to dry out. The bark can be harvested in the summer or autumn (when hydrocyanic acid content is least). Bark can be dried but does not store well for longer than one year.

Therapeutic use

Traditional

The cherry has a long history of use in Europe; bark, gum and fruit stalks all used for coughs and colds,[215] though records are sparse. The resin forming on the trunk of the cherry was used as a chew, and could be dissolved in wine to be used medicinally for gallstones and kidney stones.[216] Alcoholic drinks were widely flavoured with cherry fruits.[217] Dried powder of bird cherry berries was used in Estonian traditional medicine for complaints related to tumours.[218] The black cherry (*P. serotina*) has a long tradition of use amongst North American tribes, especially for upper respiratory infections and throat disorders, using an infusion, decoction or syrup of the bark. Another use of the leaves was an astringent wash for sores.

Medicinal actions and uses

Cherry bark is expectorant, antitussive, astringent, anti-spasmodic, anti-inflammatory, bitter and sedative. The fruits contain anthocyanins. The leaves and fruit stalks are astringent, diuretic and tonic. The main use of the bark is as a remedy for coughs, particularly easing irritated dry coughs.

Clinical applications and research

Ripe fruits of the bird cherry show high anti-oxidant activity,[219] but the fruit stalk stems actually have the highest anti-oxidant activity, having higher phenolic compound levels.[220] The fruits of black cherry (*P. serotina*) have also been shown to contain high levels of phenolic compounds which are anti-oxidant and antihypertensive.[221]

Sample preparations and dosage

Cherry bark can be used to make a syrup for a persistent cough, by making an infusion in cold water and then adding to an equal quantity of honey (see recipe p.91). A decoction of bark or fruit stalks, simmered 10-15 minutes, can be used to treat cystitis and bronchial complaints. Tincture of cherry bark can be taken from 1 to 2ml three times daily.

Constituents and commerce

Key constituents

The bark contains cyanogenic glycosides (prunasin and amygdalin), flavonoids, benzaldehyde, volatile oils, plant acids, tannins and minerals, also pentacyclic triterpenes (mainly betulin and betulinic acid). Prunasin, a cyanogenic glycoside, is hydrolysed in preparations to form hydrocyanic acid which is antitussive. This process is hindered by heat, so a cold infusion is a better method for making preparations. Cherry fruits are rich in anthocyanins, quercetin, hydroxycinnamates, carotenoids, fibre, vitamins and minerals, and form part of preventative health diets.

Commerce

Cherry bark is an ingredient in many over-the-counter cough syrups, drops and lozenges. It can also be found in hair products.

Safety

Cyanogenic glycosides are converted into hydrocyanic acid in the body and very large doses of cherry bark would be toxic. However, low levels of these glycosides are present in many rose family plants and these are readily detoxified in the body. Long-term use is not advised.

Other uses

A good wildlife plant for bees, birds, moths and mammals. Cherry timber is highly valued.

Pseudotsuga menziesii, Douglas fir

A North American conifer with gloriously soft and aromatic needles, ideal for teas and inhalations in respiratory and other complaints.

SCIENTIFIC NAME   *Pseudotsuga menziesii* (Mirb.) Franco
FAMILY   Pinaceae
ALTERNATE NAMES   Oregon pine, false hemlock
PARTS USED   Leaves, bark and resin

Description

Douglas fir is a tall conical-shaped evergreen conifer growing fast with a single trunk up to 60m tall (in the UK, larger in the US) and 10m wide. Young trees have smooth grey bark which ages to become thick, corky, deeply ridged and red-brown. Red-brown buds produce fragrant, citrus-like, soft, dark green flat leaves. Female cones, 7-10cm long, are produced from March to May and the cones ripen September to November, hanging from branches and recognisable by their three-pronged bracts (like a mouse's back legs and tail). Seed is produced from trees of 10 years or older.

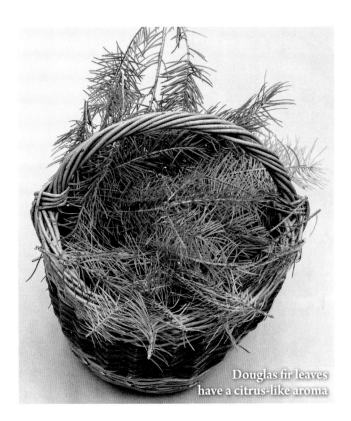
Douglas fir leaves have a citrus-like aroma

Habitat

Douglas fir is found in western North America, from Mexico to the Canadian Rockies, from sea level to mountains. It is widely planted throughout the world as a forestry timber tree, and naturalised in Europe.

Related plants

Although called a fir, the Douglas fir is not part of the *Abies* genus.

Cultivation and harvest

Cultivation

The Douglas fir does best in full sun and acid, moist, well-drained soil. It will tolerate some shade and the soil can be poor or fertile but it does not tolerate chalky or waterlogged soils. It is cold hardy, to USDA zone 5a (UK zone 7), and can tolerate strong winds. Slow growing when young but can then increase at over 1m per year. Typical of a conifer, pollarding is not feasible, as the main leader should not be stopped, but at Holt Wood we have found that with careful selection of branches it is possible to reduce height and shape the tree.

Pests and diseases

Resistant to honey fungus, young growth can be damaged by late frosts. Fast growth means that branches are liable to break in wind and so this tree is not ideal to plant near buildings and fences.

Propagation

Seed can be sown in the autumn in a cold frame. When seedlings are large enough to handle, prick them out into individual pots and grow them on in light shade

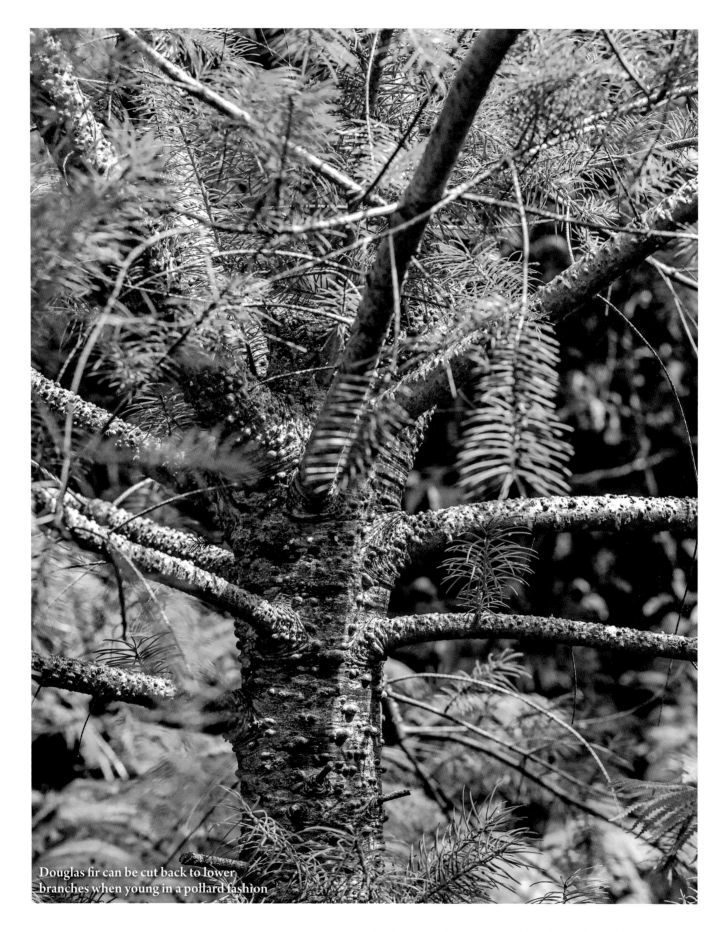

Douglas fir can be cut back to lower branches when young in a pollard fashion in the cold frame for at least their first winter. Plant in permanent positions in late spring or early summer, after the last expected frosts.

Harvesting

The leaves can be harvested at any time of year though there is some variation in the essential oil constituents. Analysis of the secondary metabolites in Douglas fir needles found that most terpenes increased significantly in concentration from mid-June to early August.[222] The bark can be harvested year round and dried for later use. The green bark of young trees is laden with blisters full of sticky resin, all designed to protect from damage. Take care when handling the trunk or bark as the resin is very sticky.

Therapeutic use

Traditional

Most parts of the Douglas fir were used by Native Americans particularly for coughs, colds and sore throats. The Sinkyone of California made Douglas fir bark tea to ease colds and as a laxative to help stomach ailments. The Shasta in Northern California used Douglas fir resin to poultice cuts. Douglas fir needles were made into tea by Isleta Puebloans in New Mexico to cure rheumatism.[223] Young shoots soaked in cold water could be used as a mouthwash or placed in the tips of shoes to prevent perspiration and athlete's foot.[224]

Medicinal actions and uses

Douglas fir is anti-inflammatory, expectorant, diuretic, antiseptic, antifungal and antiviral. It provides a remedy for respiratory complaints, and helps to deal with all kinds of infections and inflammations.

Clinical applications and research

Research evidence is remarkably limited. Based on other studies of essential oils in conifers, the active components, such as pinenes[225] and terpinolene,[226] have been shown to have antimicrobial, antiviral and anti-inflammatory effects.

Sample preparations and dosage

Use 2 tsp of fresh needles per cup of boiling water and steep for 15 minutes, then strain and drink. Inhale an

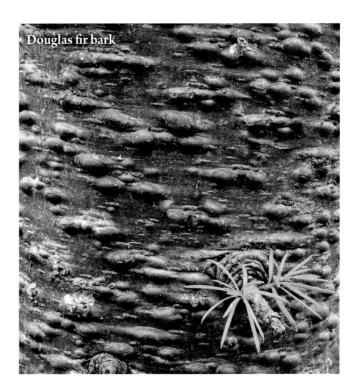

Douglas fir bark

infusion of needles or resin for coughs and colds. The aromatic needles can be infused in oil, honey, vinegar and brandy. A hydrosol can be distilled from the needles and used as an antiseptic wash.

Constituents and commerce

Key constituents

Cones, needles and wood contain monoterpenes (including alpha- and beta-pinenes, sabinene, alpha-terpinolene and alpha-terpineol).[227]

Commerce

Douglas fir is primarily cultivated for timber, and young trees are sold as Christmas trees.

Safety

No adverse effects are reported. However, the essential oil should not be used internally or around the face and eyes. Data is lacking so avoid use in pregnancy or breastfeeding.

Other uses

A valuable timber tree. Young leaves are rich in vitamin C. Incense and smudge sticks.

Ribes nigrum, Blackcurrant

A familiar shrub widely cultivated in Europe with aromatic buds and leaves and purple-black berries, providing benefits in dealing with viral complaints and stress and longer-term reduction in degenerative diseases.

SCIENTIFIC NAME *Ribes nigrum* L.

FAMILY Grossulariaceae

PARTS USED Buds, fruit and leaves

Description

The blackcurrant is a deciduous multi-stemmed shrub growing to 1.8m tall and 1.8m wide. It is in flower from April to May and the flowers are hermaphrodite and pollinated by bees or self-fertile.

Habitat

Blackcurrant grows in forests throughout Europe and northern and central Asia, and is now widely cultivated for fruit.

Related plants

Many cultivars of the blackcurrant are known; a compact variety is 'Ben Sarek'. 'Titania' is a Scandinavian variety with large berries and resistance to mildew and rust, said to have a long season of ripening from midsummer to September.[228]

Cultivation and harvest

Cultivation

Hardy to USDA zone 4 (UK zone 3), this plant grows on most soils and prefers a slightly acid, well-drained but moist soil. It can grow in semi-shade. This plant needs feeding to maintain fruit production. Up to a third of the older stems are removed each year to encourage new growth from the base, and fruiting is best from second year growth.

Pests and diseases

Susceptible to honey fungus. Aphids may cause the leaves to curl. Mildew may occur if the plant becomes congested. Big bud can be seen in swollen buds in spring which should be removed.

Propagation

Seed can be sown in the autumn in a cold frame. Stored seed requires three months' cold stratification at between 0-5°C (32-41°F). Prick out the seedlings into individual pots when they are large enough to handle and grow them on in a cold frame for their first winter, planting them out in late spring of the following year. Blackcurrant is readily grown from cuttings of half-ripe wood, 10-15cm with a heel, taken in July/August. Cuttings of mature wood can be taken November to February.

Harvesting

The buds are harvested in early spring as they start to swell. The leaves are harvested during early summer, and can be used fresh or dried.[229] Fruit is picked when ripe in summer.

Therapeutic use

Traditional

Traditionally, all parts of the blackcurrant have found a medicinal use, including roots and bark for fevers and swellings. The leaves were used as a poultice for wounds and insect bites, as a gargle for sore throat and as a diuretic infusion for bladder complaints, dropsy and rheumatism. The fruit juice was used in preparations for sore throats, colds and flu. The fruits have been used for diarrhoea.

Medicinal actions and uses

Blackcurrant has anti-inflammatory, astringent, anti-oxidant, antibacterial and antiviral effects. The leaves are diuretic and diaphoretic and used in urinary and

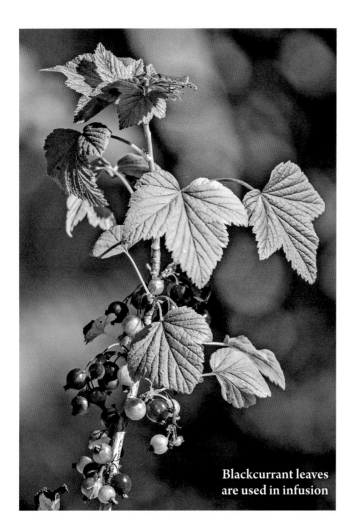
Blackcurrant leaves are used in infusion

hypertension.[233] A randomised placebo-controlled study of patients with glaucoma found that blackcurrant anthocyanins (equivalent to 50mg per day) slowed down deterioration in vision.[234]

Sample preparations and dosage

The leaves can be taken in infusion as a tea (1 tsp per cup), or as a tincture (2-3ml three times daily, see recipe p.93). The infusion serves as a gargle for sore throat. The fruits can be juiced and made into a syrup. The buds can be macerated in glycerin[235] with a suggested dosage up to 1ml three times daily.

Constituents and commerce

Key constituents

High levels of polyphenols are found in the buds (including catechins and flavonols), as well as terpenes.[236] Flavonol glycosides (including quercetin and kaempferol) are found in the leaves[237] reflecting anti-oxidant potential. Depending on harvest time, the leaves vary in levels of hydroxycinnamic acids, flavonoids (proanthocyanidins) and monoterpenes.[238]

Commerce

Blackcurrant leaf extracts are sold for use in joint pain and urinary complaints as herbal infusion or powdered extract. Blackcurrant seed oil is a source of gamma-linolenic acid and sold for its anti-inflammatory properties.

Safety

Blackcurrant leaf preparations should only be used by adults according to the European Medicines Agency. Take professional advice on consuming blackcurrant preparations alongside medications such as antipsychotics and anticoagulants.

Other uses

Highly edible and nutritious fruit, a good source of minerals and vitamins, especially vitamin C. Used to make wine and flavour spirits.

arthritic complaints.[230] Blackcurrant buds have a high level of anti-inflammatory flavonoids.[231] The buds are thought to have further anti-inflammatory effect by increasing the secretion of cortisol by the adrenal glands, and are used in treatment of stress-related conditions.

Clinical applications and research

Extracts of blackcurrant leaves have been shown to have antiviral effects, particularly useful in preventing viral infection at an early stage.[232] Blackcurrant juice is an excellent source of anthocyanins with anti-oxidant activity, of interest in combatting a range of degenerative diseases, including cancer, diabetic complications and

Rosa canina, Dog rose

A pretty shrub with arching stems and scented flowers, with astringent leaves and anti-inflammatory fruits full of vitamin C, used to combat pain and support the circulation and immune system.

SCIENTIFIC NAME *Rosa canina* L.

FAMILY Rosaceae

ALTERNATE NAMES Briar rose, wild briar

PARTS USED Fruits, flowers and leaves

Description

The dog rose is a climbing deciduous shrub with arching thorny branches growing to 3.5m by 3m at a fast rate. The leaves are pinnate with toothed margins. Hermaphrodite flowers are produced in June and July and pollinated by bees and other insects as well as being self-fertile. The pinkish-white flowers give rise to hips which ripen to scarlet red in the autumn.

Habitat

Found in hedges, woods and scrubland in Europe from southern Norway to southwest Asia and northern Africa. Also naturalised in many other parts of the world including America and Australasia.

Related plants

R. rugosa is a rose of Asian origin that readily forms thickets and is often used for hedging. Eglantine rose (*R. rubiginosa*) is characterised by an apple-like scent of the leaves. Roses have been much bred for centuries for fragrance and the flowers used for distillation. The Damask rose (*R. damascena*) is a hybrid form grown for fragrance, closely related to the Provence or cabbage rose (*R. centifolia*). These roses all have a similar range of polyphenolic compounds.[239]

Cultivation and harvest

Cultivation

Dog rose is hardy to USDA zone 3 (UK zone 3). It can grow in most soils but prefers moist, well-drained soil. It is ideal for a sunny woodland edge where it will flower and fruit better than in a shady spot.

Pests and diseases

Susceptible to honey fungus.

Propagation

Seed is sown as soon as it is ripe in a cold frame and sometimes germinates in spring though it may take a further year. Stored seed can be sown after cold stratification for six weeks at 5°C (41°F). Prick out the seedlings into individual pots when they are large enough to handle. Plant out in the summer or grow on in a cold frame for the following winter and plant out in late spring. Cuttings of half-ripe wood with a heel can be taken in July and placed in a shaded frame. Overwinter the plants in the frame and plant out in late spring. Pencil-thick cuttings of mature wood of the current season's growth can be planted in a cold frame in early autumn. Division of suckers in the dormant season. Layering.

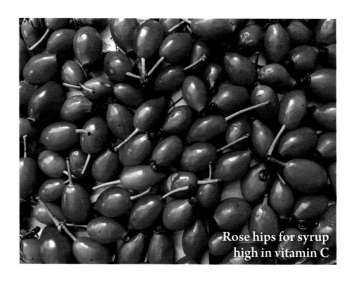

Rose hips for syrup high in vitamin C

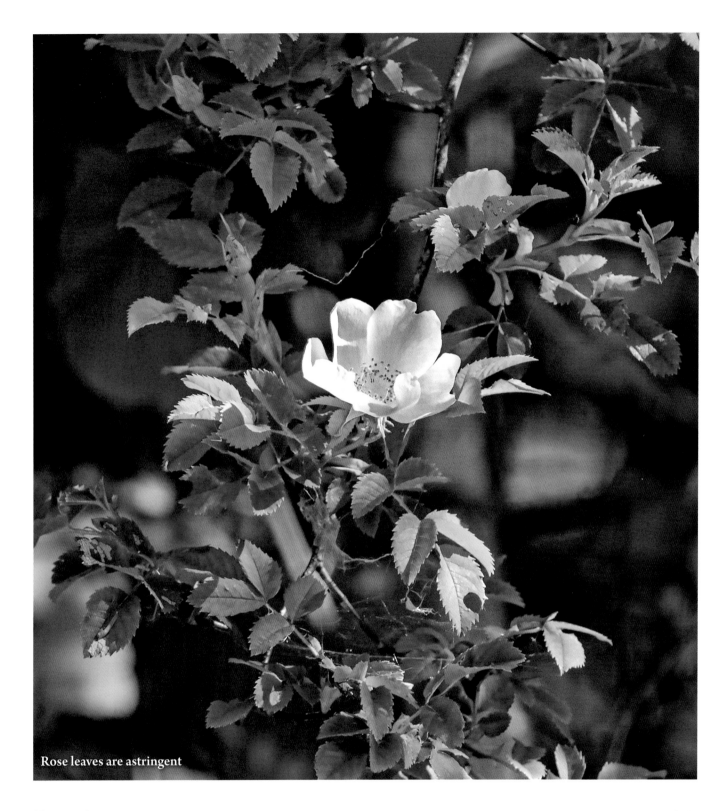

Rose leaves are astringent

Harvesting

The leaves can be harvested fresh or to dry for use in infusions. The delicate flowers can be harvested fresh for distillation or for infusion in oil. For drying, the petals need to be completely free of moisture and placed in a single layer. The rose hips can be harvested as they fully redden after the first frosts. *R. rugosa* fruits can also be used and are larger and earlier than *R. canina*. If drying or using hips fresh for tea then cut them into halves and scrape out the inside hairy parts and seeds.

Therapeutic use

Traditional

Roses have longstanding traditional use as food and medicine from China to the Mediterranean, particularly for digestive and respiratory complaints. Rose hips were used in the UK during World War II since they are a rich source of vitamin C.[240]

Medicinal actions and uses

The leaves are both antimicrobial and astringent.[241] Rose hips are anti-oxidant, anti-inflammatory, immune stimulant, astringent, carminative, diuretic, laxative, antiscorbutic and tonic. An infusion from the flowers is slightly astringent and is used as a lotion for inflamed skin or as a mouthwash. Rose flower essential oil and methanolic extracts have significant antibacterial effects. Preparations of the hips are taken internally in the treatment of colds, influenza, minor infectious diseases, scurvy, diarrhoea and gastritis.

Clinical applications and research

Clinical research has provided evidence for the use of rose hips in osteoarthritis. Pain reduction was found to be significant in arthritis patients after three months of taking rose hip fruit and seed powder.[242] Another study reported improvements in skin moisture and elasticity after eight weeks of consumption of rose hips, and suggested that there was increased stabilisation of cell membranes which improved skin cell longevity.[243] Some research has shown that rose hips can help to prevent infections such as cystitis. Rose hips were given in a trial of women after Caesarean section and found to reduce urinary tract infection, when given at a dose of 1000mg per day for 20 days.[244] Extracts based on distillation of rose flowers have been used in painful complaints and skin conditions. *R. damascena* oil used topically can reduce the pain intensity of certain types of migraine.[245] Another study has showed the antimicrobial and anti-inflammatory activity of *R. damascena* hydrosol which supports use on the skin.[246]

Sample preparations and dosage

A decoction of chopped rose hips can be made by simmering 2.5 tsp in 1 cup of water for 10 minutes, or take 5-10g daily of rosehip seed and fruit powder. Rose hips are commonly used to make rose hip syrup, though the hairy inner parts must be removed first. Rose flower petals and leaves can be used in infusions as a tea or skin wash.

Constituents and commerce

Key constituents

Rose leaves are rich in tannins. Rose petals contain rugosin B and tellimagrandin I. Rose hips contain vitamins A, C, E, essential fatty acids, carotenoids and flavanoids (including catechins and flavonones) and other polyphenols (including hydroxybenzenes and hydroxycinnamic acids).

Commerce

Much of the rose hip supply derives from wild-harvesting in eastern and southern Europe, as well as cultivated plantations elsewhere, including South America. Various quality grades are applied to harvests and the levels of vitamin C can vary with altitude and climate as well as biotype.[247] Although dog rose is widely harvested, other species may be used, for example, an anti-ageing liquid preparation 'Long-Life CiLi' is based on the fruits of *R. roxburghi* of China.

Safety

The inner fruit covering of the seeds contains fine hairs which can irritate the mouth and stomach if not removed. Rose hips and other rose preparations are generally well tolerated, and adverse reactions are generally related to the large amount of vitamin C (laxative effects) or to allergies. Take professional clinical advice if on anticoagulants, anticancer or antiviral medications and if immune system stimulation is contraindicated.

Other uses

Hedging. Wildlife.

Rosmarinus officinalis, Rosemary

A well-known evergreen shrub of Mediterranean origin which can prove effective in anxiety, memory loss and Alzheimer's disease.

SCIENTIFIC NAME   *Rosmarinus officinalis* L.

FAMILY   Lamiaceae

PARTS USED   Leaves, flowers and stems

Description

Rosemary is an evergreen shrub growing to 2m by 1.5m. It has fragrant needle-like leaves. Bluish-purple flowers are produced in early spring from March and continue through the year till autumn in a sheltered position. Flowers are hermaphrodite and pollinated by bees.

Habitat

Rosemary is a southern European plant that grows in dry and rocky places. It is widely cultivated for ornamental purposes as well as for commerce.

Related plants

Many ornamental varieties are available including a creeping form of rosemary ('Prostratus'), or more upright forms for hedging. Cultivars of rosemary can be selected for desirable essential oil constituents. These chemotypes can be selected for maximum production such as 1,8-cineole used for the respiratory system, or for verbenone and the mildest form for use on skin and

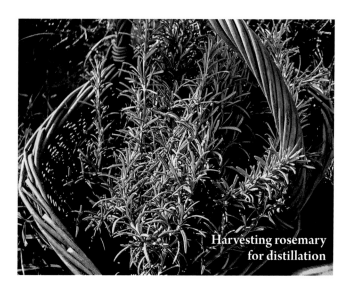

Harvesting rosemary for distillation

hair, or for camphor which is tonic and stimulating and suitable for use with the muscular system.

Cultivation and harvest

Cultivation

Rosemary is a fairly hardy evergreen perennial to USDA zone 6 (UK zone 6), which grows well in a range of soils, including very alkaline. It can only grow in sun and not in shade. Rosemary tolerates maritime exposure, and withstands drought. Rosemary can be readily pruned and it can be grown in a pot.

Pests and diseases

Rosemary is little troubled by insects. If scale insects or rosemary beetle are seen they can be removed by hand.

Propagation

Seed can be sown in spring in a cold frame, although they may be slow to germinate. Prick out seedlings when large enough to handle and grow on in a cold frame or greenhouse for the first winter. Then plant out in late spring. Cuttings of young shoots in spring or half-ripe wood can be taken with a heel in July-August. Remove the lower leaves from a cutting of 10-15cm and insert directly into the soil. Plants can also be layered.

Harvesting

The leaves are harvested as flowers open, for use fresh or dried. Drying should be carried out at less than 40°C (104°F) to reduce loss of volatile oils and maintain colour. Flowering tops are used for distillation of rosemary hydrosol and essential oil. The volatile constituents can vary with the time of harvest: younger leaves contain equal parts of camphor and 1,8-cineole while camphor is greater in older leaves.[248]

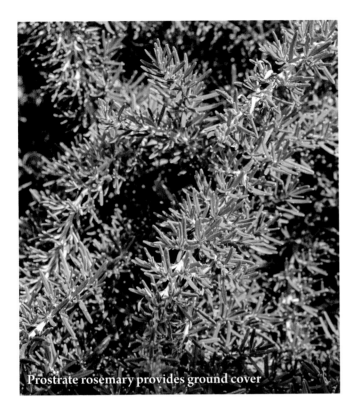
Prostrate rosemary provides ground cover

content helps with lipid-scavenging and the anti-inflammatory and anti-oxidant effects help in reducing risk of cardiovascular disease.[249] There is also potential of rosemary for use in neurodegenerative disorders such as Alzheimer's disease where there is a loss of cholinergic neurons, since diterpenes and other constituents in rosemary can reduce the damaging effects of oxidative stress.[250]

Sample preparations and dosage

Leaf infusion for digestive complaints, 2g in 150ml water, up to three times daily, also as a mouthwash or bath additive. Tincture of herb, 1-5ml three times daily. Distilled water of rosemary can be used as a deodorant, freshener and skin tonic. Essential oil diluted (1%) in carrier oil can be rubbed on the chest in bronchial complaints, or diffused on a saucer in the sickroom.

Constituents and commerce

Key constituents

Rosemary leaves contain phenolic acids (rosmarininc, chlorogenic, caffeic acids), diterpenoids (carnosolic acid and rosmaquinones), triterpenoids (oleanolic acid, ursolic acid), flavonoids (apigenin, luteolin), volatile oils (1,8-cineole, a-pinene, a-terpineol, camphor, camphene, borneol, bornyl acetate) and tannins.[251]

Commerce

Rosemary is cultivated in many countries including France, Spain, India and North Africa. Up to 1.5kg fresh herb can be harvested from each plant after several years.[252] Pharmacopoeia standards require the dried leaves to contain a minimum of 1.2% essential oil.

Safety

Avoid rosemary in pregnancy and breastfeeding. It is not recommended for children under 12 years. The essential oil should not be taken internally and should not be applied undiluted to the skin.

Other uses

Culinary flavouring. Used as a natural preservative as anti-oxidant in cosmetics and foods. Hedging. Shampoo. Insect repellent.

Therapeutic use

Traditional

Rosemary has been used since classical times in Europe, China and India, as a stimulating herb. It has been traditionally thought to strengthen memory, and also been used as a carminative for digestive disorders, and for cardiovascular, liver and nervous complaints. Externally it has been used as an analgesic for stiff joints and sore muscles, as an antiseptic and for promoting hair growth.

Medicinal actions and uses

Rosemary is anti-inflammatory, anti-oxidant, antibacterial, antispasmodic, astringent, bitter, carminative, diaphoretic, emmenagogue, expectorant and stimulant. Due to its stimulating qualities it is used in treating anxiety and depression. Rosemary can be used internally for digestive complaints and externally for rheumatism.

Clinical applications and research

Rosemary has been much researched as an anti-oxidant food preservative but little researched for potential medicinal use despite longstanding experience of its effects. More research is needed into the use of rosemary in the management of dyslipidaemia since the flavonoid

Rubus idaeus, Raspberry

A prickly fruiting shrub providing delicious fruits and offering astringent leaves for complaints such as diarrhoea and for painful periods or preparing for childbirth.

SCIENTIFIC NAME *Rubus idaeus* L.

FAMILY Rosaceae

PARTS USED Fruit and leaves

Description

Raspberry is a deciduous shrub growing to 1.5m tall by 1.5m wide. Fresh stems or canes are produced every year. Flowers are produced from June to August. The flowers are hermaphrodite and pollinated by bees and insects or are self-fertile. The red, sweet fruits ripen from July to September. Fruits are produced on stems in their second year, and after fruiting the woody stem dies.

Habitat

In addition to cultivation, raspberry grows wild in Europe and temperate Asia, in moist hedgerows and woodland edges.

Related plants

Many named varieties of raspberry are cultivated for the fruits. Raspberry is related to the blackberry (*R. fruticosus*) and many of the applications are similar, since blackberry leaves are also rich in phenolic compounds.[253] In the US, other *Rubus* species such as black raspberry (*R. occidentalis*) and thimbleberry (*R. parviflorus*) can also be harvested for fruits and leaves.

Cultivation and harvest

Cultivation

Raspberry is hardy to USDA zone 4 (UK zone 3). It can grow in part shade or sun and prefers moist, slightly acidic soil that is well drained. The canes have shallow roots and are best in a sheltered area which is not windy. When planted up to 1m apart, it can be well mulched to discourage competing plants, or surrounded with

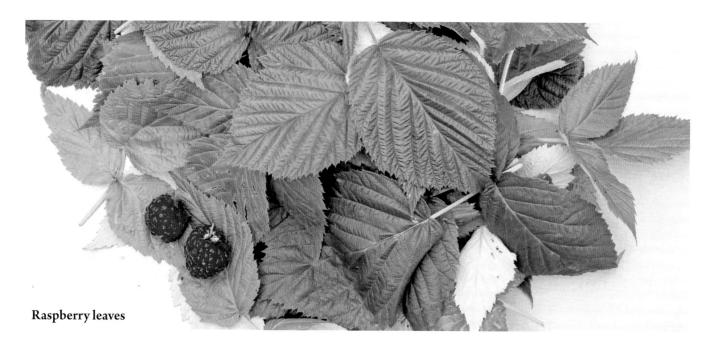

Raspberry leaves

ground cover plants such as strawberries. The canes may need shortening and/or support. Each year the previously fruiting canes can be cut out to encourage new stems.[254]

Pests and diseases

Susceptible to honey fungus. Raspberries imported to US have been subject to periodic bans due to infection from South American sources with the *Cyclosporia* parasite.

Propagation

Stored seed requires one month cold stratification at 3°C (37°F). Grow on and plant out seedlings into their permanent positions in late spring of the following year. Cuttings of half-ripe wood can be taken in July/August. Tip layering in July. Division in early spring or in the autumn.

Harvesting

The leaves are harvested in the late spring from one-year-old plants just before flowering and well dried in a single layer for later use. Use gloves to protect from prickles.

Therapeutic use

Traditional

Raspberry leaf and fruits have been long used for wounds, colic, diarrhoea and many other complaints from stomach bleeds to menstrual problems and from emotional disturbances to exhaustion. Raspberry leaves have been traditionally used as a tea to stimulate and ease labour.

Medicinal actions and uses

Raspberry leaves are anti-inflammatory, astringent, haemostatic, and used in menstrual irregularities and pregnancy.[255] A tea made from the leaves is used in the treatment of diarrhoea, painful periods and sore throat.[256] Raspberry leaf is regarded as a tonic for the uterus. The leaves can be used during the last three months of pregnancy and during childbirth, but should not be used earlier. Externally, the leaves and roots are used as a poultice and wash to treat sores, conjunctivitis, minor wounds, burns and varicose ulcers. The fruit is antiscorbutic and diuretic, and used in cough cures.

Clinical applications and research

There has not been sufficient research into the efficacy of raspberry leaf as a uterine tonic.[257] A study of raspberry leaf cells in an oil-soluble extract was found to promote skin hydration and suggested potential in skin care preparations.[258]

Sample preparations and dosage

Raspberry leaf tea is made from infusing 30g dried leaves in 500ml of boiling water. This infusion can be used as a gargle for sore throat or wash for wounds. Raspberry leaf tincture is taken 4-8ml three times daily. A raspberry leaf vinegar is an alternative to tea or tincture (see recipe p.94).

Constituents and commerce

Key constituents

Raspberry leaves contain hydroxybenzoic acids, hydroxycinnamic acids and ellagitannins which are also found in the berries. Tannins in the leaf range from 2.6-6.9%, and a greater quantity of flavonoids is found in the leaf than in the fruits. Polyphenols in the young leaf shoots are anti-oxidant, antimicrobial and cytotoxic.[259] Raspberry fruits are rich in phenolic compounds, similar to the levels in strawberries though less than levels in redcurrants and blackcurrants.[260]

Commerce

Red raspberries are the fourth most significant fruit product in the world, grown mainly in eastern Europe, Russia and the US. Raspberry leaves are often wasted by-products of fruit harvest. Raspberry leaf tablets are sold over the counter for use from 32 weeks of pregnancy until childbirth.

Safety

Adverse effects with raspberries are minimal and appear to be associated with contamination, so it is advised to wash fruits.

Other uses

Edible fruits. Wildlife.

Salix daphnoides, Violet willow

A slender and attractive tree, with reddish stems and furry white spring buds, having longstanding use of the bark and leaves to relieve back and joint pain.

SCIENTIFIC NAME *Salix daphnoides* Vill.

FAMILY Salicaceae

PARTS USED Bark and leaves

Description

Violet willow is a large shrub or small tree growing to 6-8m in height and 2-3m wide. Supple branches carry leaves which are narrow and hairless. The leaf buds are characterised by a single scale. It flowers in early spring. The flowers are dioecious and only one sex is found on each tree. They are pollinated by bees and the seeds ripen in June. There is often variation in the species as well as hybridisation.

Habitat

Violet willow is native to central Europe, and widely naturalised elsewhere due to cultivation. It grows in wetlands and alongside rivers, doing well in sandy or pebbly areas.

Related plants

White willow (*S. alba*) is the traditional willow of herbal medicine and is fast growing to 25m. There are some 500 species in the *Salix* genus, and many are high in salicin content, the concentration measured in milligrams per gram dry weight as reported from the UK National Willow Collection at Rothamsted Research.[261] Violet willow is recorded as providing 24.70mg/g salicin. Apart from white willow (*S. alba*) species containing between 8.4-12.21mg/g, another widely available species to consider is purple willow (*S. purpurea*) at 29.25mg/g. In North America, the black willow (*S. nigra*) is generally used.

Cultivation and harvest

Cultivation

Violet willow is hardy to USDA zone 5 (UK zone 5). It is fairly fast growing in sandy areas but does not tolerate competing plants well and needs weed-suppressing mulch. Suited to a wide range of soils, it prefers a sunny position and cannot grow in the shade. It prefers moist soil of neutral to acid pH. Willows have aggressive roots and should be planted well away from buildings and drains. Willow responds well to coppicing or pollarding in early spring. At Holt Wood, we mainly pollard and harvest the branches of violet willow after two or three years. The pollard branches of white willow are more vigorous in growth and are harvested every 1-2 years.

Pests and diseases

Willow is susceptible to honey fungus.

Propagation

Fresh seed has a very short viability, and is immediately surface sown. Cuttings of mature wood of pencil thickness can be taken in the dormant period, November to February, to be rooted in a sheltered outdoor bed or planted straight into their permanent positions. Cuttings of half-ripe wood are taken in June to August.

Harvesting

The bark of 2-3-year-old willow branches is harvested during the spring, when it readily peels off, and is dried for later use. Leaves can be harvested in late spring and used fresh or dried for later use. Drying recommendations vary; rapid drying in an airy room is best to reduce degradation of phenolic components. Twigs can also be harvested whole and cut into small pieces of 3-4mm.[262]

Therapeutic use

Traditional

Willow has been used since ancient times to treat pain and fever. The Assyrians used a decoction of willow

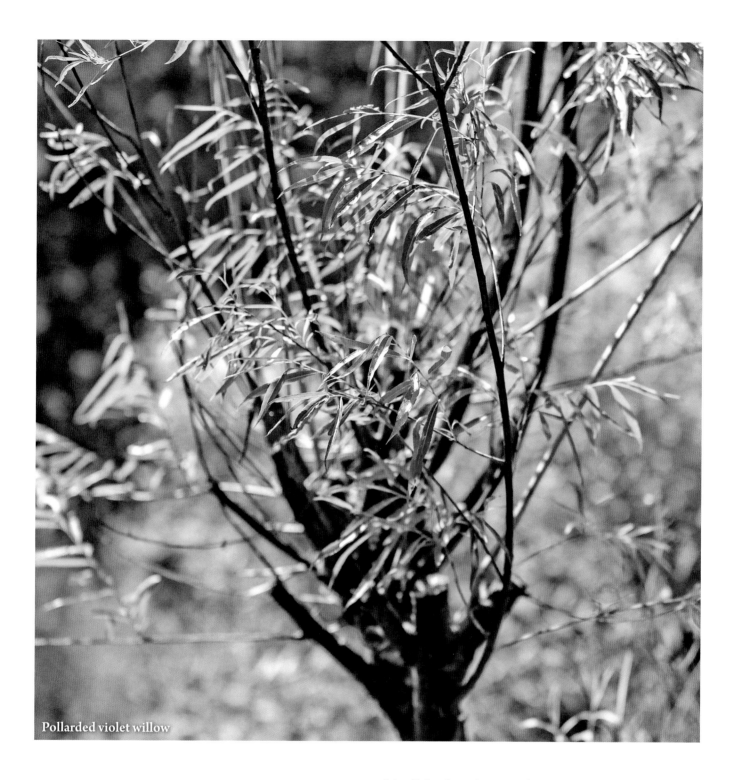

Pollarded violet willow

leaves for joint pains, and Native American healers also relied on willow for its analgesic properties. Willow leaf tea was advised for painful childbirth in ancient Greece. Willow bark has been used to relieve sore throat, fever and headache associated with upper respiratory tract infections and influenza.

Medicinal actions and uses

Willow bark is antipyretic, analgesic, anti-inflammatory, antiseptic, astringent, tonic and bitter. The salicin content is hydrolysed in the intestinal mucosa to the aglycone saligenin which is then absorbed and oxidised in the blood and liver to give salicylic acid, which has an anti-inflammatory effect. Salicylic acid has little activity on platelet function in the blood unlike the manufactured aspirin acetylsalicylic acid.[263] Willow bark is used mostly as an anti-inflammatory for symptomatic relief in back pain, joint pain, headache and toothache.[264] An infusion of leaves can be used for calming in nervous insomnia, and in the bath for rheumatism.

Clinical applications and research

Despite a long history of use, relatively few studies have been published that confirm the effects of willow.[265] The anti-inflammatory effects of a water-based extract of willow (23-26% salicin and high polyphenol content) have been confirmed, showing that the effects are not due to salicin alone, but due also to other polyphenols, flavonoids and proanthocyanidins.[266] A small number of clinical studies have been conducted that support the use of willow bark extracts in chronic lower back and joint pain and osteoarthritis. For example, one study showed a moderate analgesic effect of 240mg salicin/day dosage given for two weeks in patients with osteoarthritis.[267] A further review of research studies has provided moderate evidence of effectiveness for the use of ethanolic willow bark extract in lower back pain.[268] Other uses have been considered for the antimicrobial leaves. A small-scale study compared a mouthwash of willow and mallow leaves with standard chlorhexidine in patients with gingivitis and found it comparable in terms of bleeding and plaque removal.[269] Willow leaves have also been explored for their antimicrobial use in wound dressing applications.[270]

Sample preparations and dosage

Willow bark tea typically consists of 1-3g of bark per cup of water, decocted for 10 minutes, drunk three to four times per day. The infusion can also be used as a gargle for a sore throat. From 2-3 powdered willow bark capsules of 400mg can be taken 3-4 times daily, or willow tincture 5-8ml three times daily.

Constituents and commerce

Key constituents

Willow bark and leaves contain glycosides, salicylates (salicin, salicortin, populin, fragilin, tremulacin), tannins, aromatic aldehydes, and acids (salidroside, vanillin, syringin, salicylic acid, caffeic and ferulic acids), salicyl alcohol (saligenin) and flavonoids.[271]

Commerce

An alternative to willow was sought in the nineteenth century, partly because willow tended to upset the stomach when used. In 1899, the new compound acetylsalicylic acid was registered and introduced commercially as 'aspirin' by the Bayer Company of Germany. This new compound rapidly replaced willow as a medication. However, in Europe, the traditional use of willow bark extract is still accepted for lower back pain and for the symptomatic relief of fever associated with the common cold, minor articular pain and headache, at a standardised daily dosage equivalent to 240mg salicin. Willow products and raw materials are commonly imported from Eastern Europe and China. A quantity of 10g of willow bark has been reported to contain about 100mg total salicin. For comparison, commercial standardised bark extracts, with 120-240mg of the salicin constituent per day, are given for up to eight weeks for the treatment of pain.

Safety

Excessive use of willow bark in inflammatory joint disease means ingestion of high levels of tannin, which can irritate digestion, and so willow bark is best combined with other digestive herbs such as turmeric and ginger. Otherwise adverse effects appear to be minimal as compared to nonsteroidal anti-inflammatory drugs including aspirin. The primary cause for concern may relate to allergic reactions in salicylate-sensitive individuals.[272] Due to the potential for Reye's syndrome arising from salicylates, children with influenza, varicella or any suspected viral infection should avoid willow bark. Take professional clinical practitioner advice if on prescription medications. Not recommended in pregnancy or breastfeeding due to lack of sufficient data.

Other uses

Violet willow can be used to help stabilise sand dunes. Willows support many insects including moth caterpillars. Used in making medicinal charcoal. Hybrids are suitable for fast-growing biomass production in short rotation coppice.

Sambucus nigra, Elder

A small tree with panicles of white flowers followed by blue-black berries, having many traditional uses including treatment of colds and influenza.

SCIENTIFIC NAME *Sambucus nigra* L.
FAMILY Adoxaceae (previously Caprifoliaceae)
ALTERNATE NAMES Black elder, European elder
PARTS USED Flowers and fruit

Description

Elder is a large fast-growing shrub, reaching 6m tall by 4m wide, with branching canes arising from the base and growing almost 2m in a year. Older plants become more tree-like. The pinnate leaves appear in early spring, and white flowers emerge in flat inflorescences in May and June and are pollinated by flies. Elder is hermaphrodite, with both sexes on the same plant. The black-purple fruits ripen in September.

Habitat

Native to Europe, northern Africa, and western and central Asia, found in moist hedgerows, roadsides, wasteland.

Related plants

Red elder (*S. racemosa*) and American elder (*S. canadensis*) are North American species, the latter often planted in Europe for flower and fruit production. Dwarf elder (*S. ebulus*) grows to 1.5m. Varieties of elder can be obtained which are prolific in flowers or fruit, and levels of polyphenols can vary in different cultivars. Although the commonest cultivar planted in Europe for fruit is 'Haschberg' and is rich in organic acids, the 'Rubini' cultivar of *S. nigra* was found to contain the highest amount of anthocyanins.[273]

Cultivation and harvest

Cultivation

Hardy to USDA zone 5 (UK zone 5), the elder is vigorous and can grow fast in most soils, in full sunlight or in light shade (though fruiting is poor in shade). Elder will grow in very chalky sites and can tolerate atmospheric pollution. It prefers moist soil. Drought can cause damage to elder

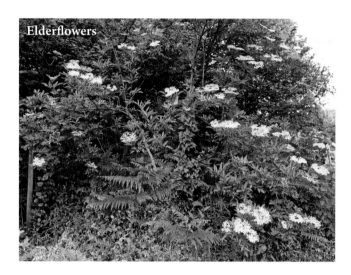

Elderflowers

trees so minimise this with mulching. Canes are short-lived, and pruning is needed to cut out old, dead or broken canes from branches, ideally leaving canes with ages ranging from 1-3 years. Alternatively, the elder can be coppiced, and cut back to ground level on a three-year cycle; fruit will be produced in the second and third years.

Pests and diseases

Resistant to honey fungus, though can be troubled with blackfly, red spider mite and verticillium wilt.

Propagation

Fresh seed is sown in a cold frame in autumn, and should germinate in early spring. Stored seed should be given two months' warm followed by two months' cold stratification. Prick out the seedlings into individual pots when they are large enough to handle. If good growth is made, the young plants can be placed in their permanent positions during the early summer. Otherwise, plant them

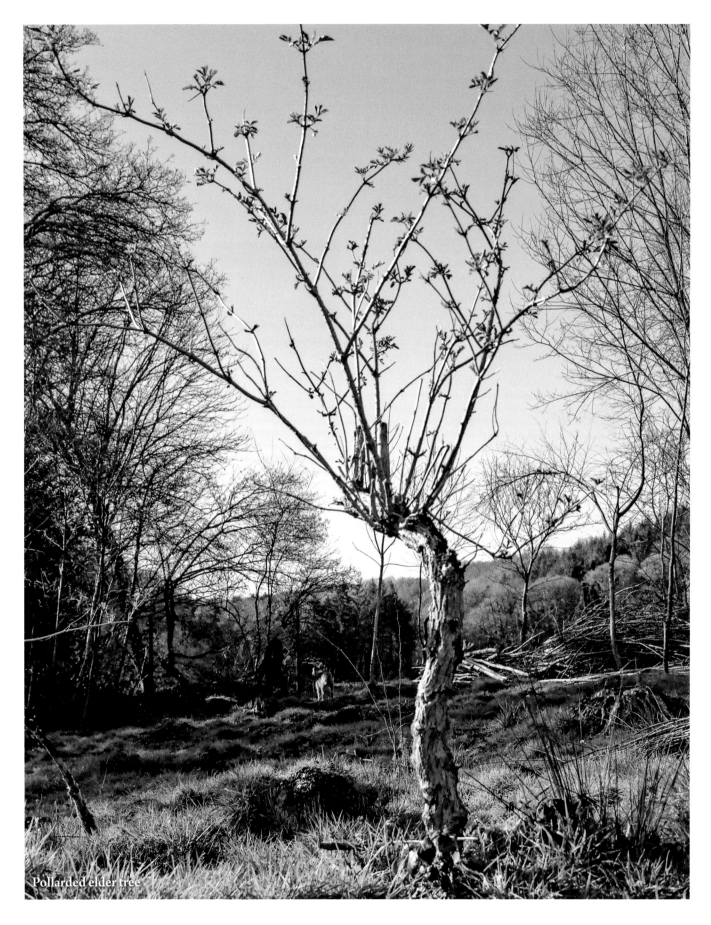

Pollarded elder tree

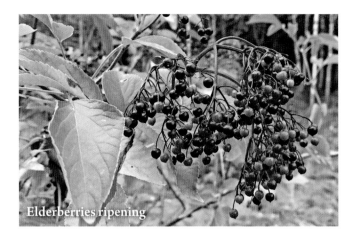
Elderberries ripening

out in spring of the following year. Cuttings of half-ripe wood, 7-10cm with a heel, can be taken in July/August. Or take 25-30cm cuttings of living canes from the previous season and plant in the ground with the top bud exposed, firm soil around, water occasionally and transplant the following spring. Division of suckers in the dormant season.

Harvesting

Flowers are harvested when open, removed from the stalks with a fork and can be dried for later use. The fruit is harvested when ripe and can be used fresh or dried for later use. If the fruit is frozen then it will readily fall off the stalks, and 3kg or more of fruit per bush may be harvested in the second year, depending on the cultivar.

Therapeutic use

Traditional

The elder tree is much associated with folklore, and has a long history of use in Europe, particularly as a purgative and emetic in driving secretions from the body. The purgative bark was used as a cure-all, and the leaves for making an ointment. Traditional uses include treatment of conjunctivitis, constipation, diabetes, diarrhoea, dry skin, headache and rheumatism.

Medicinal actions and uses

Elderflowers are anti-inflammatory, diaphoretic, diuretic, expectorant, anti-oxidant, anticatarrhal, antibacterial, antiviral and laxative.[274] The flowers can be used as a diaphoretic for fever and chills, for symptomatic treatment of the common cold[275] and as an expectorant

for inflammation of the upper respiratory tract.

Clinical applications and research

Elder fruit syrup and juice are popular for treating colds and influenza, leading to a reduction in upper respiratory symptoms.[276] One study showed that elderberry extract significantly reduced duration and severity of cold symptoms in air travellers.[277] Antiviral properties have been shown for the fruit of elder though more research is needed.

Sample preparations and dosage

Elderflowers can be used fresh in infusion, 1 tsp to a cup three times daily for respiratory complaints and hayfever. The flowers can be infused in vinegar. Elderberry tincture is taken from 5-25ml per day. Elderberries can be made into a syrup, used at 2 tsp up to four times daily.

Constituents and commerce

Key constituents

The flowers contain flavonoids (kaempferol, astagalin, quercetin, rutin, isoquercitrin, hyperoside), as well as triterpenes, sterols, phenolic acids and glycosides.[278] Elder fruits contain flavonoid glycosides (hyperoside, isoquercitrin, rutin) and anthocyanin glycosides (chrysanthemin, sambucin, sambucyanain). Toxic alkaloids (sambucine and conicine) and cyanogenic glycosides (sambunigrin) are mainly found in the bark, leaves and stems.

Commerce

Elder is widely cultivated in Europe and preparations of elderberry such as Sambucol are sold over the counter for relief of flu symptoms.

Safety

Although there is safe and longstanding use in many cultures, it is advised to avoid elder preparations in pregnancy or breastfeeding. Avoid consumption of uncooked or unripe berries, leaves, bark or stem due to alkaloid and cyanogenic glycoside content.

Other uses

Nesting for many birds. Wine making. Hedging.

Thuja occidentalis, Arbor vitae

An evergreen conifer from North America with aromatic foliage, traditionally prized for purification and having antiseptic and antiviral properties.

SCIENTIFIC NAME   *Thuja occidentalis* L.

FAMILY   Cupressaceae

ALTERNATE NAMES   American white cedar, tree of life

PARTS USED   Leafy twigs

Description

Arbor vitae is an evergreen tree growing to 15m tall by 5m wide, possibly taller in damp nutrient-rich soils. It is monoecious with male and female flowers growing on the same plant and is wind pollinated. It has flat scale-like leaves and small cones. On older trees the bark sheds in long ragged strips.

Habitat

Indigenous to eastern North America, growing in moist and rocky soils. It is widely cultivated as an ornamental or hedging plant.

Related plants

Western red cedar (*T. plicata*) is used to produce an essential oil for insect repellent and topical cosmetic uses.[279] There are ornamental arbor vitae varieties, including 'Smaragd' or 'Emerald Green', a semi-dwarf compact shrub to 4m spreading to 1m. An Asian species of the cypress family, *Platycladus orientalis* (previously known as *T. orientalis*), is used in traditional Chinese medicine.

Cultivation and harvest

Cultivation

Arbor vitae is hardy to USDA zones 3 (UK zone 2) and will grow in full sun to part shade. It can be grown on most soils, and grows best in moist well-drained soils. Arbor vitae can be used to form a hedge as it is tolerant of regular trimming. Whole branches can be harvested close to the main stem.

Pests and diseases

The young leaves are eaten by deer.

Propagation

Fresh ripe seed is sown in the autumn in a cold frame. Stored seed germinates best if given a short period of cold stratification. When they are large enough to handle, prick the seedlings out into individual pots and grow them on in the greenhouse for their first winter. Plant out into their permanent positions in late spring or early summer, after the last frosts. Cuttings of half-ripe wood, 5-8cm with a heel, can be taken in July/August in a shaded frame, and overwintered in a frame. Cuttings of almost ripe wood, 5-10cm with a heel in September.

Harvesting

The leafy young twigs can be harvested in spring and used fresh in infusion or dried for later use. An essential oil can be distilled from the leafy twigs.

Therapeutic use

Traditional

Traditionally, arbor vitae was considered purifying and used by Native Americans for colds, fever, cough, headache, skin disorders, swollen extremities and rheumatic problems.[280]

Medicinal actions and uses

Antimicrobial, antiviral, anti-inflammatory, diaphoretic, diuretic, emmenagogue, immunostimulant and laxative. The essential oil is antiseptic, expectorant and rubefacient.

A tea of the leaves has been used internally for respiratory problems, and externally as a wash for swollen feet or burns. The tincture has been used to treat fungal skin infections and warts. The powdered leaves can be used as an insect repellent.

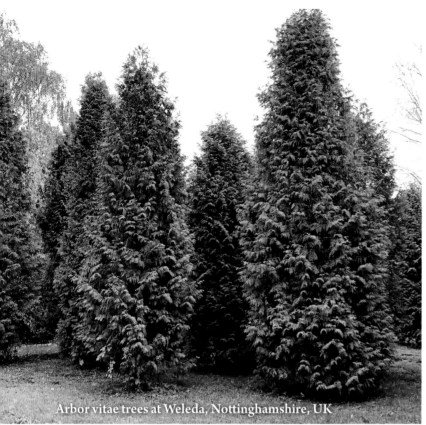
Arbor vitae trees at Weleda, Nottinghamshire, UK

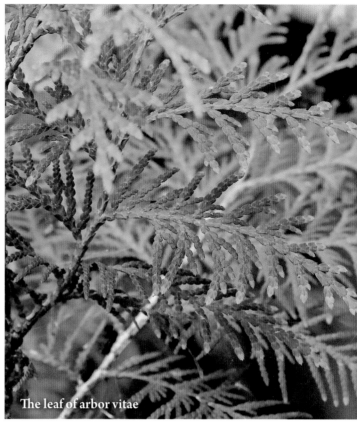
The leaf of arbor vitae

Clinical applications and research

Limited studies have been carried out. Arbor vitae is part of a herbal product, Esberitox, used in viral upper respiratory tract infection, supported by randomised controlled trials for reducing common cold symptoms.[281] Thujone, a toxic constituent of the essential oil, has been investigated for possibilities of use against brain tumour cells.[282]

Preparations and dosage

The leaf can be infused in oil for external use in skin complaints such as warts. Arbor vitae leaf tincture, which is high in alcohol (90%), contains significant amounts of thujone, and is only for external use. A tincture with a lower proportion of alcohol (30%) is safer for internal use, 1-2ml three times per day.[283]

Constituents and commerce

Key constituents

Fresh leaves contain essential oils (1-4%), sugars, polysaccharides, minerals and are high in vitamin C.

The essential oil contains monoterpenes including thujone, isothujone, fenchone, sabines and pinenes.

Commerce

Esberitox is promoted for the common cold and contains arbor vitae, purple coneflower (*Echinacea purpurea* and *E. pallida*) and wild indigo root (*Baptisia tinctoria*) extracts.

Safety

Not for use in pregnancy. Not for long-term use. Large doses of fresh arbor vitae leaves and twigs are irritant to the gastrointestinal tract, uterus, liver and kidney. The essential oil is not for internal use.

Other uses

Shelter belt formation and hedging. Incense smudge sticks. Disinfectant and moth repellent. Floristry wreaths. Timber.

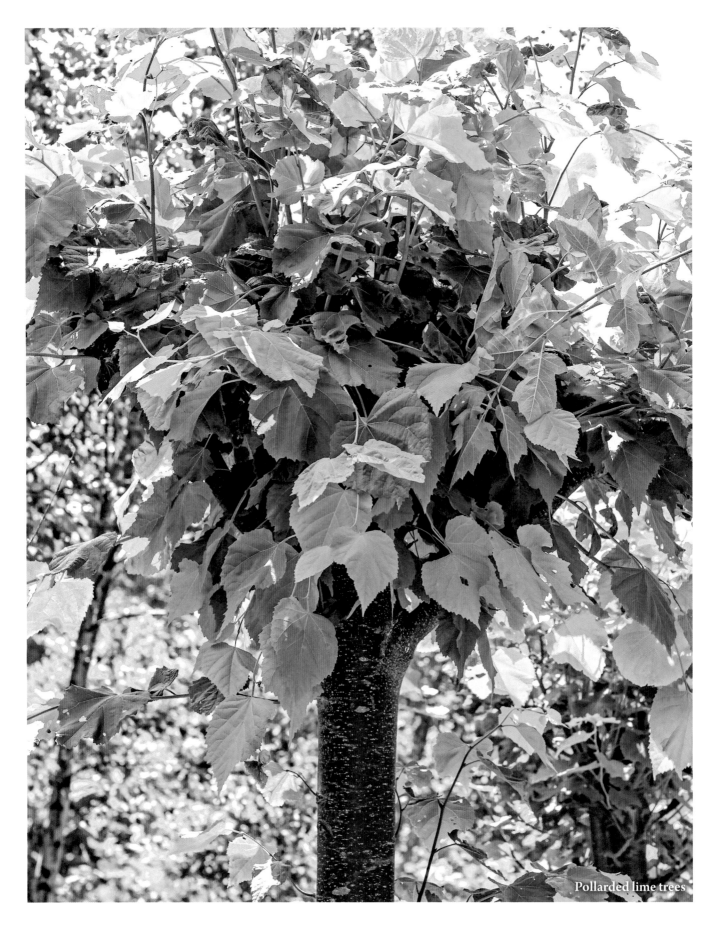
Pollarded lime trees

Tilia cordata, Small-leaved lime

A handsome medium to large tree with edible leaves and honey-scented flowers providing gentle sedative action and circulatory support.

SCIENTIFIC NAME   *Tilia cordata* Mill.

FAMILY   Malvaceae

ALTERNATE NAMES   Linden

PARTS USED   Flowers and leaves

Description

The small-leaved lime is a medium to large deciduous tree growing to 30m by 12m at a fast rate. Heart-shaped green leaves have toothed margins. It flowers in June-July and the yellowish-green fragrant flowers are borne in clusters. The flowers are hermaphrodite and pollinated by bees.

Habitat

The small-leaved lime is native throughout Europe.

Related plants

Flowers are also obtained from the large-leaved lime (*T. platyphyllos*). Lime trees hybridise freely and the common lime (*Tilia × europea*) is a hybrid of *T. cordata* and *T. platyphyllos* suitable for poorer soils. *Tilia × europea* is vigorous and readily produces suckers at the base. In the US, basswood (*T. americana*) can be harvested for flowers and leaves.

Cultivation and harvest

Cultivation

Lime is hardy to USDA zone 3 (UK zone 3). The small-leaved lime will grow in a range of soils though it prefers moist well-drained soil that is somewhat alkaline. It can grow in semi-shade and tolerates strong winds. This tree produces heavy shade. Lime can be readily coppiced or pollarded. Traditional pleaching involves pruning lime trees alongside each other to form a raised hedge. Trees begin flowering from 15-20 years of age.

Pests and diseases

The leaves can be infested with aphids which produce a sticky honey dew. Resistant to honey fungus.

Propagation

Fresh seed should be sown immediately in a cold frame before the seed coat hardens. It may germinate in the following spring though it could take 18 months. Stored seed is stratified for five months at high temperatures (10°C (50°F) at night, up to 30°C (86°F) by day) followed by five months' cold stratification in a refrigerator. When they are large enough to handle, prick the seedlings out into individual pots and grow them on in the greenhouse for their first winter. Plant them out into their permanent positions in late spring or early summer, after the last frosts. Layering in spring, just before the leaves unfurl, takes 1-3 years. Suckers, when formed, can be removed with as much root as possible during the dormant season and replanted immediately.

Harvesting

Collect the clusters of lime flowers when some of them are open (recognisable with their stamens), while others may still be closed, including the small leaves or bracts on the flowers. Hang in bunches to dry. Lime flowers are said to develop narcotic properties as they age and so they should only be harvested when young. Take care when harvesting as the nectar-rich flowers are attractive to bees.

Therapeutic use

Traditional

Lime flowers have traditionally been used widely in Europe,[284] especially as a diaphoretic to promote perspiration. They have been used for a soothing tea and as a mild sedative to treat headaches and in insomnia and epilepsy. The leaves are mucilaginous and were used in poultices.

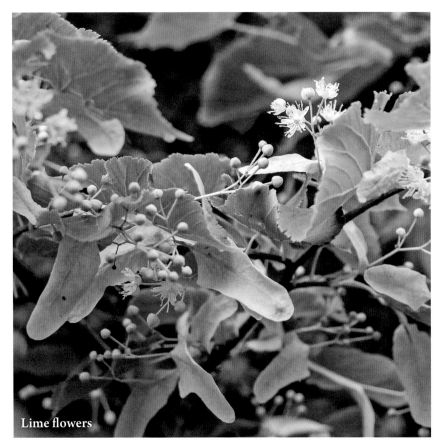
Lime flowers

Medicinal actions and uses

Lime flowers are antispasmodic, diaphoretic, diuretic, sedative and vasodilatory. The leaves are demulcent and anti-oxidant. Lime flowers are a popular domestic remedy for colds and catarrhal ailments. Lime flower tea is also used in the treatment of hypertension, hardening of the arteries, indigestion and nervous complaints.[285]

Clinical applications and research

Little significant clinical research has been carried out and lime flower use is based on tradition and knowledge of the constituents. The sedative activity of the flowers is probably due to flavonoid derivatives of quercetin and kaempherol.[286] The anti-inflammatory effects of procyanidins in the flowers have been identified to support the traditional use of lime flowers in treating colds and sore throats.[287] Both the flowers and leaves have been found to be rich in anti-oxidant polyphenols[288] supporting further use in neurological degeneration related to oxidative stress such as Parkinson's disease and Alzheimer's disease.

Sample preparations and dosage

Herbal tea daily dose of 3-6g dried flowers, or use around five fresh blossoms for a cup of tea and infuse for five minutes. Tincture of limeflowers dose of 1-3ml three times daily.

Constituents and commerce

Key constituents

Lime flowers contain 1% flavonoids (particularly heterosides with quercetin and with kaempferol) alongside polysaccharides, condensed tannins, phenylcarboxylic acids, amino acids, saponins, volatile oils and proanthocyanidins. Farnesol, a sesquiterpene, is considered to be a significant constituent of the flowers, having antispasmodic properties.

Commerce

The European Medicines Agency acknowledges well-established use of lime flowers (*T. cordata* and *T. platyphyllus*) for relief of symptoms of the common cold and mental stress. Lime flowers are widely available in teabags or sold whole loose for infusions throughout Europe and the US. Harvesting takes place in Bulgaria, Romania, Turkey, and other parts of Eastern Europe as well as China.

Safety

Lime flower preparations are generally regarded as safe. However, if the flowers are harvested when too old they may produce symptoms of intoxication.

Other uses

Wildlife plant especially for bees. Edible buds and leaves. Hedge or shelterbelt.

Vaccinium myrtillus, Bilberry

A deciduous low-growing shrub with leaves and edible fruit providing a rich source of anthocyanins beneficial for circulation, visual and urinary complaints.

SCIENTIFIC NAME *Vaccinium myrtillus* L.

FAMILY Ericaceae

ALTERNATE NAMES European blueberry, whortleberry, blaeberry, whinberry

PARTS USED Fruit and leaves

Description

Bilberry is a low-growing deciduous shrub reaching a height of 0.5m and width of 0.3m. Flowering is from April to June with small, dark blue fruits ripening July to September. The plant is hermaphrodite and pollinated by insects.

Habitat

Bilberry is found in Europe on heaths, moors and in coniferous woods from southern Iceland to Spain, extending as far as northern Asia.

Related plants

A number of related plants have similar actions including the evergreen lingonberry (*V. vitis-idaea*) particularly found in Scandinavian countries and cranberry (*V. macrocarpon*) native to the US.[289]

Cultivation and harvest

Cultivation

Hardy to USDA zone 3 (UK zone 3). This plant prefers well-drained soils and must have lime-free (pH 4.5-6)

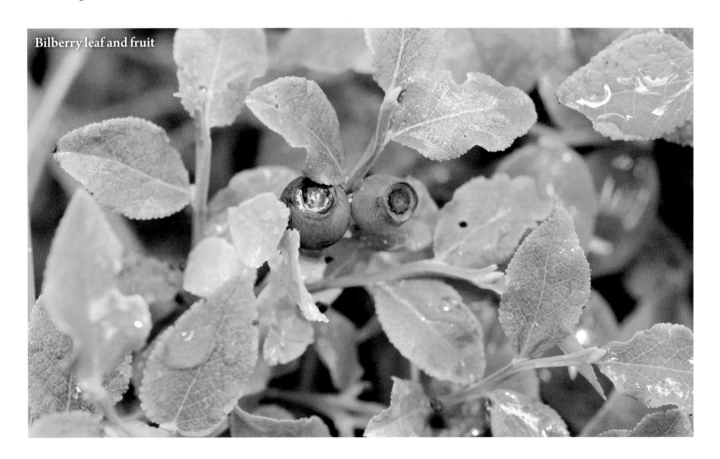

Bilberry leaf and fruit

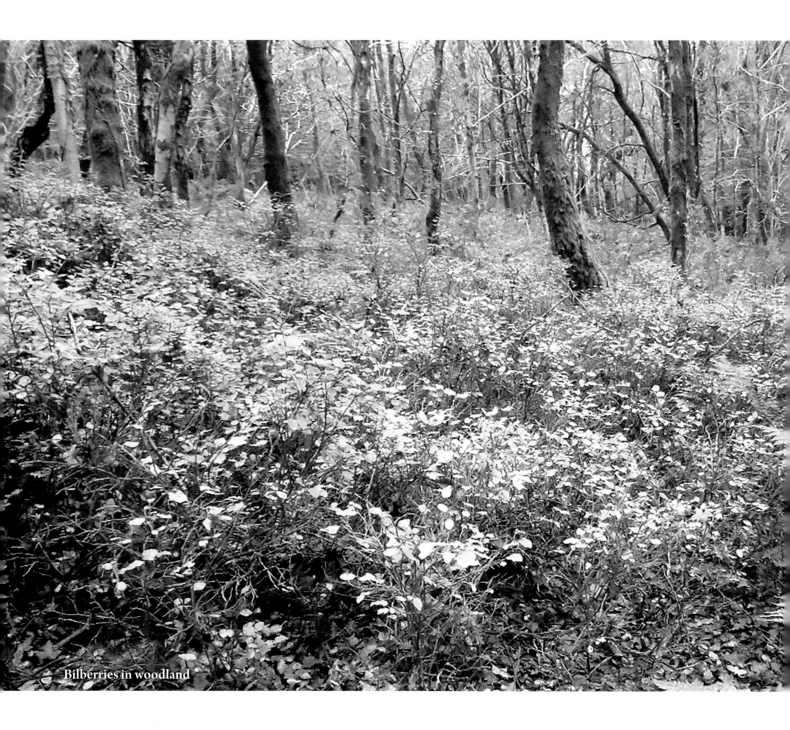

Bilberries in woodland

soil. It can grow in semi-shade, though fruits better in a sunny position, and it tolerates strong winds. Bilberry dislikes root disturbance so is best grown in a pot until planting in a permanent position. It is a freely suckering shrub which tolerates some grazing and quickly regenerates after being burnt.

Pests and diseases
Resistant to honey fungus.

Propagation
Seed can be sown late winter in a greenhouse in a lime-free potting mix and lightly covered. Stored seed needs three months' cold stratification. Once they are about 5cm tall, prick the seedlings out into individual pots and grow them on in a lightly shaded position in the greenhouse for at least their first winter. Plant them out into their permanent positions in late spring or early

summer. Cuttings of half-ripe wood, 5-8cm with a heel, can be taken in August, but are slow to root. Cuttings of mature wood can be taken in late autumn. Division of suckers in spring or early autumn. Layering can take 18 months.

Harvesting

Fruits are harvested when ripe and blue-black in August or September and can be used fresh, frozen or dried. The green leaves can be harvested in early summer (June) and dried for later use.

Therapeutic use

Traditional

Bilberry fruits have been widely used for many centuries as remedies for a range of complaints, from urinary conditions to dysentery and diarrhoea. The leaves have also been used in a decoction as a wash for ulcers and eczema.

Medicinal actions and uses

Both fruit and leaves are highly anti-oxidant, antitumour, anti-inflammatory, antimicrobial and hypoglycaemic. The leaves are antiseptic, astringent, diuretic and tonic and can be used in diarrhoea and urinary complaints. The fresh fruit can be used to benefit peripheral circulatory disorders in the legs and elsewhere.

Clinical applications and research

The fruit can be used in eye complaints; a study of a preparation based on fresh frozen bilberries (Mirtoselect), showed significant improvement of symptoms in cases of dry eye, including volume of tear secretion.[290] Antimicrobial effects have also been shown. The leaf extract was found effective against *Staphylococcus aureus*, including the methicillin-resistant *S. aureus* (MRSA).[291] Antimicrobial effects are evident in the action of extracts against *Salmonella* species, and growth inhibition of gram-positive organisms such as *Bacillus* and *Clostridium*.[292] Bilberry juice, like cranberry juice, inhibits adhesion of *Streptococcus pneumoniae* to human bronchial cells.[293] The anti-oxidant effects of anthocyanins which are found in bilberry fruits and leaves are thought to benefit a number of cardiovascular conditions.[294] A randomised clinical trial for patients after a heart attack showed

that eight weeks of bilberry extract (equivalent to 480g fresh daily) significantly improved walking distance and blood fats.[295] However, further research is needed into the association of anthocyanins with reduction in risks of developing cardiovascular disease and type 2 diabetes.[296]

Sample preparations and dosage

Take bilberry leaves, 5-10g in infusion daily. Bilberry leaf tincture (66% alcohol) is given at 2-4ml twice daily. Dried bilberry fruits can taken at 20-60g per day, fresh fruits may be juiced.

Constituents and commerce

Key constituents

Bilberry fruit contains a variety of phenolic compounds, including flavonols (quercetin, catechins) and anthocyanins (delphinidins and cyanidins) in addition to tannins, ellagitannins and phenolic acids. Bilberry leaves contain similar amounts of phenols (including hydroxycinnamic and hydroxybenzoic acids).

Commerce

Frozen bilberries are widely available, sourced from Eastern Europe and Scandinavia, and sold as a popular herbal supplement. Commercial bilberry extracts may be standardised to 25% anthocyanidin content (equivalent to 36% anthocyanins).[297] However, when commercial bilberry extracts were analysed in a research study, many were found to contain a lower anthocyanin content than that declared, and were adulterated with mulberry and chokeberry.[298]

Safety

The leaves should not be used medicinally for more than three weeks at a time. Avoid in pregnancy or breast-feeding. No adverse effects have been reported from fruit consumption. However, anticoagulant effects suggest caution in use in cases of bleeding disorders.

Other uses

Green dye plant. Edible fruit. Flavouring for conserves, wine and spirits.

Viburnum opulus, Cramp bark

A vigorous shrub or small tree, with showy white flowers, having stem bark with antispasmodic properties useful in painful periods, and other cramps and colicky pains.

SCIENTIFIC NAME   *Viburnum opulus* L.

FAMILY   Adoxaceae (previously called Caprifoliaceae)

ALTERNATE NAMES   Water or swamp elder, snowball tree, guelder rose, European cranberry

PARTS USED   Bark

Description

Cramp bark is a deciduous shrub growing fast up to 3-5m tall and 2-3m wide with grey hairless angled twigs and scaly buds. The opposite leaves are palmately lobed. The flowers open in June-July in flat umbel-like clusters. Globular shiny red fruits ripen in September-October and are intensely bitter. The main stems have terminal flower buds and new growth made by the side branches gives a bushy form. Cramp bark has rich autumn colours as the leaves turn red or yellow in autumn.

Habitat

Cramp bark is a shrub found in damp hedgerows, woodlands, fens and scrubland throughout most of Europe and north and west Asia.

Related plants

V. opulus var. 'Compactum' is worth considering in smaller gardens as it has a more compact habit. *V. opulus* var. 'Sterile' or 'Roseum' has globular shaped heads of sterile flowers, much planted in gardens as an ornamental. This is the original Guelder rose first cultivated near Guelders in Holland. The wayfaring tree (*V. lantana*) has bark which is said to have similar antispasmodic properties and grows in drier conditions. The highbush or American cranberry (*V. opulus* var. *americanum*) is found in northern US and Canada. Black haw (*V. prunifolium*) is native to dry woods in eastern and southern North America and has similar herbal uses to cramp bark.[299]

Cultivation and harvest

Cultivation

Cramp bark thrives in moist soils and will grow in both moderately acid and alkaline soils. The shrub will survive in shade although it is more productive of flowers and fruits in lighter conditions. It is hardy to USDA zone 3 (UK zone 3) and is not frost tender. Cramp bark regenerates quickly after cutting and is a good candidate for coppice production, and the plants can be closely spaced about 1-1.2m apart.

Pests and diseases

Cramp bark foliage is browsed by deer, attacked by aphids, flea beetle and caterpillars, although it will usually recover. The berries stay on the bush for some time as they are not palatable to birds.

Propagation

Gather the berries as they begin to turn red and place in a well-drained medium until late winter. Bruising the berries will help to ensure the skin and thin pulp rot away more quickly. Sow the cleaned seed in February or March outside in a cold frame. Seedlings can be transplanted the following spring and grown on for 1-2 years before planting in permanent sites. Seeds that have dried out since gathering may take longer to germinate, with 2-3 months' warm stratification (20-30°C/68-86°F) followed by cold stratification for 1-2 months (5°C/41°F). Soft summer cuttings can be placed under mist in a well-drained medium. Alternatively firmer

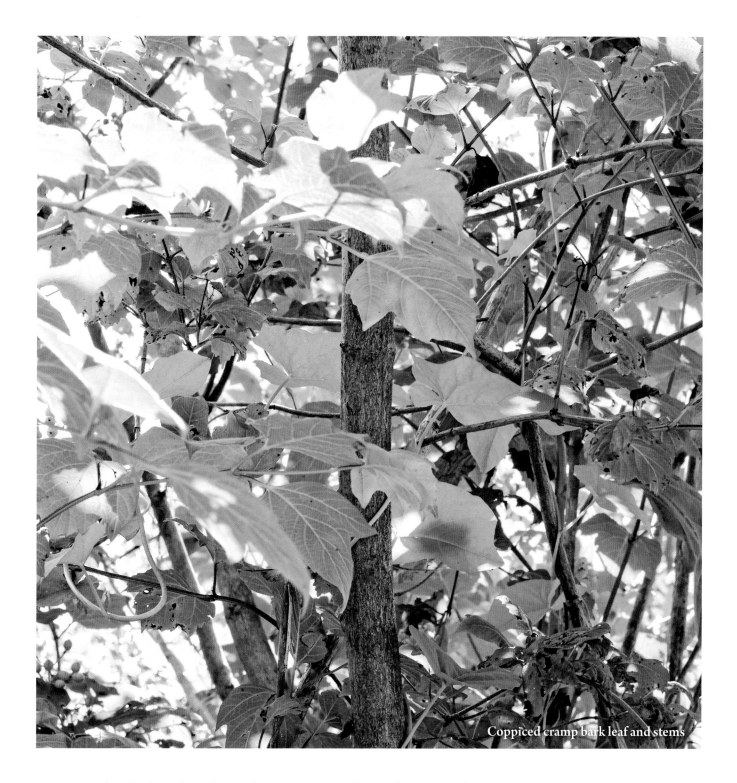
Coppiced cramp bark leaf and stems

cuttings with a heel can be taken in late summer, and rooted in soil in a cold frame. Layering is possible.

Harvesting
The bark can be harvested any time of year, but it is usually taken in spring or early summer. Can be used fresh or dried for later use.

Therapeutic use

Traditional
Cramp bark may have longstanding use, but relatively few records show this. It was mentioned by Chaucer, and John Gerard described rose elder or 'Gelders rose' in his herbal of 1597,[300] though he was unable to say

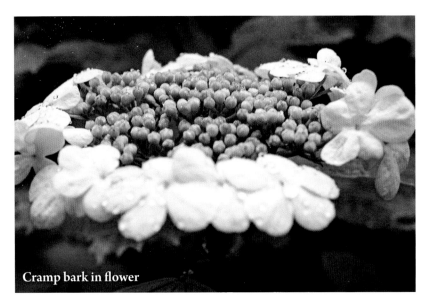
Cramp bark in flower

functional foods and one study argues for the fruits of *V. opulus* as having high anti-oxidant activity, due to the contents of flavonoids and vitamin C which were assayed at 4.89g/kg and 1.64g/kg, respectively.[305]

Sample preparations and dosage

Dried cramp bark can be taken as powder in capsules, 6-12g/day (see p.96). Cramp bark tincture dose: 3-5ml three times daily in water.

Constituents and commerce

Key constituents

Cramp bark contains viburnin (bitter glycoside), valeric and isovalerianic acids, salicin, tannins, iridoid glycosides (penstemide, patrinoside and others), coumarins (scopoletin, aesculetin), triterpenes (oleanolic and ursolic acids), hydroquinones (arbutin, methylarbutin, and traces of free hydroquinone) and resin.

Commerce

Cramp bark is sold as tablets or in tincture form. There is concern about threats from overharvesting and loss of habitat to the American species (*V. opulus* L. var. *americanum*) in its natural habitat,[306] and there is a good rationale for using alternatives such as the European variety.

Safety

There are no reported harmful effects in pregnancy or breastfeeding, and no contraindications, warnings, adverse reactions or interactions are recorded. Given the medicinal indications, it would be appropriate to seek professional advice on use where medication is already taken to lower blood pressure. The berries, although attractive, are incredibly bitter and in large quantities can produce diarrhoea, nausea and vomiting.[307]

Other uses

Dye or ink can be made from the berries. We have tried making cramp bark fruit jelly at Holt Wood but found it inedible.

what it was used for. Records show the use of *Viburnum* species in North America by Native Americans and colonists to alleviate a range of female conditions from menstrual pain to threatened miscarriage.[301]

Medicinal actions and uses

Cramp bark is antispasmodic, astringent, mildly sedative, astringent, hypotensive and a peripheral vasodilator. Any condition of spasm is likely to be helped by this bark, especially where pain arises from tension: cramps, menstrual pain, headache, muscle spasm, backache, high blood pressure, restless legs, rheumatic pain, Raynaud's syndrome and poor circulation in hands and feet. Further indications for internal use are anxiety, heavy menstrual bleeding, high blood pressure, irregular periods, insomnia and threatened miscarriage.

Clinical applications and research

Despite established use there has been limited clinical research, though a Turkish study found that patients with urinary stones given cramp bark required fewer painkillers and less additional treatment. An in vitro study found that 'viopudial' isolated from *V. opulus* had antispasmodic effects on smooth muscle.[302] Water extracts of leaf and branch of both *V. opulus* and *V. prunifolium* have anti-oxidant properties.[303] The iridoid glucosides contribute to the muscle relaxant properties.[304] Other parts of this plant deserve attention as

Vitex agnus-castus, Chaste tree

A very ornamental, slender Mediterranean shrub with fragrant foliage and flowers, historically used for women's complaints from painful periods to menopause.

SCIENTIFIC NAME   *Vitex agnus-castus* L.

FAMILY   Lamiaceae

ALTERNATE NAMES   Agnus castus, monks pepper, chasteberry

PARTS USED   Berries and leaves

Description

Chaste tree forms a medium-sized shrub, multi-branched, and grows to 3m tall by 3m wide. Chaste tree flowers in later summer bearing fragrant purplish flowers in racemes followed by dark reddish-black berries. The palmate opposite leaves are strongly aromatic.

Habitat

Chaste tree is native to southern Europe and central Asia. It has become naturalised in southern parts of the US.

Related plants

Chinese chaste tree or cut-leaf chaste tree (*V. negundo*) is hardy to USDA zones 6-9 (UK zone 8) and has similar constituents and effects.[308] It is used extensively in Asian and Chinese traditional medicine for coughs and colds and as an inhalation for sinus problems.

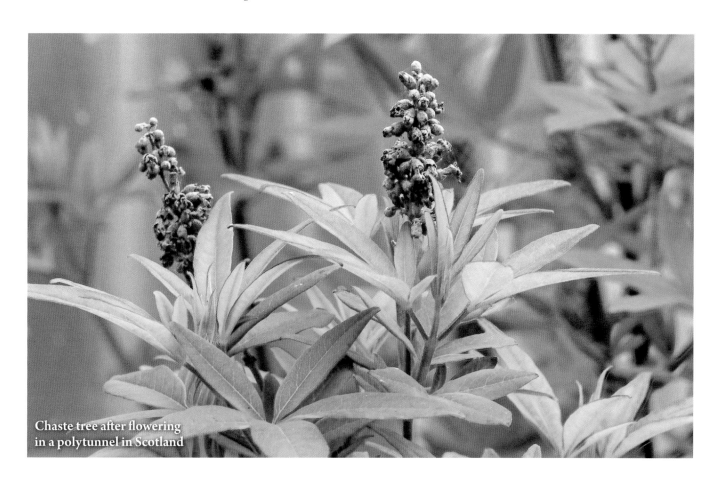

Chaste tree after flowering in a polytunnel in Scotland

Cultivation and harvest

Cultivation

Chaste tree needs full sun, good drainage and protection from cold winds. It is hardy to USDA zone 8a (UK zone 7) and cannot grow in shade. Chaste tree succeeds in dry soils and is intolerant of waterlogging. It may grow in milder locations but flowers may be produced so late in the season that seeds are not viable. If cut down by frost it may still regrow from the base. If it does flower then the old flowering shoots can be pruned in late February-March. In warmer areas chaste tree may reproduce from seed prolifically, and can be regarded as invasive.

Pests and diseases

Resistant to deer.

Propagation

Stored seeds should be scarified and soaked for 24 hours, then cold stratified for three months. Sow the seed in March indoors. Prick out the seedlings into individual pots when they are large enough to handle and grow them on in the greenhouse for their first winter. Plant them out into their permanent positions in early summer of the following year. Cuttings of half-ripe wood, 5-8cm with a heel, can be taken in July/August. Cuttings of mature wood can be taken in November and placed in a cold frame.

Harvesting

Chaste tree leaves can be harvested before flowering gets under way and used fresh or dried for later use. Berries are harvested when ripe and can be used fresh or dried.

Therapeutic use

Traditional

Chaste tree has been used for thousands of years for its beneficial effect on women's complaints including menstrual irregularities and lack of milk production. It has also been used by men to suppress libido and treat acne. Traditionally, both the leaves and fruits were used.

Medicinal actions and uses

Chaste tree leaf is anti-inflammatory, antibacterial, expectorant, digestive, tonic and antifungal. Chaste tree fruit has an ability to normalise a hormonal imbalance of oestrogen and progesterone. Thus it has been used in restoring absent menstruation, regulating heavy periods, restoring fertility after the pill, relieving premenstrual tension and easing the change of the menopause.[309] Other uses include: reduction of flatulence, suppression of appetite and induction of sleep. Sometimes the effects of chaste tree appear slowly, taking 2-3 months to develop, and are contradictory, for example, it is variously claimed to increase or reduce breastmilk, and it is likely that the level of dosage is important in determining the effects. Low doses increase prolactin levels and high doses decrease prolactin levels, increasing and decreasing breastmilk respectively.

Clinical applications and research

Extracts of chasteberry leaf were found to be antifungal in a study based on *Candida albicans*.[310] However, most modern research has focused on the fruits and women's conditions. Systematic reviews have been carried out of randomised, controlled trials investigating use of chaste tree seeds.[311] Despite some methodological limitations, the results from randomised, controlled trials to date suggest benefits for chaste tree seed extracts in the treatment of premenstrual problems and hyperprolactinaemia. Further research has been recommended.[312]

Sample preparations and dosage

Tincture of chaste tree berries, typically 0.5-1ml, is usually taken once a day in the morning. Tincture of chaste tree leaves can be taken 2-3ml three times daily. An infusion of leaves can be drunk as a tea or used as an inhalation or as a mouthwash for toothache.

Constituents and commerce

Key constituents

Chaste tree contains flavonoids (casticin, orientin, apigenin and penduletin), iridoids, alkaloids (viticin) and diterpenes.[313] The leaves contain lesser quantities of significant constituents than the berries.

Commerce

Commercial products of chaste tree are standardised to the content of the flavonoid casticin and contain a minimum of 0.08% in dried ripe fruit and powdered extracts.

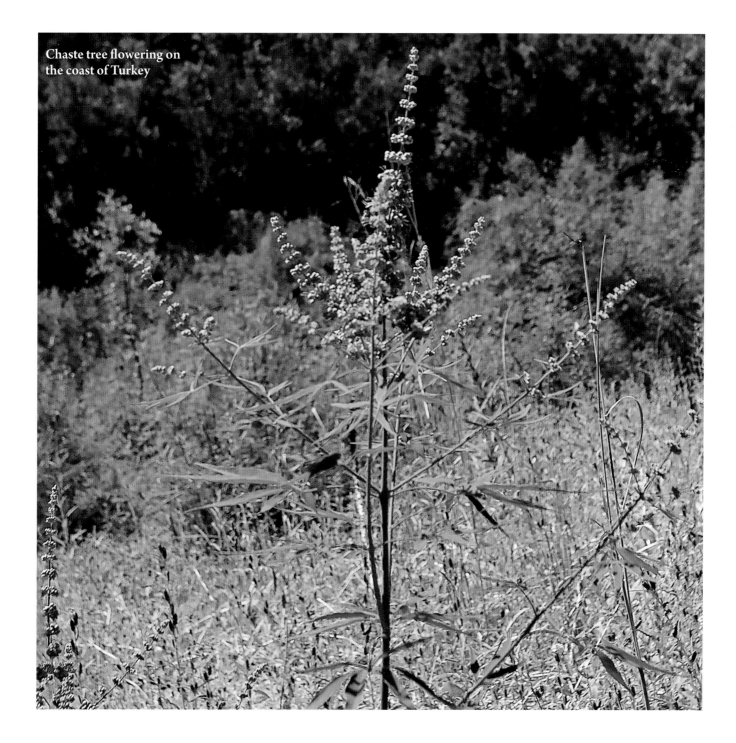

Chaste tree flowering on the coast of Turkey

Safety

Side effects reported are mild such as digestive upset, headache and itching and these effects cease on stopping intake of chaste tree. Chaste tree is not recommended during pregnancy and could inhibit milk production. Medical advice should be sought if taken alongside medications such as bromocriptine, apomorphine, some antipsychotics and some antiemetics.

Other uses

Attracts butterflies. Ornamental flowers can be dried. The bendy canes can be used as basket weaving material. Insect and mosquito repellent.

Zanthoxylum americanum, Prickly ash

A deciduous shrub from northern America with spicy leaves and berries which are used to support the circulation and immune system.

SCIENTIFIC NAME   *Zanthoxylum americanum* Mill.

FAMILY   Rutaceae

ALTERNATIVE NAMES   Northern prickly ash, common prickly ash, toothache tree

PARTS USED   Leaf, bark and fruit

Description

A deciduous shrub with pinnately compound leaves and thorny branches growing up to 4m tall and 4m wide. Prickly ash has short stout spines and pinnate leaves of 5-11 oval leaflets. All parts are pungent and aromatic. Inconspicuous flowers are produced in May-June followed by small black fruits which ripen September-October.

Habitat

The prickly ash is native to central and eastern North America. As an understorey shrub in damp woods and on riverbanks in the wild, it forms dense thickets and can grow in partial shade.

Related plants

A close relative, the southern prickly ash (*Z. clava-herculis*), has similar actions. Oriental varieties include the Chinese Szechuan pepper (*Z. bungeanum*) or Japanese pepper tree (*Z. piperitum*). A study of different species found that different habitats affected the chemical components of volatile and non-volatile oils.[314] Higher volatile oil levels in winged prickly ash (*Z. armatum*) were seen in a warmer and more arid climate.

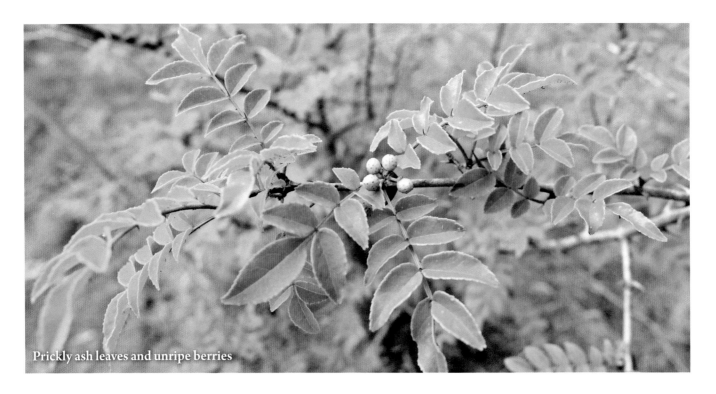

Prickly ash leaves and unripe berries

Cultivation and harvest

Cultivation

Prickly ash should be planted in well-drained soil that does not dry out. It does well in rocky, calcareous soils. It can grow in sun or on a woodland edge. It does not need frost protection, being hardy to USDA zone 4 (UK zone 3). It is fairly slow growing, at Holt Wood we manage this bush somewhat like a gooseberry bush, each year cutting out crossing branches and aiming for an open goblet kind of shape. For berry production, some advisers say that both male and female plants are needed.

Pests and diseases

Not troubled by insects or diseases, though may need protection from slugs and voles when young.

Propagation

Scarify and soak seed in hot tap water, leaving to stand 24 hours, then cold stratify for four months or sow outside in autumn for spring germination, and keep moist. Germination may be slow, and plants should be kept in a cold frame for the first winter. Cuttings of half-ripe wood may be taken in July/August and rooted in pots in a cold frame. Suckers with roots may also be potted up.

Harvesting

Leaf and bark can be harvested in spring when pruning and berries are harvested when ripe in the autumn. Take care when harvesting as the branches and twigs are thorny.

Therapeutic use

Traditional

Members of the *Zanthoxylum* family can be found in both temperate and tropical climates, and have long been used for the aromatic spicy foliage, bark and seeds which stimulate secretions. In traditional Chinese medicine the prickly ash treats cold and dampness. In Nigeria the root of Senegal prickly ash (*Z. zanthoxyloides*) is used as a chewing stick. The description of 'toothache tree' in North American usage probably arises from the numbing and tingling sensation experienced when chewing a leaf or seed.

Medicinal actions and uses

Prickly ash actions are carminative, diuretic, diaphoretic, circulatory stimulant, sialogogue, antibacterial, antiviral and antifungal.[315] Prickly ash is used mainly in Western herbal medicine for its circulatory stimulant properties, in complaints such as leg cramps and rheumatism.

Clinical applications and research

Some research studies have been carried out, showing anti-inflammatory, antifungal, antiviral and antibacterial effects of various parts of the plant and the distilled essential oil.[316] More recent studies suggest that *Zanthoxylum* species may have a role to play in anti-cancer drug development.[317]

Sample preparations and dosage

Fresh young leaves and twigs can be used to make a tincture to be given 2-5ml three times daily. The bark can also be used in this way. The bark and berries can be dried and then powdered for capsules. Where increased digestive activity is needed the tincture can be given as 20 drops in hot water, or 1-3g of bark as a decoction three times daily.

Constituents and commerce

Key constituents

Prickly ash contains terpenoid essential oils, flavonoids, isoquinoline alkaloids (lauriflorine and nitidine), alkylamides, coumarins, resins and tannins.

Commerce

Prickly ash is accepted as a natural food flavouring source by the Council of Europe.

Safety

The safety of use of prickly ash in pregnancy has not been established, and it should be avoided due to the alkaloid content. Avoid in conditions with gastrointestinal reflux or ulcers.

Other uses

A culinary spice, the berries are used like pepper.

APPENDIX 1

Useful conversion measures

	Imperial	Metric
Length	1 inch = 2.54cm	1cm = 0.39 inches
	1 foot = 30.48cm	30cm = 11.8 inches
	1 yard = 91.44cm	100cm = 39 inches
Area	1 acre = 0.4 hectares	1 hectare = 2.47 acres
Temperature	-10°C = 14°F	0°F = -18°C
	0°C = 32°F	
	30°C = 86°F	
	40°C = 104°F	212°F = 100°C
Volume	1 fluid ounce = 28.4ml	1ml = approx 20 drops
	1 pint = 568.2ml	5ml = approx 1 teaspoon
	1 gallon = 4.5 litres	15ml = approx 1 tablespoon
		1 litre = 1.76 pints
Weight	1 ounce = 28.4g	1g = 0.04 ounces
	1 pound = 453.6g	1kg = 2.2 pounds

APPENDIX 2

Glossary of useful terms

adaptogen	helps the body to increase stamina and respond to stress
agroecology	an ecological approach to farming with awareness of ecosystems and sustainability
agroforestry	land use system integrating trees and their harvest with agriculture
ague	historical term for illness with alternating fever and chills
alkaloids	nitrogen-containing organic compounds often affecting the nervous system
alterative	restores to normal health
alternate	leaves arranged singly at different points along a stem
analgesic	relieves pain
anodyne	relieves pain
anthelmintic	active against intestinal worms
anthocyanins	chemicals responsible for pigments giving red, blue and purple colours
anthraquinones	derivatives of anthracene and often highly coloured
anti-anaemic	helps to counteract anaemia
antibiotic	inhibits growth of, or kills, bacteria
anticatarrhal	reduces the production of phlegm
anticoagulant	reduces blood clotting
antidiabetic	prevents or alleviates diabetes
antihypertensive	counteracts hypertension
antihypoxic	increases peripheral and cerebral blood flow
anti-inflammatory	reduces heat, redness, swelling and pain
antimicrobial	destroys or inhibits multiplication of microorganisms
anti-oxidant	prevents or reduces damage due to free radicals or oxidation
antiproliferative	reduces proliferation of cancerous cells
antipsychotic	drug used in treating psychotic illness
antipyretic	prevents or alleviates fever
antiscorbutic	prevents or cures caused scurvy due to lack of vitamin C
antispasmodic	prevents or reduces spasm
antithrombotic	prevents the formation of blood clots
antitussive	suppresses coughing
anxiolytic	reduces anxiety
apical dominance	ability of a growing shoot to suppress lower buds from developing
astringent	drying effect by contracting tissues and reducing secretions
axillary	arising in the angle of a leaf or bud
benzoic acid	antifungal preservative occurring naturally in some plants
bid	Latin for 'bis in die' meaning twice a day
biochar	kind of charcoal which provides soil improvement
biomass	plant material used as fuel
biotype	individuals of the same species having different characteristics
bitter	has a stimulating effect on digestive system
cambium	thin layer of active growth just under the bark
cardioactive	can influence heart function
cardiotonic	has a tonic effect on the heart
cardiovascular	of the heart and blood vessels
carminative	relieves digestive wind or flatulence
carotenoids	plant pigments giving yellow, orange and red colours to plants
cathartic	stimulates bowel evacuation, stronger than purgative or laxative
cerebrovascular	of the blood vessels of the brain
cholagogue	increases flow of bile from the gallbladder
cognitive	relating to mental processes of thinking, learning and memory
conifer	trees or shrubs that are typically evergreen with needle-like leaves and cones

coppice	cutting stems down to the ground so that a tree or shrub sprouts from the base or stool
coumarins	chemicals which reduce coagulation of blood and are found in some plants
cultivar	a named variety often associated with breeder's rights, indicated by quotes, and usually propagated by grafting
cytokines	proteins released by the immune system that provide signals to cells
cytotoxic	kills cells and used for treatment of cancer cells
deciduous	trees which shed their leaves and have a dormant period
decoction	an extract made by boiling plant parts such as bark and roots
decongestant	decreases congestion of the sinuses
dehisce	bursting open of seed pod to eject contents
demulcent	has a soothing effect on the lining of digestive or urinary tracts
diaphoretic	increases perspiration and has a cooling effect in fevers
digestive	stimulates digestive function
dioecious	having male and female reproductive organs situated on separate plants
distillation	extraction of plant material by use of steam
diuretic	increases the flow of urine
division	splitting the roots of a perennial plant as a means of propagation
dormancy	prevents germination of seed or further growth of a plant until conditions are favourable
dropsy	a historical term for fluid accumulation likely due to failing heart function
drupe	fleshy fruit with a central seed-containing stone
eleutherosides	constituents of Siberian ginseng with anti-inflammatory and other antistress effects
emetic	causes vomiting
emmenagogue	stimulates menstruation and should be avoided in pregnancy
endocrine	relating to glands and the secretion of hormonal messengers

essential fatty acid	fatty acids which cannot be synthesised by the body such as linolenic acid
essential oil	oil obtained from plants by distillation which is often highly aromatic
ester	an organic compound made by replacing hydrogen with another organic group
expectorant	helps to bring up phlegm in the respiratory system
febrifuge	reduces body temperature in fevers
flavonoids	large class of plant pigments including flavanols and flavonols
galactagogue	increases the production of milk when breastfeeding
glycan	glycan is another term for polysaccharide
glycerin	colourless sweet liquid with emollient and laxative effects, also called glycerol
glycoside	compound of a simple sugar and another compound, common in plants
gram-positive	a staining technique used for identification of bacteria
guild	a group of plant species that support each other in beneficial ways thereby aiding self-maintenance
haemostatic	causes bleeding to stop
hepatoprotective	prevents damage to the liver
herbaceous	non-woody plants that die back to the ground in winter
hermaphrodite	refers to a flower having both male and female organs
hydrolat	another term for hydrosol
hydrosol	aromatic water extract with essential oils produced when a plant is steam distilled
hypoglycaemic	lowers blood sugar
hypolipidaemic	lowers blood fat levels
hypotensive	lowers blood pressure
inflorescence	a complete flowerhead including stem, stalk, bracts and flowers
infusion	an extract prepared by soaking plant material in hot or cold water
inhalation	preparation inhaled from a steam or spray
iridoid	a kind of monoterpenoid found in plants
ischaemic	refers to a restricted blood supply causing a shortage of oxygen

lanceolate	describes leaf with a narrow oval shape tapering to a point
latex	milky fluid found in many plants which exudes and coagulates when the plant is cut
laxative	promotes bowel movement and used in constipation
layering	propagation of a plant by fastening down a stem to form roots
lignans	a group of polyphenols in plants with anti-oxidant effects
lymphatic	relating to the lymph fluid containing white blood cells
maceration	process of extraction involving soaking of plant material in a liquid
metabolic	relating to the body processes of a living being
methanolic	dissolved in methanol
metrorrhagia	abnormal bleeding from the uterus
misting	spraying a plant with a fine cloud of water droplets
monoamine oxidase	enzyme involved in nerve transmission in the body
monoecious	both female and male flowers can be found on the same plant
monoterpenes	terpenes with two isoprene units many of which are aromatic such as limonene and pinene
mucilage	viscous substance containing poly-saccharides that is protective and soothing
mulch	material spread over or around plants to prevent weeds and/or enrich the soil
multidrug resistant bacteria	bacteria causing infections that are resistant to antibiotics
mycorrhiza	soil-dwelling fungus associated with plant roots so that each have mutually beneficial effects related to moisture and nutrition
napthaquinones	phenolic constituents in plants with antiviral and antifungal activity
narcotic	addictive substance affecting mood or behaviour
naturalise	refers to a plant that is established and can reproduce in a country where it is not native
neurodegenerative	relates to degeneration of the nervous system, especially the neurons in the brain
nitrogen-fixing	draws nitrogen from the air
oedema	excess of swelling due to watery fluid accumulation
overstorey	the uppermost canopy formed by the tallest trees in a forest
oxidative stress	imbalance of free radicals and anti-oxidants which leads to cell and tissue damage
oxytocic	stimulates uterine contractions and should be avoided in pregnancy
palmate	describes a compound leaf having three or more leaflets radiating from one point
parabens	a group of synthetic compounds used as preservatives
percolation	making a fluid extract using powdered herb to maximise extraction of constituents
pH	soil indicator of acidity and alkalinity indicates acidity of the soil if below neutral level of 7, or alkalinity if above
pharmacopoeia	an official publication listing pharmaceutical substances and relevant standards
phenolic acids	naturally occurring acids found in many plants especially in the seeds and skins of fruits
phenoxyethanol	a solvent chemical used widely as a preservative in body care products
phytoestrogens	naturally occurring compounds in plants with some oestrogenic effects
phytosterol	naturally occurring sterols in plants that are similar in structure to cholesterol
pinnate	describes a compound leaf with leaflets arranged on either side of a stem and often opposite each other
podophyllotoxinin	a plant extract used to stop cell division and treat viral skin complaints such as warts
pollard	cutting stem or trunk of a tree at a certain height to encourage desired growth
polyphenols	organic chemicals consisting of multiple phenol units such as tannins
polysaccharides	carbohydrates made of long chains of sugar molecules bonded together

potentiate	can increase the power of a drug or reaction
poultice	soft moist application of plant material to relieve soreness or inflammation
proanthocyanidins	polyphenols found especially in grapes, red wine and purple and black fruits
provenance	refers to the location from which a plant or its ancestors derive
purgative	stronger than a laxative and promotes bowel evacuation
purines	organic compounds often found in meats
raceme	flower cluster with flowers on stalks along the stem
radicals	reactive molecules involved in oxidative damage
resin	exudate from trees such as conifers which is often aromatic and flammable
rhizome	horizontal underground stem which can put out shoots
rootstock	stem with roots that can be used for grafting another plant in fruit tree propagation
rubefacient	used for topical application to produce irritation and increased blood flow
saponins	compounds which make foam when shaken with water and can be toxic if they get into the bloodstream
scarification	treatment of seeds to help germination, such as abrading or nicking the hard seed coat
secoiridoids	terpenoid plant compounds produced as a defence against predators or infection
secondary metabolite	organic compound produced in plants or fungi which is not directly involved in growth or reproduction
sedative	promotes calm and reduces excitability
sesquiterpenes	class of terpenes containing three isoprene units often produced by plants as a defence
sialogogue	promotes the production of saliva
softwood	in propagation refers to young pliable growth of stems suitable for cuttings
species	group of plants that can interbreed
stomachic	promotes the appetite or assists digestion
stratification	refers to seed treatment with warm or cold temperatures to overcome dormancy
sucker	a shoot springing from the base of a tree
synergy	refers to complementary constituents having a greater effect when combined than alone
tannins	class of astringent or drying polyphenolic molecules widespread in plants
temperate	climate of the middle latitudes with seasonal and moderate characteristics
terpenes	terpenoid molecules which form a large group of volatile organic compounds in plants
tid	Latin for 'ter in die' meaning three times a day
tincture	a medicinal preparation made by extracting material in ethanol and water
tonic	has a supportive and enhancing effect either for the whole body or on particular organs or systems
topical	of a preparation that is applied directly to a part of the body
triglycerides	compounds formed from glycerol and fatty acids which are the main constituents of natural fats and oils
triterpenes	class of chemical compounds with six isoprene units including steroids and saponins
umbel	flower cluster with stalks of similar length
variety	a distinct genetic individual within a species, such as an heirloom variety propagated by seed
vascular	relating to vessels, especially those that carry blood
vasoconstrictor	causes narrowing of blood vessels
vasodilator	promotes the widening of blood vessels
vermifuge	destroys worms
volatile	easily evaporates at normal temperatures
vulnerary	promotes skin repair of wounds
whip	seedling tree not yet showing side shoot growth
wind rock	caused by high winds loosening roots of unsecured trees and shrubs
woody	woody plants have hard stems with buds surviving over winter

Herbaceous medicinal plants

Common name (Latin name), family	Description	Height and habit	Site preference	Parts used	Actions and uses	Possible preparations	Precautions to note
Agrimony, (*Agrimonia eupatoria*) Rosaceae	Vulnerary herb with anti-inflammatory and diuretic properties.	Hardy perennial herb up to 60cm with spikes of small yellow flowers.	Dry thickets, hedgebanks, sides of fields. Needs sun.	Leaves harvested before flowering and dried.	Astringent gargle for sore throat, and tea for diarrhoea.	Infusion, decoction	
Angelica, (*Angelica archangelica*) Apiaceae	Aromatic tall herb traditionally used for circulatory and digestive disorders.	A European biennial plant to 1.5m.	A hardy biennial plant preferring a moist fertile soil, growing in sun or light shade.	Root and seeds. The root is harvested in the first autumn. Seeds are harvested in the second year.	Antispasmodic, carminative, diaphoretic, diuretic and tonic. Used for flatulence and indigestion, and can also help poor circulation.	Infusion, decoction	Avoid in pregnancy. Furocoumarins can increase skin sensitivity, so avoid strong sunlight.
Astragalus, (*Astragalus membranaceus*) Fabaceae	Important Chinese herb (Huang Qi) with tonic properties.	Hardy perennial plant to 0.3m high.	Sandy neutral or alkaline well-drained soil. Needs full sun.	Root. Harvest 4-year-old root in autumn for drying.	Diuretic and immune stimulant with uses in lowering blood pressure and blood sugar.	Tincture, decoction	Caution as this plant may be toxic due to glycosides.
Avens, (*Geum urbanum*) Rosaceae	A fragrant astringent herb used for mouth, throat and digestive complaints.	Hardy perennial plant to 0.5m high.	Can grow in shady woodland in moist but well-drained soil.	Root. Harvest in spring for drying.	Anti-inflammatory, antiseptic and astringent, used for digestive complaints such as diarrhoea and externally for skin spots and eruptions.	Infusion	
Bergamot, (*Monarda didyma*) Lamiaceae	An aromatic herb used for teas, particularly useful in digestive and urinary complaints.	Hardy perennial plant to 0.9m high.	Can grow in shady woodland in moist soil.	Leaves, fresh or dried.	The plant is carminative and diuretic, used for digestive complaints such as colic or urinary disorders.	Infusion	
Bistort, (*Polygonum bistorta*) Polygonaceae	A plant used in digestive and other complaints to contract tissue and staunch blood flow.	Hardy perennial plant to 0.5m high.	Can grow in sun or light shade, preferring moist acid soil.	Leaves and root. The root is gathered in early spring and dried.	Astringent and also diuretic and laxative. It is used for internal or external bleeding, diarrhoea, excessive menstruation.	Decoction of root, infusion of leaves as a wash or gargle	
Bittersweet, (*Solanum dulcamara*) Solanaceae	A scrambling climbing plant with history of use in skin and other diseases.	Hardy perennial climber to 2.5m high, found in hedgerows and moist woods.	Can grow in light shade, preferring moist soil.	Roots and 2-3-year-old stem, harvested after leaf fall and dried.	Alterative, anodyne, emetic and purgative, used in skin diseases and arthritis.	Decoction of stem or root	Not for internal use without practitioner advice due to alkaloid content.
Black cohosh, (*Actae racemosa*) Ranunculaceae	A North American woodland plant widely sold over the counter for menopausal disorders.	Hardy perennial to 1.5m high, found in deciduous moist woods.	Prefers to grow in shade, in moist rich soil.	Root, harvested in autumn and dried.	Sedative and emmenagogue, has traditional use for women's complaints including painful periods and menopause.	Dried root or root in tincture of water and alcohol	May cause liver damage so take with clinical advice, and avoid in pregnancy.

Common name (Latin name), family	Description	Height and habit	Site preference	Parts used	Actions and uses	Possible preparations	Precautions to note
Black peppermint, (*Mentha × piperita vulgaris*) Lamiaceae	Black peppermint is an aromatic herb generally considered as a herb for digestive complaints.	Black peppermint is a hardy perennial that grows to 0.5m in ditches and wasteground.	Grows in moist fertile soil, in sun or part shade. Roots can be invasive.	Leaves and stems harvested before flowers open, fresh or dried.	Antiseptic, antispasmodic, carminative, diaphoretic and tonic. Is used in digestive problems including flatulence and irritable bowel.	Infusion	Avoid in pregnancy.
Blue flag, (*Iris versicolor*) Iridaceae	An attractive blue-flowered iris with traditional use to detoxify the body.	Hardy perennial plant growing to 0.6m with spreading roots.	Can grow in sun or shade, prefers heavy rich wet soil.	Root, harvested late summer or early autumn and dried.	The root is alterative, anti-inflammatory, diuretic and strongly laxative.	Decoction, tincture	Blue flag root can cause nausea and should not be taken in pregnancy.
Bogbean, (*Menyanthes trifoliatum*) Menyanthaceae	A pond plant providing bitter and tonic effects in chronic conditions.	Hardy European perennial plant growing to 0.3m in marshy ground.	Bogbean cannot grow in shade and is a plant of the water margins.	Leaves harvested in late spring and dried for use.	Bitter, astringent, anti-inflammatory, diuretic and tonic effects, with applications in debilitated and rheumatic disorders.	Infusion, tincture	Excess can cause nausea and vomiting and should not be given if digestion is irritated.
Burdock, (*Arctium lappa*) Asteraceae	Burdock is a large-leaved plant, the root of which provides a detoxifying remedy in both Chinese and Western traditions.	Burdock is a hardy biennial that grows to 2m and is widespread in meadows, waste ground and woodlands.	Prefers moist well-drained soils and can grow in sun or light shade.	Root, harvested from one-year-old plant in mid-summer and dried.	Alterative, cholagogue, demulcent, diaphoretic, diuretic. Leaves and seeds can be used as poultices for burns and sores.	Decoction	
Cleavers, (*Galium aparine*) Rubiaceae	Cleavers is a scrambling plant which has a reputation as a lymphatic cleanser.	Cleavers is an annual and grows to 1.2m by 3m and is widespread in hedgerows and cultivated land.	Suitable for any soils and can grow in sun or light shade.	Whole plant, harvested in May or June before running to seed, and can be juiced or dried.	Alterative, diuretic, lymphatic. Used internally and externally to treat skin complaints, and as a spring tonic.	Infusion, juice	
Comfrey, (*Symphytum officinale*) Boraginaceae	Comfrey is a tallish plant which has a reputation for healing wounds.	A hardy perennial that grows to 1.2m in moist and grassy environments.	Prefers moist soils and can grow in sun or light shade.	Leaves harvested when young and before flowering. The roots are harvested in autumn. Can be dried although beware mould.	Astringent, demulcent, vulnerary and is used to treat skin complaints and wounds.	Infused oil	Comfrey contains pyrrolizidine alkaloids and should be used externally only.
Curled dock, (*Rumex crispus*) Polygonaceae	Curled dock root is used as a tonic and to promote elimination.	Hardy perennial that grows to 0.6m in moist grass and waste ground.	Prefers moist and acid soils and can grow in sun or light shade.	Root is harvested in spring and can be dried.	Alterative, astringent, laxative and tonic. Used for skin complaints and mild constipation.	Tincture	High in oxalic acid and caution advised in conditions such as arthritis and gout.
Dandelion, (*Taraxacum officinale*) Asteraceae	Dandelion is a common plant of both waste and cultivated land, and has uses in liver complaints and urinary disorders.	Dandelion is a hardy perennial to 0.5m, forming a rosette in moist grass and waste ground.	Grows anywhere though prefers moist soils and can grow in sun or light shade.	Root is harvested in autumn when two years or older, and can be used fresh or dried. Leaves can also be used.	Cholagogue, diuretic, laxative and tonic, and is used internally for gallbladder, liver and urinary disorders.	Infusion, tincture	

Common name (Latin name), family	Description	Height and habit	Site preference	Parts used	Actions and uses	Possible preparations	Precautions to note
Elecampane, (*Inula helenium*) Asteraceae	Elecampane is a tall sunflower-like plant traditionally used in respiratory ailments.	Hardy perennial that grows to 1.5m in fields and waste ground.	Prefers moist soils and can grow in sun or light shade.	Root is harvested in autumn, two years or older, and can be dried.	Antiseptic, bitter, cholagogue, diaphoretic, diuretic, expectorant and tonic, and the aromatic root can be used in coughs, bronchitis as well as digestive disorders and fungal infections.	Syrup, decoction, powder, tincture	Not for use in pregnancy, not suitable for use if allergic to the daisy family.
Feverfew, (*Tanacetum parthenium*) Asteraceae	Feverfew is a daisy-like plant traditionally used in fevers, headache and rheumatic disorders.	Hardy perennial that grows to 0.6m on rocky slopes and waste ground.	Prefers well-drained soils and can grow in sun but not in shade.	Leaves gathered as flowering begins and can be dried.	Anti-inflammatory, bitter and vaso-constrictive effects which make it useful in treatment of migraine.	Powdered dry leaf, infusion	Not for use in pregnancy, not for use if allergic to the daisy family.
Gipsywort, (*Lycopus europaeus*) Labiatae	Gypsywort is a plant of shallow water.	Hardy perennial growing to 1.0m in marshland and by rivers and streams.	A plant of the water edge which can grow in sun and in part shade.	The herb is gathered as flowering begins and can be dried.	Astringent, hypoglycaemic and sedative, and it is used in excessive menstruation and in treating hyperthyroidism.	Infusion, tincture	Not for use in pregnancy, take advice if a thyroid condition.
Globe artichoke, (*Cynara scolymus*) Asteraceae	Globe artichoke has bitter tasting leaves of value in a range of digestive disorders and diabetes.	Hardy perennial growing to 1.5m in cultivation, not known in the wild.	Prefers moist soil and can only grow in sun and not in shade.	The leaves are gathered just before flowering begins and can be used fresh or dried.	Bitter, cholagogue, diuretic, hypoglycaemic and used in chronic liver and gallbladder complaints.	Infusion, tincture	
Goat's rue, (*Galega officinalis*) Fabaceae	Goat's rue herb is a meadow plant traditionally used in fevers and infections.	A Southern European hardy perennial herb which grows to 1.2m in marshy fields and woodland.	Prefers moist soils and can grow in poor soils and in sun or light shade.	Leaves and flowering tops, harvested when coming in to flower and dried.	Diaphoretic, diuretic, galactagogue and hypoglycaemic. Used in digestive problems and to promote lactation.	Infusion, tincture	
Goldenrod, (*Solidago virgaurea*) Asteraceae	Goldenrod is a herb with many uses including digestive and urinary complaints.	Hardy perennial grows to 0.6m in grassland and dry woods.	Needs good drainage and can grow in sun or light shade.	Leaves and flowering tops, harvested in summer and dried.	Antifungal, anti-inflammatory, astringent, digestive and diuretic. Used internally in cystitis and other urinary tract disorders. Externally can be used as a mouthwash or vaginal douche.	Infusion, tincture	
Ground ivy, (*Glechoma hederacea*) Lamiaceae	Ground ivy is a ground cover herb with use in treating sinusitis and other catarrhal complaints.	Hardy perennial providing ground cover up to to 0.2m in waste ground and damp woodland edges.	Prefers moist soil and can grow in sun or light shade.	Leaves and flowering stems, harvested in May and dried.	Anticatarrhal, astringent, digestive, diuretic and tonic. Mainly used in ear, throat and chest problems due to catarrh.	Infusion, tincture	Not for use in pregnancy.
Heartsease, (*Viola tricolor*) Violaceae	Heartsease is a ground cover herb with traditional uses in treating nervous and skin complaints.	Hardy perennial plant that grows to 0.2m in waste ground and grassland.	Prefers acid or neutral soil and can grow in sun or light shade.	The herb is harvested in summer and dried.	Alterative, anti-inflammatory, diuretic, expectorant, laxative and vulnerary, and is used mainly in skin complaints such as eczema.	Infusion, tincture	

Common name (Latin name), family	Description	Height and habit	Site preference	Parts used	Actions and uses	Possible preparations	Precautions to note
Hops, (*Humulus lupulus*) Cannabinaceae	Hops have traditional uses in treating nervous and skin complaints.	A hardy perennial climbing plant which grows to 6m. Is drought tolerant.	Prefers rich soil in a sheltered position and can grow in sun or light shade.	Female cones or strobiles are harvested in summer as they start to ripen, and dried.	Bitter, antiseptic, diuretic and sedative, and used to increase digestive secretions and in sleeplessness. Also used to increase milk production in nursing mothers.	Tincture	Avoid in pregnancy.
Lady's mantle, (*Alchemilla xanthochlora*) Rosaceae	Lady's mantle is an attractive plant traditionally used in women's complaints.	Hardy perennial ground cover up to 0.3m in damp meadows and on mountain rock ledges.	Grows in most soils, in sun or light shade.	Leaves and flowering stems harvested as the plant comes into flower, and can be dried.	Alterative, astringent, diuretic and emmenagogue. Used externally and internally for excessive menstruation, vaginal discharge and wounds.	Infusion, tincture	
Lemon balm, (*Melissa officinalis*) Lamiaceae	Lemon balm is a lemon-scented plant traditionally used for its sedative and digestive properties.	Hardy perennial plant of Southern Europe growing to 0.6m in waste ground. Tolerates drought.	Grows best in moist well-drained soil, in sun or light shade.	Leaves harvested before the plant comes into flower. Can be dried or frozen for later use.	Antispasmodic, anti-inflammatory, antiviral, carminative, diuretic, relaxant. Used in dyspepsia, anxiety and sleeplessness.	Infusion, tincture	Avoid during pregnancy.
Liquorice, (*Glycyrrhiza glabra*) Fabaceae	Liquorice root has been widely used in inflammatory and respiratory complaints.	Hardy perennial that grows to 1.2m along riverbanks in Southern Europe and is a nitrogen fixer.	Grows well in deep moist free-draining soil, in sun or light shade, does not stand up to wind.	Rhizomes around the main tap root are harvested in autumn between 3–4 years old.	Anti-inflammatory, demulcent, expectorant, laxative and tonic. The root or its extract are used in many conditions from arthritis to asthma.	Decoction, tincture, powder	Encourages water retention and should be avoided in high blood pressure. Not for use in pregnancy.
Marsh mallow, (*Althaea officinalis*) Malvaceae	Marsh mallow is a tall plant with soothing demulcent properties.	A hardy perennial plant of salty marshes and ditches near the sea and grows to 1.2m.	Can grow in most soils including saline soil, in sun and light shade.	Leaves harvested when starting to flower and root harvested from 2-year-old plants, can be dried for later use.	Demulcent. Used to soothe inflammation in complaints of the digestive, urinary and respiratory systems, such as gastritis, cystitis and bronchitis.	Cold infusion, tincture, syrup	
Marigold, (*Calendula officinalis*) Asteraceae	Marigold has resinous flowers and leaves and is widely used in treating skin conditions.	A Southern European annual plant that can be found on waste and cultivated land and grows to 0.6m.	Grows in most soils, best in sun.	Flowers are harvested when fully open and before seeding. Leaves can be used fresh or dried.	Antiseptic, astringent, cholagogue, diaphoretic, stimulant and vulnerary. Used in external preparations for bites, stings, sprains, fungal infections, wounds etc.	Infusion, infused oil	
Meadowsweet, (*Filipendula ulmaria*) Rosaceae	Meadowsweet is a plant with anti-inflammatory properties due to aspirin-like constituents.	Hardy perennial found in moist meadows and wet woods and grows to 1.2m.	Prefers moist soils, growing in sun and in partial shade.	Flowers, stems and leaves harvested in summer and dried for later use.	Anodyne, antibacterial, antacid, anti-inflammatory, astringent. Is a useful treatment for hyperacidity, heartburn, gastritis and diarrhoea.	Infusion, tincture	

Common name (Latin name), family	Description	Height and habit	Site preference	Parts used	Actions and uses	Possible preparations	Precautions to note
Motherwort, (*Leonurus cardiaca*) Lamiaceae	Motherwort is an aromatic herb with traditional uses in women's complaints.	Hardy perennial of waste land and hedgebanks and grows to 1.0m.	Can grow in most soils including poor soil, preferring good drainage, in sun and in partial shade.	Flowering herb harvested in August, used fresh or dried.	Antispasmodic, astringent, bitter, emmenagogue, sedative effects. Used for nervous complaints and problems of menstruation, childbirth and menopause.	Tincture	Not for use in pregnancy or heavy periods.
Mugwort, (*Artemisia vulgaris*) Asteraceae	Mugwort is a bitter herb with traditional uses in digestive and women's complaints.	Hardy perennial that grows to 1.2m on wasteland and hedgebanks.	Can grow in most well-drained soils in sun and in partial shade.	Flowering herb is used fresh or dried.	Bitter, anthelmintic, antibacterial, antispasmodic, cholagogue, emmenagogue and laxative. Used to stimulate digestion and in dysmenorrhoea.	Tincture, powder	Not for use in pregnancy. Should not be taken for long periods.
Mullein, (*Verbascum thapsus*) Scrophulariaceae	Mullein is a tall plant used traditionally in chest complaints and treating skin wounds.	Hardy biennial tall plant up to 1.8m on waste ground.	Does best in dry soils in sun, and can grow in alkaline soils.	Leaves and flowers are harvested in summer and used fresh or dried.	Anti-inflammatory, antiseptic, demulcent, diuretic and expectorant. Used in chest complaints and to make an infused oil for ear drops.	Tincture, infused oil	Not for use internally if on anticoagulant medication.
Nettle, (*Urtica dioica*) Urticaceae	Nettle is a nourishing herb with traditional uses as a cleansing tonic and blood purifier.	Hardy perennial widely found on wasteland and in woods and grows to 1.2m.	Grows in moist fertile soil in sun and in partial shade. Can be invasive.	Leaves, root, seed. Young leaves harvested in spring before flowering and dried; caution to wear gloves as the leaves have stinging hairs.	Alterative, astringent, diuretic, galactagogue, hypoglycaemic and tonic. The leaves are used in anaemia, arthritis, skin conditions. Root and seed are used in prostate and urinary disorders.	Infusion, tincture	
Passionflower, (*Passiflora incarnata*) Passifloraceae	Passion flower is a climbing plant with sedative properties.	Grows to 6m in North American fields and thickets.	Grows best in well-drained soil, in sun or part shade and a sheltered position.	Leaves and stems harvested while growing and after some berries have matured and dried.	Antispasmodic, astringent, diaphoretic, diuretic and sedative and can be used for neuralgia, insomnia, premenstrual tension.	Infusion, tincture	Avoid in pregnancy.
Sage, (*Salvia officinalis*) Lamiaceae	Sage is an aromatic herb traditionally used as a digestive remedy.	Hardy perennial of Southern Europe that grows to 0.6m in dry stony places.	Prefers a well-drained alkaline soil, in sun and dislikes shade.	Leaves harvested before flowers open, used fresh or dried.	Antiseptic, antispasmodic, astringent, carminative, cholagogue and stimulant. Used for night sweats, excess salivation, anxiety or depression. Also a mouthwash or gargle for sore throats.	Infusion, tincture	Avoid in pregnancy. Avoid large doses or long periods of use.
Schisandra, (*Schisandra chinensis*) Schisandraceae	Schisandra is a Chinese traditional medicine remedy used for many ailments as a tonic and restorative.	A hardy deciduous plant of Northern China that grows to 9m by streams on forest edges.	A climber that grows in moist well-drained soil, in part or full shade.	Berries harvested when ripe, and dried.	Adaptogenic, adrenal tonic, anti-inflammatory, astringent, cholagogue, expectorant, hepatic, hypotensive, immune stimulant, sedative and tonic. A restorative in treating stress and nervous complaints.	Tincture	

Common name (Latin name), family	Description	Height and habit	Site preference	Parts used	Actions and uses	Possible preparations	Precautions to note
Self-heal, (*Prunella vulgaris*) Lamiaceae	Self-heal is a low-growing plant and traditionally used as a wound herb.	Hardy perennial plant of grassland and woodland edges growing to 0.2m, good ground cover.	Prefers moist soil, in sun or light shade. Will spread readily in moist ground.	Whole herb harvested midsummer, and used fresh or dried.	Alterative, antibacterial, astringent, carminative, diuretic, styptic and vulnerary. Used as a poultice for wounds, ulcers, sores. Also internal use for disorders such as diarrhoea and sore mouth.	Infusion, poultice	
Sheep's sorrel, (*Rumex acetosella*) Polygonaceae	Sheep's sorrel is a dock-like plant used as an aid to detoxification.	Hardy perennial plant of acid grassland and heaths growing to 0.3m.	Prefers moist soil, in sun or light shade. Will grow in acid soil and tolerates maritime exposure.	Leaves and root used fresh or dried.	Astringent, diaphoretic, diuretic and laxative. Used in remedies for detoxification.	Decoction, infusion	The leaves are rich in oxalic acid and large doses should be avoided.
Skullcap, (*Scutellaria lateriflora*) Lamiaceae	Skullcap is a restorative remedy used in nervous disorders.	Hardy perennial North American herb of meadows and swampy woods growing to 0.6m.	Grows best in moist soil and sun.	Leaves harvested in early summer and used fresh or dried.	Astringent, antispasmodic, diuretic, sedative and tonic. Used for anxiety, insomnia and withdrawal from tranquilisers.	Infusion, tincture	Avoid in pregnancy.
St John's wort, (*Hypericum perforatum*) Hypericaceae	St John's wort has a long tradition of use as a remedy for skin problems, more recently sold over the counter for depression.	Hardy perennial plant grows to 0.9m in open woods and hedge banks.	Prefers well-drained soil, in sun or very light shade.	Flowering tops, leaves and stems.	Analgesic, antiseptic, antidepressant, anti-inflammatory, antiviral, sedative and vulnerary. An oil infused with flowers in late summer is used for skin complaints, such as shingles. Internally, for anxiety and depression.	Infusion, tincture, infused oil	Internal use not appropriate with other medications since liver enzymes are increased.
Valerian, (*Valeriana officinalis*) Valerianaceae	Valerian is an aromatic plant of woodland with sedative effects.	Hardy perennial plant of moist woodland and grassland to 1.5m.	Prefers a rich moist soil, in light shade.	Root harvested before flowering and can be used fresh or dried.	Antispasmodic, diuretic, hypotensive, sedative due to valepotriates. Used in anxiety, insomnia, nervous tension and painful menstruation.	Powder, tincture	Avoid in pregnancy and not recommended for long-term use.
Vervain, (*Verbena officinalis*) Verbenaceae	Vervain is a wiry upright plant with traditional use for nervous disorders.	Hardy perennial plant that grows to 0.6m on wasteground, in hedgerows and walls.	Prefers a well-drained soil, growing best in sun and does not tolerate shade.	Leaves and stems harvested as flowering begins and can be used fresh or dried for later use.	Analgesic, antispasmodic, astringent, emmenagogue and tonic. Has uses in treating headache and nervous exhaustion.	Tincture	Avoid in pregnancy and breastfeeding. Avoid large doses.
White deadnettle, (*Lamium album*) Lamiaceae	White deadnettle is a herb traditionally used for women's complaints.	Hardy perennial plant that grows in woodland edges to 0.6m.	Prefers a well-drained soil, and can grow in light shade.	Flowering tops are harvested in the summer and can be used fresh or dried for later use.	Antispasmodic, astringent, diuretic, and vulnerary. White deadnettle is used in treating vaginal discharge and excessive menstrual flow, as well as urinary complaints.	Infusion	

Common name (Latin name), family	Description	Height and habit	Site preference	Parts used	Actions and uses	Possible preparations	Precautions to note
Wild carrot, (Daucus carota) Apiaceae	Wild carrot is an aromatic herb used in urinary and other complaints.	Hardy biennial that grows to 1m in both cultivated and wasteland.	Prefers a well-drained slightly alkaline soil, growing in sun or light shade.	Roots are harvested in the first autumn, sliced and dried. Whole herb can be harvested in July and dried.	Carminative, diuretic, emmenagogue and tonic. Used for stimulating the flow of urine in cystitis, kidney disorders and oedema. The root and seeds can induce uterine contractions and are used in delayed menstruation.	Infusion, decoction	Avoid in pregnancy. Contains furocoumarins which can increase skin sensitivity to light, so avoid strong sunlight if using this plant.
Wild garlic, (Allium ursinum) Alliaceae	Wild garlic is a pungent woodland herb used in promoting digestion and in respiratory complaints.	Hardy perennial and spreading ground cover plant of damp woodlands growing to 0.3m.	Needs a moist well-drained soil, growing in shade.	Root bulbs are harvested and dried. Leaves can be harvested in spring and dried.	Antibiotic, anthelmintic, antispasmodic, diaphoretic, diuretic, hypotensive and tonic. The bulbs or leaves are used to treat diarrhoea, indigestion, threadworms, and in asthma and bronchitis.	Juice, tincture	
Wood betony, (Stachys officinalis) Lamiaceae	Wood betony has traditional use for wounds and nervous complaints.	Hardy perennial that grows to 0.6m in grassland, hedgebanks and open woods.	A plant for moist well-drained soil, growing in sun or light shade.	Leaves and flowering tops can be harvested in summer and dried.	Antiseptic, astringent, carminative, diuretic, emmenagogue, sedative and tonic. Used for premenstrual complaints and nervous tension.	Infusion, tincture	
Wormwood, (Artemisia absinthum) Asteraceae	Wormwood is strongly bitter and traditionally used in digestive complaints.	Hardy perennial plant that grows in wasteland and rocks to 1m.	Prefers a well-drained soil, growing in sun or very light shade.	Leaves and flowering shoots can be harvested as the plant begins to flower, and dried.	Anthelmintic, antiseptic, antispasmodic, carminative, cholagogue, emmenagogue and stimulant. The bitter taste of the leaves is used to stimulate digestion and to ease wind and bloating.	Tincture	Avoid in pregnancy and breastfeeding. Contains thujone and only small doses should be taken.
Yarrow, (Achillea millefolium) Asteraceae	Yarrow is an anti-inflammatory herb used in many disorders.	Hardy perennial plant offering spreading groundcover on dry grassland growing to 0.6m.	Prefers well-drained poor soil, and will grow in sun or light shade. Is highly drought tolerant.	Flowering plant can be harvested in summer, and dried.	Anti-inflammatory, antiseptic, antispasmodic, astringent, carminative, cholagogue, emmenagogue, vasodilator and stimulant. Used as tea in colds, fever, arthritic or menstrual pain. Externally, can be used to stop bleeding and treat wounds.	Infusion, poultice, tincture	

European climate zones

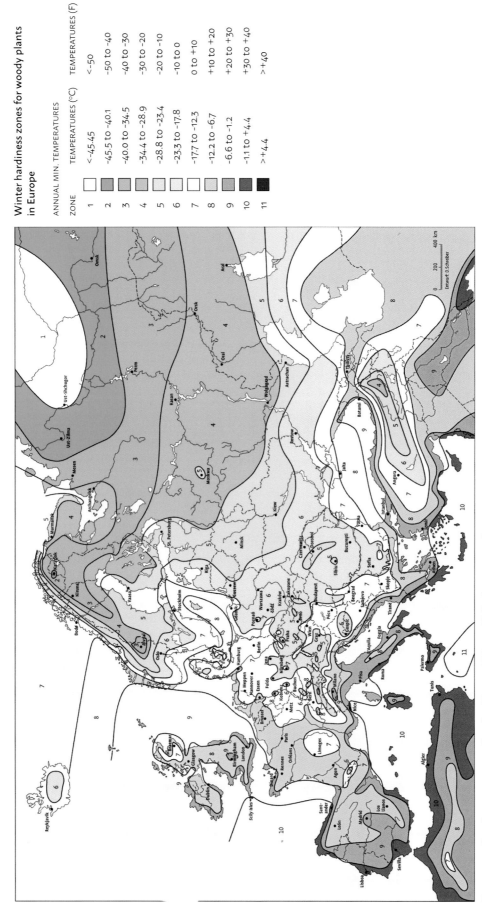

Winter hardiness zones for woody plants
in Europe

ANNUAL MIN. TEMPERATURES

ZONE	TEMPERATURES (°C)	TEMPERATURES (F)	
1	<-45.45	<-50	
2	-45.5 to -40.1	-50 to -40	
3	-40.0 to -34.5	-40 to -30	
4	-34.4 to -28.9	-30 to -20	
5	-28.8 to -23.4	-20 to -10	
6	-23.3 to -17.8	-10 to 0	
7	-17.7 to -12.3	0 to +10	
8	-12.2 to -6.7	+10 to +20	
9	-6.6 to -1.2	+20 to +30	
10	-1.1 to +4.4	+30 to +40	
11	>+4.4	>+40	

European hardiness zones. Credit: Eugen Ulmer KG, Stuttgart, Germany

APPENDIX 5

US climate zones

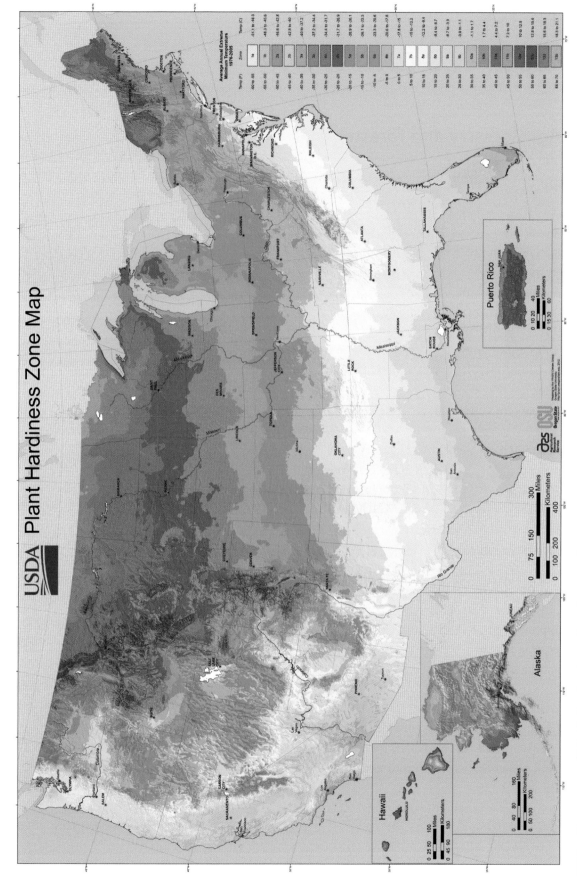

US hardiness zones (2012). Credit: Agricultural Research Service, US Department of Agriculture, USA

Resources and links

(A) Agroforestry and forestry

Europe

Agroforestry Research Trust
Publishes articles on forest gardening, offers courses and maintains a network of active practitioners of agroforestry.
www.agroforestry.co.uk

European Agroforestry Federation
Seeks to promote agroforestry, and the use of trees on farms in Europe. Organises conferences and has a newsletter.
www.eurafagroforestry.eu

Forest Research
This is the research agency part of the UK Forestry Commission, with information about research and scientific services related to forestry, including tree health.
www.forestresearch.gov.uk

Small Woods Association
A UK organisation for small woodland owners, workers and supporters, providing a magazine, training days and woodland visits.
https://smallwoods.org.uk

UK Forestry Commission
Issues licences for tree felling, provides information about pests and diseases, also offers grants to UK woodland owners for various improvements and planting.
www.gov.uk/government/organisations/forestry-commission

Woodland Trust
Has a mission in UK to plant trees, protect and restore ancient woodland. May provide some funding for planting schemes and hedges.
www.woodlandtrust.org.uk

North America

Association for Temperate Agroforestry
Seeks to promote wider adoption of agroforestry by landowners in temperate regions of North America, and holds conferences and provides a newsletter.
www.aftaweb.org

National Agroforestry Center
Provides much useful information including details of US events, research and training related to agroforestry.
www.fs.usda.gov/nac/

New Crops and Organics
US site with extensive information and research about medicinal herbs and non-timber forest products, co-ordinated by Jeanine Davis at North Carolina State University.
https://newcropsorganics.ces.ncsu.edu/herb/medicinal-herbs-and-non-timber-forest-products/

Worldwide

World Agroforestry
Works to support food security and environmental sustainability through agroforestry. Hosts publications and science reports relevant to a wide range of agroforestry enterprises.
http://new.worldagroforestry.org

(B) Conservation and climate issues

Europe

Botanic Gardens Conservation International

Many botanic gardens have medicinal plants, and these gardens provide an important resource for conservation. The organisation has databases on tree distributions and assessments of conservation issues for individual plants.
www.bgci.org

Plantlife

A body that works in UK and internationally to preserve wild flowers, plants and fungi.
www.plantlife.org.uk/uk

The Plant List

This is an online working list of all known plant species and provides the up-to-date agreed scientific name for each species. It is searchable by genus or species.
www.theplantlist.org

The Red List

A listing of European medicinal plants on the worldwide threatened species list.
https://www.iucnredlist.org/resources/allen2014

North America

CABI Invasive Species Compendium

Detailed coverage of invasive species; gives good coverage of the extent and status of plants that are problematic in USA providing detailed datasheets (including prevention and control) and research articles.
www.cabi.org/ISC

Sustainable Herbs Program

This programme in the USA provides awareness-raising with regard to the sourcing of herbs, partnered with the American Botanical Council.
https://sustainableherbsproject.com

United Plant Savers

The United Plant Savers maintain a Species At Risk List.
https://unitedplantsavers.org/species-at-risk-list

Worldwide

FairWild

Has a mission to promote a fair and sustainable future for wild plant resources and people, and encourage sustainable businesses.
www.fairwild.org

Global Trees Campaign

This is a partnership between Flora and Fauna International and Botanic Gardens Conservation International. Resources aimed at conservation of trees worldwide and primarily giving advice on monitoring endangered species.
www.globaltrees.org

(C) Herbal medicine information and training

Europe

British Herbal Medicine Association
Promotes standards in herbal medicine manufacturing in the UK and is keen to support quality supplies from growers.
https://bhma.info

College of Practitioners of Phytotherapy
Professional herbalist body in the UK with membership of trained herbal practitioners, code of ethics and insurance.
http://thecpp.uk

European Herb Growers Association
Organisation of herb growers and producers in Europe which provides good practice guidelines for agriculture and wild harvest.
www.europam.net

European Herbal and Traditional Practitioners Association

An umbrella organisation for traditional and herbal practitioner professional bodies that are seeking better recognition and regulation.
http://ehtpa.eu/about-us

National Institute of Medical Herbalists

Professional herbalist body in the UK with membership of trained herbal practitioners, code of ethics and insurance.
www.nimh.org.uk

North America

American Herbal Products Association

A national trade association for the herbal product industry in the USA, bringing together growers, producers, manufacturers and marketers. Provides guidance on regulatory and technical issues.
www.ahpa.org

American Herbalists Guild

Professional herbalist body in USA which provides a list of registered members.
www.americanherbalistsguild.com

Dr Duke's Phytochemical and Ethnobotanical Database

Detailed and searchable online database of most medicinal plants incorporating information on individual chemical constituents.
https://phytochem.nal.usda.gov/phytochem/

Native American Ethnobotany Database

An online database including plants used by Native American peoples for foods, drugs, dyes and fibres.
http://naeb.brit.org

PubMed

This online database hosted by the US National Library of Medicine provides abstracts for scientific research articles and is searchable by plant names and conditions. Many of the articles listed are freely available as full texts.
https://pubmed.ncbi.nlm.nih.gov

United Plant Savers Goldenseal Sanctuary

An inspiring botanical sanctuary project in Ohio, USA providing a focus for herbal cultivation training and forest farming projects.
www.goldensealsanctuary.org

(D) Organic and other organisations offering information and certification

Europe

Biodynamic Association

Holistic approach to agriculture with a certification system for both biodynamic and organic operations.
http://bdcertification.org.uk

EcoCert

A certification body for sustainable development, widely used in Europe.
www.ecocert.com

Organic Research Centre

Supply a newsletter and useful publications on research relating to organic agroforestry and agriculture.
www.organicresearchcentre.com

Soil Association

Well-established organic certification body with support for farmers and producers.
www.soilassociation.org

Worldwide

Rainforest Alliance

An international organisation acting against deforestation and supporting ethical supply chain commitments, offering certification for organic and other standards.
www.rainforestalliance.org

(E) Permaculture information and training

Europe

European Permaculture Network
A network of national and regional organisations in Europe.
https://permaculture-network.eu

Permaculture Association
The Permaculture Association provides networking opportunities, information about events and projects, and course details.
www.permaculture.org.uk

Permaculture Magazine
Regular publication with articles on all aspects of permaculture including herb cultivation.
www.permaculture.co.uk

Plants For A Future (PFAF)
Plants For A Future provides a detailed listing of many useful plants, incorporating a wide range of references. It is keyword searchable to help locate particular kinds of plants.
https://pfaf.org/user/Default.aspx

North America

Permies
Well-used online forum for all things to do with permaculture, lots of practical tips. Includes subscribers in USA and Europe.
https://permies.com

Worldwide

The Permaculture Research Institute
Provides regular articles on permaculture in a wide range of contexts worldwide.
https://permaculturenews.org

(F) Suppliers of plants and seeds

Europe

Agroforestry Research Trust
An educational and research organisation founded by Martin Crawford in 1992 and has since developed a comprehensive catalogue of good quality plants and seeds for sale.
www.agroforestry.co.uk

B&T World Seeds
Based in France but able to ship to most places, and a huge range of seeds which can be priced in small or large quantities. Plus guidance online available about germinating different plants.
http://b-and-t-world-seeds.com

Ivywood Botanicals
Based in Sligo, Eire, a retail outlet for the supply of a range of herb plants, and also provides training for growers in quality standards.
www.ivywood.ie

Poyntzfield Herb Nursery
A plant nursery based in Scotland, UK, supplying an extensive range of hardy herbs as seeds and bare-root plants, including unusual species for aromatic, culinary, medicinal and wildlife use.
www.poyntzfieldherbs.co.uk

North America

Prairie Moon Nursery
Minnesota-based supplier of native plants as seeds or bare-root with books and tools.
www.prairiemoon.com

Richters
Ontario-based growers and sellers of herbs with extensive range of seeds, plants, books and herb supplies including dried herbs and oils.
www.richters.com

Strictly Medicinal Seeds
Oregon-based large supplier of seeds, plants, books and useful equipment such as screens and tincture press.
https://strictlymedicinalseeds.com

Endnotes

Introduction, pp. 1-9

1. Hart R. (1991) *Forest Gardening*, Bideford: Green Books.

2. Whitefield P. (2002) *How to Make a Forest Garden*, East Meon, Hampshire: Permanent Publications.

3. Crawford M. (2010) *Creating a Forest Garden: Working with Nature to Grow Edible Crops*, Totnes, Devon: Green Books, p17.

4. Jacke D and Toensmeier E. (2005) *Edible Forest Gardens: Ecological Design and Practice for Temperate Climate Permaculture*, White River Junction, VT: Chelsea Green Publishing.

5. Smith J, Pearce BD and Wolfe MS. (2013) Reconciling productivity with protection of the environment: Is temperate agroforestry the answer? *Renewable Agriculture and Food Systems* 28: 80-92; Woodland Trust. (2018) Agroforestry in England: benefits, barriers and opportunities, www.woodlandtrust.org.uk/publications/2018/06/agroforestry-in-england/ (accessed 25 March 2019).

6. Weiseman W, Halsey D and Ruddock B. (2014) *Integrated Forest Gardening: The Complete Guide to Polycultures and Plant Guilds in Permaculture Systems*, White River Junction, VT: Chelsea Green Publishing, p13.

7. Weiseman et al. (2014) p11.

8. Crawford (2010) pp33-37 outlines the effects of climate change; The environmental challenges for individual trees are outlined in Hirons AD and Thomas PA. (2018) *Applied Tree Biology*, Hoboken, NJ: John Wiley, pp351-384.

9. Huang Y, Chen C and Castro-Izaguirre N. (2018) Impacts of species richness on productivity in a large-scale subtropical forest experiment. *Science* 362: 80-83.

10. Conway P. (2001) *Tree Medicine: A Comprehensive Guide to the Healing Power of Over 170 Trees*, London: Piatkus, pp91-92.

11. High Level Panel of Experts on Food Security and Nutrition. (2017) Sustainable forestry for food security and nutrition, Rome, Italy: Food and Agriculture Organization of the United Nations (FAO), summary p4, available at www.cifor.org/library/6549; A forest is defined by the FAO as land having trees over 5m tall, with at least 10% canopy cover and an area of more than 0.5 hectares; see FAO (2016) *Global Forest Resources Assessment: How Are the World's Forests Changing*, Rome: FAO.

12. Kanninen M, Murdiyarso D, Seymour F, et al. (2007) *Do Trees Grow on Money? The Implications of Deforestation Research for Policies to Promote REDD*, Situ Gede, Indonesia: Centre for International Forestry Research.

13. Willis KJ. (2017) *State of the World's Plants 2017*, Kew: Royal Botanic Gardens.

14. Spathelf P, Van Der Maaten E, Van Der Maaten-Theunissen M, et al. (2014) Climate change impacts in European forests: The expert views of local observers. *Ann For Sci* 71: 131-137.

15. Rothamsted Research. (2005) *Climate Change and Land Management*, Harpenden: Rothamsted Research.

16. Broadmeadow MSJ, Ray D and Samuel CJA. (2005) Climate change and the future for broadleaved tree species in Britain. *Forestry* 78: 145-161.

17. Willis (2017) p22.

18. Jenkins M, Timoshyna A and Cornthwaite M. (2018) *Wild at Home: Exploring the Global Harvest, Trade and Use of Wild Plant Ingredients*, Cambridge: Traffic International, available at www.traffic.org/site/assets/files/7339/wild-at-home.pdf (accessed 29 June 2019).

19. Convention on International Trade in Endangered Species of Wild Fauna and Flora (CITES) Secretariat. (2018) Non-timber forest products: CITES implementation for medicinal plant species. Document submitted to the Seventieth Meeting of the Standing Committee, 1-5 October 2018. Available at: https://cites.org/sites/default/files/eng/com/sc/70/Inf/E-SC70-Inf-36.pdf (accessed 7 March 2019).

20. FAO. (2018) *The State of the World's Forests, 2018 – Forest Pathways to Sustainable Development*, Rome: FAO, p500; Laird SA, McLain R and Wynberg RP. (eds) (2010) *Wild Product Governance: Finding Policies that Work for Non-timber Forest Products*, London: Earthscan.

21. Schippmann U, Leaman DJ and Cunningham AB. (2002) Impact of cultivation and gathering of medicinal plants on biodiversity: global trends and issues. Biodiversity and the Ecosystem Approach in Agriculture, Forestry and Fisheries. Satellite event on the occasion of the Ninth Regular Session of the Commission on Genetic Resources for Food and Agriculture. Rome, 12-13 October 2002, p8; Shackleton CM and Pandey AK. (2014) Positioning non-timber forest products on the development agenda. *For Policy Econ* 38: 1-7.

22. Schippmann et al. (2002).

23. Vines G and Behrens J. (2004) *Herbal Harvests with a Future: Towards Sustainable Sources for Medicinal Plants*, Salisbury: Plantlife International.

24. Rao MR, Palada MC and Becker BN. (2004) Medicinal and aromatic plants in agroforestry systems. *Agroforestry Systems* 61-62: 107-122. For organisations related to agroforestry in USA and Europe see Appendix 6(A).

25. Vance NC and Thomas J. (October 1997) *Special Forest Products: Biodiversity Meets the Marketplace*, Washington DC: US Department of Agriculture, Forest Service.

26. Davis JM. (2012) Assisting farmers to produce high-quality medicinal herbs. *HortScience* 47: 976-978.

27. Chamberlain JL, Bush R and Hammett AL. (1998) Non-timber forest products: The other forest products. *Forest Products Journal* 48: 10-19; Milliken W and Bridgewater S. (2001) *Flora Celtica: Sustainable Development of Scottish Plants*, Edinburgh: Edinburgh Development Consultants/ Royal Botanic Garden/ Scottish Executive Central Research Unit.

28. van Bemmel K, Grimm K, van der Maas S, et al. (2017) *The Potential of Permaculture Principles in the Agrifood Transition*, Den Bosch, The Netherlands: HAS Research Group: New Business Models for Agrifood Transition. For organisations related to permaculture see Appendix 6(E).

29. Booker AAA, Frommenwiler DA, Scotti F, et al. (2018) St John's

wort (*Hypericum perforatum*) products – an assessment of their authenticity and quality. *Phytomedicine* 40: 158-164.

30 A list of products granted traditional herbal registration in the UK is at www.gov.uk/government/publications/herbal-medicines-granted-a-traditional-herbal-registration-thr (accessed 25 July 2019).

31 Newmaster SG, Grguric M, Shanmughanandhan D, et al. (2013) DNA barcoding detects contamination and substitution in North American herbal products. *BMC Medicine* 11: 222.

32 Palhares R, Drummond M, dos Santos Alves Figueiredo Brasil B, et al. (2015) Medicinal plants recommended by the World Health Organization: DNA barcode identification associated with chemical analyses guarantees their quality. *PLoS One* 10: e0127866.

33 Lange D. (2006) International trade in medicinal and aromatic plants: Actors, volumes and commodities. In: Bogers RJ, Craker LE and Lange D (eds) *Medicinal and Aromatic Plants*, Netherlands: Springer, pp155-170.

34 Jenkins et al. (2018).

35 The Standard International Trade Classification, first established in 1950, classifies most medicinal and aromatic plants as 'Plants and parts of plants (including seeds and fruits) of a kind used primarily in perfumery, in pharmacy, or for insecticidal, fungicidal or similar purposes, fresh or dried, whether or not cut, crushed or powdered'. The code used is 292.4. The European Union uses another more recently introduced system of 'Harmonized Commodity Description and Coding'. The code used is HS 1211.

36 Bodeker G, Ong CK, Grundy C, et al. (eds) (2005) *WHO Global Atlas of Traditional, Complementary and Alternative Medicine*, Kobe, Japan: WHO Centre for Health and Development.

37 International Trade Center (ITC). (March 2017) *Market Insider for Medicinal Plants*, Geneva, Switzerland: ITC.

38 Ressmann AK, Kremsmayr T, Gaertner P, et al. (2017) Toward a benign strategy for the manufacturing of betulinic acid. *Green Chem* 19: 1014-1022.

39 Smith T, Kawa K, Eckl V, et al. (2018) Herbal supplement sales in US increased 8.5% in 2017, topping $8 billion. *HerbalGram* 119: 62-71.

40 Grand View Research. (2019) Organic personal care market size, share and trends analysis report, www.grandviewresearch.com/industry-analysis/organic-personal-care-market (accessed 29 June 2019).

41 Karjalainen E, Sarjala T and Raitio H. (2010) Promoting human health through forests: Overview and major challenges. *Environ Health Prev Med* 15: 5.

42 Jenkins et al. (2018); Osemeobo GJ. (2005) Living on the forests: Women and household security in Nigeria. *Small-scale Forest Economics, Management and Policy* 4: 343-358.

43 Species at risk in Europe have been identified, Allen D, Bilz M, Leaman DJ, et al. (2014) *European Red List of Medicinal Plants*, Luxembourg: Publications Office of the European Union. For further sources of information see Appendix 6(B).

44 Schippmann et al. (2002) p10.

45 Self-help advice books have had a resurgence, for example see Wong J. (2009) *Grow Your Own Drugs: Easy Recipes for Natural Remedies and Beauty Treats*, London: Collins.

46 Smith et al. (2018).

47 Sustainability report for Pukka Herbs is at www.pukkaherbs.com/media/76571305/pukka-sustainability-report-2017.pdf; and for Weleda is at www.weleda.co.uk/content/files/pdfs/Weleda-Annual-Sustainability-Report2017.pdf (both accessed 19 July 2019).

48 The International Code of Botanical Nomenclature ensures that all plants are classified with the binomial system giving first the genus name and second the species name. The most up-to-date accepted list of binomial names is the Plant List found at www.theplantlist.org (accessed 29 June 2019).

49 The Plants for a Future database is at www.pfaf.org (accessed 29 June 2019).

50 PubMed is hosted at www.ncbi.nlm.nih.gov/pubmed and provides access to abstracts of published scientific research studies.

Chapter 1: Medicinal Uses, pp.10-26

1 Thomas P. (2000) *Trees: Their Natural History*, Cambridge: Cambridge University Press, p1.

2 In the UK, many trees and shrubs were in use in medieval times for healing purposes; see Pollington S. (2008) *Leechcraft: Early English Charms Plant Lore and Healing*, Hockwold-cum-Wilton: Anglo-Saxon Books, pp493-507; Hooke D. (2013) *Trees in Anglo-Saxon England: Literature, Lore and Landscape*, Woodbridge: Boydell.

3 Allen DE and Hatfield G. (2004) *Medicinal Plants in Folk Tradition: An Ethnobotany of Britain & Ireland*, Portland, Oregon: Timber Press.

4 Elkes R. (1651) *Approved Medicines of Little Cost, to Preserve Health and also to Cure those that are Sick Provided for the Souldiers Knap-sack and the Country Mans Closet*, London: Printed for Robert Ibbitson and are to be sold by Tho: Vere at the Angel in the Old-Baily, p1.

5 For example: Hussain T, Rafay M, Manj IA, et al. (2017) Desert dwelling trees: Forage suitability and ethnobotany, Pakistan. *J Biodivers Endanger Species* 5: 194; Dolatkhahi M, Dolatkhahi A and Nejad JB. (2014) Ethnobotanical study of medicinal plants used in Arjan – Parishan protected area in Fars Province of Iran. *Avicenna J Phytomed* 4: 402-412.

6 For example in Tanzania: Luoga EJ, Witkowski ETF and Balkwill K. (2000) Differential utilization and ethnobotany of trees in Kitulanghalo Forest Reserve and surrounding communal lands, Eastern Tanzania. *Economic Botany* 54: 328-343.

7 For example in Austria: Vogl S, Picker P, Mihaly-Bison J, et al. (2013) Ethnopharmacological in vitro studies on Austria's folk medicine: An unexplored lore in vitro anti-inflammatory activities of 71 Austrian traditional herbal drugs. *J Ethnopharmacol* 149: 750-771.

8 Newman D and Cragg G. (2007) Natural products as sources of new drugs over the last 25 years. *J Nat Prod* 70: 461-477.

9 Pennachio M, Jefferson LV and Havens K. (2010) *Uses and Abuses of Plant-derived Smoke: Its Ethnobotany as Hallucinogen, Perfume, Incense, and Medicine*, Oxford: Oxford University Press.

10 Chapter 2 of Conway (2001) provides a brief history of trees in medicine. A more detailed description of introductions is in Bean WJ. (1980) *Trees and Shrubs Hardy in the British Isles*, London: John Murray, pp3-21. For a detailed overview of the past use of individual plants see Grieve M. (1980) *A Modern Herbal: The Medicinal, Culinary, Cosmetic and Economic Properties, Cultivation and Folklore of*

Herbs, Grasses, Fungi, Shrubs and Trees with All Their Modern Scientific Uses, 1931 edition, London: Penguin.

11 Bean WJ. (1976) *Trees and Shrubs Hardy in the British Isles*, Eighth edition, London: John Murray.

12 Based on Gerard J. (1633) *The Herball or Generall Historie of Plantes*, London: Printed by Adam Islip Ioice Norton and Richard Whitakers.

13 Bean (1980) p13.

14 World Health Organization (WHO). (2013) *WHO Traditional Medicine Strategy: 2014-2023*, Hong Kong: WHO.

15 See Appendix 6(C) for details of clinical herbal practitioner organisations.

16 Gardner Z and McGuffin M. (eds) (2013) *American Herbal Products Association's Botanical Safety Handbook,* 2nd ed, Boca Raton: CRC Press; Mills S and Bone K. (2013) *Principles and Practice of Phytotherapy*, Edinburgh: Churchill Livingstone; Williamson E, Driver S and Baxter K. (2009) *Stockley's Herbal Medicines Interactions*, London: Pharmaceutical Press; European Medicines Agency (April 2018) HMPC Monographs: Overview of recommendations for the uses of herbal medicinal products in the paediatric population, available at: www.ema.europa.eu/en/documents/other/hmpc-monographs-overview-recommendations-uses-herbal-medicinal-products-paediatric-population_en.pdf (accessed 13 March 2019).

17 Wagner H and Ulrich-Merzenich G. (2009) Synergy research: Approaching a new generation of phytopharmaceuticals. *Phytomedicine* 16: 97-110.

18 Sadowska B, Paszkiewicz M, Podsędek A, et al. (2014) *Vaccinium myrtillus* leaves and *Frangula alnus* bark derived extracts as potential antistaphylococcal agents. *Acta Biochim Pol* 61: 163-169.

19 Riva A, Togni S, Franceschi F, et al. (2017) The effect of a natural, standardized bilberry extract (Mirtoselect®) in dry eye: A randomized, double blinded, placebo-controlled trial. *Eur Rev Med Pharmacol Sci* 21: 2518-2525.

20 Ferlemi A and Lamari F. (2016) Berry leaves: An alternative source of bioactive natural products of nutritional and medicinal value. *Anti-oxidants (Basel)* 5: E17.

21 Rasolofoson R, Hanauer M, Pappinen A, et al. (2018) Effects of forests on children's diets in developing countries: A cross-sectional study. *Lancet Planet Health* 2: S15.

22 For example, Abreu AC, Coqueiro A, Sultan AR, et al. (2017) Looking to nature for a new concept in antimicrobial treatments: Isoflavonoids from *Cytisus striatus* as antibiotic adjuvants against MRSA. *Sci Rep* 7: 3777.

23 Zenãoa S, Aires A, Dias C, et al. (2017) Antibacterial potential of *Urtica dioica* and *Lavandula angustifolia* extracts against methicillin resistant *Staphylococcus aureus* isolated from diabetic foot ulcers. *J Herb Med* 10: 53-58.

24 Seca AML and Pinto DCGA. (2018) Plant secondary metabolites as anticancer agents: Successes in clinical trials and therapeutic application. *Int J Mol Sci* 19: E263.

25 Walsh V and Goodman J. (2002) From Taxol to Taxol(R): The changing identities and ownership of an anti-cancer drug. *Med Anthropol* 21: 307-336.

26 Seca and Pinto (2018).

27 Pinto-Garcia L, Efferth T, Torres A, et al. (2010) Berberine inhibits cell growth and mediates caspase-independent cell death in human pancreatic cancer cells. *Planta Med* 76: 1155-1161.

28 Pickhardt M, Gazova Z, von Bergen M, et al. (2005) Anthraquinones inhibit tau aggregation and dissolve Alzheimer's paired helical filaments in vitro and in cells. *J Biol Chem* 280: 3628-3635.

29 Dr Duke's Phytochemical and Ethnobotanical Database, https://phytochem.nal.usda.gov/phytochem/search/list (accessed 13 February 2019).

30 Alves RRN and Rosa IML. (2007) Biodiversity, traditional medicine and public health: Where do they meet? *J Ethnobiol Ethnomed* 3: 14.

31 Coutts C and Hahn M. (2015) Green infrastructure, ecosystem services, and human health. *Int J Environ Res Public Health* 12: 9770; Rouquette JR and Holt AR. (2017) *Research Report: The Benefits to People of Trees Outside Woods*, Grantham: Woodland Trust/ Natural Capital Solutions.

32 Hickman C. (2013) *Therapeutic Landscapes: A History of English Hospital Gardens Since 1800*, Manchester: Manchester University Press, p14.

33 Sarajevs V. (2011) *Health Benefits of Street Trees*, Forest Research. Available at www.forestresearch.gov.uk/research/health-benefits-of-street-trees (accessed 30 June 2019).

34 Kardan O, Gozdyra P, Misic B, et al. (2015) Neighbourhood green space and health in a large urban centre. *Sci Rep* 5: 11610.

35 Coutts and Hahn (2015).

36 Li Q, Morimoto K, Koboyashi M., et al. (2008) Visiting a forest, but not a city, increases human natural killer activity and expression of anti-cancer proteins. *Int J Immunopathol Pharmacol* 21: 117-127.

37 Mao GX, Cao YB, Lan XG, et al. (2012) Therapeutic effect of forest bathing on human hypertension in the elderly. *J Cardiol* 60: 495-502; also on reducing depression in an arboretum see Berman MG, Kross E, Krpan KM, et al. (2012) Interacting with nature improves cognition and affect for individuals with depression. *J Affect Disord* 140: 300-305.

38 Lee J-Y and Lee D-C. (2014) Cardiac and pulmonary benefits of forest walking versus city walking in elderly women: A randomised, controlled, open-label trial. *Eur J Integr Med* 6: 5-11.

39 Ideno Y, Hayashi K, Abe Y, et al. (2017) Blood pressure-lowering effect of Shinrin-yoku (Forest bathing): A systematic review and meta-analysis. *BMC Complement Altern Med* 17: 409.

40 Oh B, Lee KJ, Zaslawski C, et al. (2017) Health and well-being benefits of spending time in forests: Systematic review. *Environ Health Prev Med* 22: 71.

41 For a readable account of secondary metabolites see Tudge C. (2005) *The Secret Life of Trees: How They Live and Why they Matter*, London: Penguin, pp352-361; for the chemistry of natural products see Dewick PM. (2009) *Medicinal Natural Products: A Biosynthetic Approach*, Chichester: John Wiley; for a complete analysis of medicinal actions of plant constituents see Ganora L. (2008) *Herbal Constituents: Foundations of Phytochemistry*, Louisville, Colorado: Herbalchem Press.

42 Yang L, Wen K-S, Ruan X, et al. (2018) Response of plant secondary metabolites to environmental factors. *Molecules* 23: E762; Crawford M. (2015) Useful chemicals from trees. *Agroforestry News* 23: 24-39.

43 British Herbal Medicine Association (BHMA) Scientific Committee. (1983) *British Herbal Pharmacopoeia*, Bournemouth: BHMA, p184.

44 Meyrick W. (1790) *The New Family Herbal: or Domestic Physician*, Birmingham: Printed by T. Pearson; and sold by R. Baldwin, London, p464; Mills SY. (1993) *Out of the Earth: The Essential Book of Herbal Medicine*, London: Arkana, p280.

45 Gagnier JJ, Oltean H, van Tulder MW, et al. (2016) Herbal medicine for low back pain: A Cochrane review. *Spine* (Phila Pa 1976) 41: 116-133.

46 Jadoon S, Karim S, Hassan Bin Asad MH, et al. (2015) Anti-aging potential of phytoextract loaded-pharmaceutical creams for human skin cell longevity. *Oxid Med Cell Longev* 2015: ID 709628.

47 Hubert J, Angelis A, Aligiannis N, et al. (2016) In vitro dermo-cosmetic evaluation of bark extracts from common temperate trees. *Planta Med* 82: 1351-1358.

48 Yatkin E, Polari L, Laajala T, et al. (2014) Novel lignan and stilbenoid mixture shows anticarcinogenic efficacy in preclinical PC-3M-luc2 prostate cancer model. *PLoS One* 9: e93764.

49 Klein R. (2004) Phytoecdysteroids. *Journal of the American Herbalists Guild* Fall/Winter: 18-28.

50 Desgagné-Penix I. (2017) Distribution of alkaloids in woody plants. *Plant Science Today* 4: 137-142.

51 Willis (2017) p29.

52 Wang H, Zhu C, Ying Y, et al. (2018) Metformin and berberine, two versatile drugs in treatment of common metabolic diseases. *Oncotarget* 9: 10135–10146.

53 See Appendix 6(C) for details of herbal medicine organisations.

Chapter 2: Designing, pp.27–44

1 There are numerous design techniques which can be used to help identify aims and further elements in the design process including mind maps, strengths/weaknesses/opportunities/threats (SWOT) analysis, SMART goals, and others. The best way to learn about these techniques is to join a permaculture training course and permaculture organisations are listed in Appendix 6(E).

2 Some useful formats for listing site features are in Remiarz T. (2017) *Forest Gardening in Practice: An Illustrated Practical Guide for Homes, Communities and Enterprises*, East Meon, Hampshire: Permanent Publications, pp231-236. Further help can be gained on permaculture training courses, details from the Permaculture Association, www.permaculture.org.uk.

3 Pritchett WL. (1979) *Properties and Management of Forest Soils*, New York: John Wiley and Sons, pp6-8.

4 Crawford M. (2015) *Trees for Gardens, Orchards and Permaculture*, East Meon, UK: Permanent Publications, p87 and p206; see also Willoughby I, Stokes V, Poole J, et al. (2007) The potential of 44 native and non-native species for woodland creation on a range of contrasting sites in lowland Britain. *Forestry* 80: 532-553.

5 Peterken GF. (1981) *Woodland Conservation and Management*, London and New York: Chapman and Hall.

6 Rotherham ID. (2017) *Ancient Woodland: History, Industry and Crafts*, Oxford: Shire Publications, p55.

7 For the UK see Hall JE, Kirby KJ and Whitbread AM. (2004) *National Vegetation Classification: Field Guide to Woodland*, Peterborough: Joint Nature Conservation Committee; also see Crawford CL. (2009) Ancient woodland indicator plants in Scotland. *Scottish Forestry* 63: 7-19. There are over 200 habitat types identified in Europe; more details at Ecosystems and habitats, https://biodiversity.europa.eu/topics/ecosystems-and-habitats (accessed 11 July 2019).

8 For UK and Europe see Barker J. (2001) *The Medicinal Flora of Britain and Northwestern Europe: A Field Guide Including Plants Commonly Cultivated in the Region*, West Wickham: Winter Press; in USA see, for example, Foster S and Duke JA. (1990) *A Field Guide to Eastern and Central North American Medicinal Plants*, Boston: Houghton Mifflin Co.

9 Whitefield (2002) pp41-43.

10 Crawford (2010) pp58-59.

11 For the UK see the online advice 'Tree felling licence: when you need to apply', www.forestry.gov.uk/england-fellinglicences (accessed 2 March 2019). In the UK, licences are issued by the Forestry Commission. Usually, you do not need a licence to fell or prune in a garden or orchard, but do need a licence if you plan to fell more than five cubic metres in a calendar quarter.

12 Nichol L. (2003) Planning legislation and small woodlands. *Smallwoods* 10: 10-11.

13 Weiseman W, Halsey D and Ruddock B. (2014) *Integrated Forest Gardening: The Complete Guide to Polycultures and Plant Guilds in Permaculture Systems*, White River Junction, VT: Chelsea Green Publishing, p24.

14 For selecting edible or other useful plants for hedges etc. see advice in Fern K. (2000) *Plants for a Future: Edible and Useful Plants for a Healthier World*, East Meon, Hampshire: Permanent Publications.

15 Clark JR, Hemery GE and Savill PS. (2008) Early growth and form of common walnut (*Juglans regia* L.) in mixture with tree and shrub nurse species in southern England. *Forestry* 81: 631-644.

16 Mosquera-Losada MR, Feirreiro-Dominguez N, Romero-Franco R, et al. (November 2017) Intercropping medicinal plants under cherry timber trees: understory planting to improve productivity of plantations, AGFORWARD, available at: www.agforward.eu/index.php/en/silvoarable-systems-in-spain.html (accessed 30 May 2018).

17 Nicoll B. (2016) *Agriculture and Forestry Climate Change Report Card Technical Paper 8. Risks for Woodlands, Forest Management and Forestry Production in the UK from Climate Change*, Roslin: Forest Research.

18 Brang P, Spathelf P, Larsen JB, et al. (2014) Suitability of close-to-nature silviculture for adapting temperate European forests to climate change. *Forestry* 87: 492-503.

19 Crawford (2010) p45.

20 Dobson FS. (1979) *Common British Lichens*, Norwich: Jarrold.

21 Fernández-Moriano C, Gómez-Serranillos MP and Crespo A. (2016) Anti-oxidant potential of lichen species and their secondary metabolites. A systematic review. *Pharm Biol* 54: 1-17.

22 Brisdelli F, Perilli M, Sellitri D, et al. (2013) Cytotoxic activity and anti-oxidant capacity of purified lichen metabolites: An in vitro study. *Phytother Res* 27: 431-437.

23 Drobnik J and Stebel A. (2018) *Brachythecium rutabulum*, a neglected medicinal moss. *Hum Ecol Interdiscip J* 46: 133-141.

24 Lindequist U, Niedermeyer THJ and Jülich W-D. (2005) The pharmacological potential of mushrooms. *Evid Based Complement Alternat Med* 2: 285-299; Wasser SP. (2014) Medicinal mushroom science: Current perspectives, advances, evidences, and challenges. *Biomed J* 37: 345-356.

25 Powell M. (2010) *Medicinal Mushrooms: A Clinical Guide*, Eastbourne: Mycology Press; Wasser (2014); Stamets P. (2005) *Mycelium Running: How Mushrooms Can Help Save the World*, New York: Ten Speed Press.

26 Weiseman et al. (2014), p27.

27 Mast Tree Network. Stump culture: Coppice for conifers, www.mast-producing-trees.org/2010/11/stump-culture-coppice-for-conifers/ (accessed 14 February 2019). At Holt Wood we have done this with Douglas fir (*Pseudotsuga menziesii*) with some success.

28 Matthews JD. (1996) *Silvicultural Systems*, Oxford: Oxford University Press.

29 Fuller RJ and Warren MS. (1993) *Coppiced Woodlands: Their Management for Wildlife*, Peterborough: Joint Nature Conservation Committee.

30 Crawford (2010) p420.

31 Scott TL. (2010) *Invasive Plant Medicine: The Ecological Benefits and Healing Capabilities of Invasives*, Rochester, VT: Healing Arts Press.

32 Department for Environment, Food and Rural Affairs (DEFRA). (2008) *The Invasive Non-native Species Framework Strategy for Great Britain: Protecting our Natural Heritage from Invasive Species*, London: DEFRA; also see the Global Compendium of Weeds, available at www.hear.org/gcw (accessed 25 March 2019).

33 Raja S and Ramya I. (2016) A review on ethnopharmacology, phytochemistry and pharmacology of *Buddleja asiatica*. *Int J Pharm Sci Res* 7: 4697-4709.

34 Watson B. (2006) *Trees: Their Use, Management, Cultivation and Biology*, Marlborough, Wilts: Crowood Press, p335.

Chapter 3: Establishing and Maintaining, pp.45-57

1 Watson (2006) p332.

2 Hugelkuktur refers to raised beds constructed in trenches with logs and other organic matter; see Holzer S. (2011) *Sepp Holzer's Permaculture: A Practical Guide to Small-scale, Integrative Farming and Gardening*, East Meon, Hampshire: Permanent Publications.

3 Watson (2006) p335.

4 Higman S, Mayers J, Bass S, et al. (2005) *The Sustainable Forestry Handbook: A Practical Guide for Tropical Forest Managers on Implementing New Standards*, London: Earthscan, p179.

5 Watson (2006) p327.

6 Evelyn J. (1670) *Sylva, or, A Discourse of Forest-trees*, London: Printed by Jo. Martyn and Ja. Allestry, p11.

7 Watson (2006) p338.

8 Phillips M. (2017) *Mycorrhizal Planet: How Symbiotic Fungi Work with Roots to Support Plant Health and Build Soil Fertility*, White River Junction, VT: Chelsea Green; Pritchett (1979) p178.

9 Holden J, Grayson RP, Berdeni D, et al. (2019) The role of hedgerows in soil functioning within agricultural landscapes. *Agric Ecosyst Environ* 273: 1-12.

10 Smith SE and Read D. (2008) *Mycorrhizal Symbiosis*, Amsterdam: Academic Press, pp613, 622.

11 Avio L, Sbrana C, Giovannetti M, et al. (2017) Arbuscular mycorrhizal fungi affect total phenolics content and anti-oxidant activity in leaves of oak leaf lettuce varieties. *Sci Hortic (Amsterdam)* 224: 265-271.

12 Pierart A, Dumat C, Maes AQ, et al. (2018) Influence of arbuscular mycorrhizal fungi on antimony phyto-uptake and compartmentation in vegetables cultivated in urban gardens. *Chemosphere* 191: 272-279.

13 Peterken GF. (2017) Lessons from a 'natural' woodland. *Smallwoods* Autumn issue: 10-13.

14 Crawford (2010) pp51-55.

15 Watson (2006) p348.

16 Low M. (2014) Biochar: How to build soil, lock up carbon and build fertility on the farm. *Permaculture Magazine*. 7 May 2014.

17 Prendergast-Miller MT, Duvall M and Sohia SP. (2014) Biochar–root interactions are mediated by biochar nutrient content and impacts on soil nutrient availability. *Eur J Soil Sci* 65: 173-185.

18 Wilson PJ. (2019) Botanical diversity in the hedges and field margins of lowland Britain. In: Dover JW (ed) *The Ecology of Hedgerows and Field Margins*, Dover: Routledge, pp35-54.

19 Rackham O. (1990) *Trees and Woodlands in the British Landscape*, London: Phoenix Gunat Publishers, pp59-66.

20 Williamson T, Barnes G and Pillatt T. (2017) *Trees in England: Management and Disease since 1600*, Hatfield: University of Hertfordshire Press.

21 Haeggström C-A. (1998) Pollard meadows: Multiple use of human-made nature. In: Kirby KJW and Watkins C. (eds) *The Ecological History of European Forests*, Wallingford: CABI, pp33-41; Rochel X. (2015) Forest management and species composition: A historical approach in Lorraine, France. In: Kirby KJ and Watkins C (eds) *Europe's Changing Woods and Forests: From Wildwood to Managed Landscapes*, Wallingford: CABI, pp279-289.

22 Watson (2006) p242.

23 Cobos R, Mateos RM, Álvarez-Pérez JM, et al. (2015) Effectiveness of natural antifungal compounds in controlling infection by grapevine trunk disease pathogens through pruning wounds. *Appl Environ Microbiol* 81: 6474–6483.

24 Williamson et al. (2017) pp183-185.

Chapter 4: Propagation and Provenance, pp.58-71

1 McVicar J. (2001) *Seeds: The Ultimate Guide to Growing Successfully from Seed*, London: Kyle Cathie Ltd in association with the Royal Horticultural Society, p233.

2 Kock H. (2008) *Growing Trees from Seed: A Practical Guide to Growing Native Trees, Vines and Shrubs*, New York: Firefly Books, p32.

3 McDonald MF and Copeland LO. (2012) *Seed Production: Principles and Practices*, Dordrecht: Springer Science and Business Media.

4   Dirr MA and Heuser CW. (2006) *The Reference Manual of Woody Plant Propagation: From Seed to Tissue Culture*, Second ed., Portland, Oregon: Timber Press, pp42-45.

5   There is discussion of composting bark in Miller JH and Jones N. (1995) *Organic and Compost-based Growing Media for Tree Seedling Nurseries*, Washington DC: World Bank, Annex V.

6   Thompson P. (1992) *Creative Propagation: A Grower's Guide*, London: BT Batsford, p148.

7   In the UK suppliers for specific plants can be located through the Royal Horticultural Society 'Find a plant' (https://www.rhs.org.uk/plants/search-Form) and entering all or part of a plant name returns results in a list or map format.

8   Watson (2006) p332.

9   Howard PH. (2009) Visualizing consolidation in the global seed industry: 1996–2008. *Sustainability* 1: 1266-1287.

10 Colley M, Navazio J and DiPietro L. (2010) *A Seed Saving Guide for Gardeners and Farmers*, Organic Seed Alliance, available at https://seedalliance.org/publications/seed-saving-guide-gardeners-farmers/ (accessed 30 June 2019); Gough R and Moore-Gough C. (2011) *The Complete Guide to Saving Seeds: 322 Vegetables, Herbs, Flowers, Fruits, Trees, and Shrubs*, North Adams, MA: Storey Publishing.

11 Antony JR and Lal SB. (2013) *Forestry Principles and Applications*, Jodhpur, India: Scientific Publishers.

12 Edlin HL. (1956) *Trees, Woods and Man*, London: Collins, p12.

13 To gather this seed the capsules need to be collected as they become brown and kept in a stout paper bag and as they dry they will pop and expel the seeds.

14 Gosling P. (2007) *Raising Trees and Shrubs from Seed*, Edinburgh: Forestry Commission.

15 Kock (2008) pp30-31.

16 Gosling (2007). At the Millennium Seed Bank, UK, seeds are dried out and stored in airtight containers at -20°C.

17 Dirr and Heuser (2006) pp2-3.

18 Broadmeadow et al. (2005) p147.

19 Williamson et al. (2017) p203.

20 Bailie A, Renaut S, Ubalijoro E, et al. (2016) Phytogeographic and genetic variation in *Sorbus*, a traditional antidiabetic medicine – adaptation in action in both a plant and a discipline. *Peer J* 4: e2645.

21 Some useful experience of propagation for field crops is given in Sturdivant L and Blakley T. (1999) *Medicinal Herbs in the Garden, Field and Marketplace*, Friday Harbour, WA: San Juan Naturals, pp129-136.

22 A basic guide to establishing a tree nursery (albeit in a tropical context) is available from the Global Trees Campaign, Stott G and Gill D. (2014) *How to Design and Manage a Basic Tree Nursery: Global Trees Campaign Brief 4*, Fauna and Flora International, http://globaltrees.org/resources/resource-type/practical-guidance/ (accessed 30 June 2019).

Chapter 5: Harvesting, pp.72-83

1   Hart (1991) p111.

2   For more on harvesting or foraging from wilder places, see Bruton-Seal J and Seal M. (2008) *Hedgerow Medicine: Harvest and Make Your Own Herbal Remedies*, Ludlow: Merlin Unwin Books; Hawes Z. (2010) *Wild Drugs: A Forager's Guide to Healing Plants*, London: Gaia.

3   Henkel A. (1909) *American Medicinal Barks*, Washington: US Department of Agriculture, p8.

4   Rohloff J, Dragland S, Mordal R, et al. (2005) Effect of harvest time and drying method on biomass production, essential oil yield, and quality of peppermint (*Mentha × piperita* L.). *J Agric Food Chem* 53: 4143-4148.

5   Sibao C, Dajian Y, Shilin C, et al. (2007) Seasonal variations in the isoflavonoids of radix *Puerarae*. *Phytochem Anal* 18: 245-250.

6   Li SL, Yan R, Tam YK, et al. (2007) Post-harvest alteration of the main chemical ingredients in *Ligusticum chuanxiong* Hort. (Rhizoma Chuanxiong). *Chem Pharm Bull (Tokyo)* 55: 140-144.

7   Higman et al. (2005) p167-169.

8   Such as Stace C. (2019) New flora of the British Isles, 4th edition, Middlewood Green, Suffolk: C&M Floristics; Rose F. (2006) *The Wild Flower Key: How to Identify Wild Plants, Trees and Shrubs in Britain and Ireland*, London: Frederick Warne; Mitchell A. (1974) *A Field Guide to the Trees of Britain and Northern Europe*, London: Collins.

9   There have been reports of contamination of some Western herbs with leaves of potentially toxic plants such as deadly nightshade (*Atropa belladonna*), foxglove (*Digitalis* species) and ragworts (*Senecio* species); Mills SY and Bone K. (2005) *The Essential Guide to Herbal Safety*, St Louis: Elsevier Churchill Livingstone, pp108-109.

10 Whitten G. (1997) *Herbal Harvest: Commercial Organic Production of Quality Dried Herbs*, Hawthorn, Victoria, Australia: Bloomings Books, pp139-140.

11 Whitten (1997) pp147-148.

12 A more detailed explanation of voucher specimen standards is available in Hildreth J, Hrabeta-Robinson E, Applequist W, et al. (2007) Standard operating procedure for the collection and preparation of voucher plant specimens for use in the nutraceutical industry. *Anal Bioanal Chem* 389: 13-17.

13 Skelton, J. (1878) *Family Medical Adviser: A Treatise on Scientific or Botanic Medicine*, 11th edn, Plymouth: Published by the author.

14 Li et al. (2007), in their study of processing of a Chinese root, found that drying at 60°C meant that some compounds were decreased, some increased and some new compounds appeared.

15 Upton R. (ed.) (1999) *Willow Bark, Salix spp. Analytical, Quality Control and Therapeutic Monograph*, Santa Cruz: America Herbal Pharmacopoeia.

16 Lonner J and Thomas M. (2003) *A Harvester's Handbook to Wild Medicinal Plant Collection in Kosovo*, Kosovo Business Support, p5.

17 Whitten (1997) pp151-153.

18 Ibid. pp155-156. Whitten also provides instructions for building a small cabinet dryer – 950 × 1500 × 2400mm to take 13 screens with

a 1000W heat source, pp173-176.

19 Scanlin D. (2014) 'Best-ever solar food dehydrator plans', *Mother Earth News*. Available at: www.motherearthnews.com/diy/tools/solar-food-dehydrator-plans-zm0z14jjzmar (accessed 6 May 2018).

20 Makanjuola SA. (2017) Influence of particle size and extraction solvent on anti-oxidant properties of extracts of tea, ginger, and tea-ginger blend. *Food Sci Nutr* 5: 1179-1185.

21 Whitten (1997) pp197-198.

22 Our model at Holt Wood is a Titan 2500W Rapid Garden Shredder, and the front panel can be removed in order to clean the cutting blade within.

23 At Holt Wood we use a FDS Continuous Feed Powdering Machine, an accessory supplied by Mayway Herbs, Oakland, California, USA, www.mayway.com/supplies/accessories (accessed 30 July 2019).

24 Whitten (1997) p204.

25 Cunningham AB. (2001) *Applied Ethnobotany: People, Wild Plant Use and Conservation*, London: Earthscan.

Chapter 6: Herbal Preparations, pp.84-104

1 There are a number of ways of calculating reduced dosages for children. For suitable herbal treatments for children you should consult a local qualified herbal practitioner; see the contact details for professional clinical practitioner organisations in Appendix 6(C).

2 These seed oils are rich in essential fatty acids such as linolenic acid and have beneficial anti-inflammatory effects on the skin.

3 Heckels F, Lawton K and Benfield B. (2019) *The Sensory Herbal Handbook: Connect with the Medicinal Power of your Local Plants*, London: Watkins Publishing.

4 In the UK, the government Excise Notice 47 governs the use of duty free spirits for manufacturing and medicinal purposes. Note that a licence to purchase duty free 96% proof alcohol has to be applied for, stating the intended use. Denatured alcohol (with additives designed for easy recognition and to prevent internal use) is used for cosmetics.

5 Green J and Green A. (2000) *The Herbal Medicine-maker's Handbook: A Home Manual*, Freedom, CA: Crossing Press.

6 For more on gemmotherapy or the use of buds and embryonic substances in herbal medicine, see Rozencwajg J. (2013) *Dynamic Gemmotherapy: Integrative Embryonic Phytotherapy*, Emryss.

7 Bradley R. (1732) *The Country Housewife and Lady's Director, in the Management of a House, and the Delights and Profit of a Farm*, Sixth ed. London: Printed for D Browne and T Woodman, p97.

8 A 'vinegar mother' contains the bacteria needed to form acetic acid. For more on the practicalities of vinegar making see Hafferty S. (2018) *The Creative Kitchen: Seasonal Plant-based Recipes for Meals, Drinks, Crafts, Body and Home Care*, East Meon, Hampshire: Permanent Publications, pp28-30; Hedley C and Shaw N. (1996) *Herbal Remedies: A Practical Beginner's Guide to Making Effective Remedies in the Kitchen*, Avonmouth: Parragon, pp27-33.

9 Cockayne TO. (1864) *Leechdoms, Wortcunning and Starcraft of Early England*, Reprint 1961. London: Longman.

10 For more on making poultices and compresses, see Cech R. (2016) *Making Plant Medicine*, Williams, OR: Horizon Herbs, pp91-102.

11 More about hydrosols in Price S and Price L. (2004) *Understanding Hydrolats: The Specific Hydrosols for Aromatherapy*, Edinburgh: Churchill Livingstone.

12 The pharmacopoeia standard for distilled witch hazel (*Hamamelis virginiana*) includes the addition of 14-15% alcohol.

13 Note that the ownership of a still for producing alcohol is prohibited in some countries.

14 Kunicka-Styczyńska A, Śmigielski K, Prusinowska R, et al. (2015) Preservative activity of lavender hydrosols in moisturizing body gels. *Lett Appl Microbiol* 60: 27-32.

15 Diouf PN, Stevanovic T and Cloutier A. (2009) Anti-oxidant properties and polyphenol contents of trembling aspen bark extracts. *Wood Sci Technol* 43: 457-470.

Chapter 7: Scaling Up the Harvest, pp.105-116

1 Some general considerations about commercial opportunities are given in Remiarz (2017) pp165-174.

2 For example, the Blue Patch sustainable marketplace (www.bluepatch.org) offering UK sourced items; the Etsy global online marketplace (www.etsy.com).

3 Bachmann J. (2002) *Woody Ornamentals for Cut Flower Growers*, Appropriate Technology Transfer for Rural Areas (ATTRA). Available at: https://attra.ncat.org/attra-pub/summaries/summary.php?pub=43 (accessed 29 May 2018). For a comprehensive treatment of cut flowers see Armitage AM and Laushman JM. (2003) *Specialty Cut Flowers: The Production of Annuals, Perennials, Bulbs, and Woody Plants for Fresh and Dried Cut Flowers*, Portland, OR: Timber Press.

4 Oaks R and Mills E. (2010) *Coppicing and Coppice Crafts: A Comprehensive Guide*, Marlborough: Crowood Press.

5 Crawford (2010) pp92-93.

6 European Innovation Partnership Agricultural Productivity and Sustainability' (EIP-AGRI) Focus Group. (2017) *Agroforestry: Introducing Woody Vegetation into Specialised Crop and Livestock Systems: Final Report*, Brussels: EIP-AGRI.

7 den Herder M, Moreno G, Mosquera-Losada RM, et al. (2017) Current extent and stratification of agroforestry in the European Union. *Agric Ecosyst Environ* 241: 1121-1132.

8 Grado S and Husak AL. (2004) Economic analysis of a sustainable forestry system in the southeastern United States. In: Alavalapati JRR and Mercer DE (eds) *Valuing Agroforestry Systems*, Kluwer, pp39-57.

9 See Tree I. (2018) *Wilding: The Return of Nature to a British Farm*, London: Picador.

10 Davis J and Scott Persons W. (2016) *Growing and Marketing Ginseng, Goldenseal and other Woodland Medicinals*, Gabriola Island, Canada: New Society Publishers.

11 See Chapter 6 on 'Forest medicinals' for an assessment of potential profits in the US in Mudge K and Gabriel S. (2014) *Farming the Woods: An Integrated Permaculture Approach to Growing Food and Medicinals in Temperate Forests*, White River Junction, VT: Chelsea Green Publishing.

12 Association for Temperate Agroforestry. Couple farms herbs and mushrooms under managed forest, www.aftaweb.org/about/what-is-

agroforestry/forest-farming/2-uncategorised/24-herbs-mushrooms-managed-farm.html (accessed 25 March 2019).

13 European Medicines Agency. Herbal products: European Union monographs and list entries, available at www.ema.europa.eu/en/human-regulatory/herbal-products/european-union-monographs-list-entries (accessed 7 March 2019). In the UK, the Human Use Regulations Act 2012 incorporates provisions from the earlier Medicines Act 1968 which allow exemptions from licensing for one-to-one consultations with a herbal practitioner.

14 US Food and Drug Administration. Dietary supplements: What you need to know, www.fda.gov/food/dietarysupplements/usingdietarysupplements/ucm109760.htm (accessed 7 March 2019).

15 Food Standards Agency. Register a food business, www.food.gov.uk/business-guidance/register-a-food-business (accessed 7 March 2019).

16 Cosmetic Product Notification Portal, https://ec.europa.eu/growth/sectors/cosmetics/cpnp_en (accessed 7 March 2019); International Nomenclature of Cosmetic Ingredients (INCI), https://ec.europa.eu/growth/sectors/cosmetics/cpnp_en (accessed 7 March 2019).

17 According to Regulation (EC) No. 1223/2009 of the European Parliament and of the Council of 30 November 2009.

18 US Food and Drug Administration. Cosmetics: Labelling regulations, www.fda.gov/Cosmetics/Labeling/Regulations/default.htm (accessed 7 March 2019).

19 Mills and Bone (2005) pp106-107.

20 Blumenthal M. (1999) Herb industry sees mergers, acquisitions, and entry by pharmaceutical giants in 1998. *HerbalGram* 45: 67.

21 Davies G and Lennartsson M. (eds) (2005) *Organic Vegetable Production: A Complete Guide*, Marlborough, Wiltshire: The Crowood Press, pp13-14. See Appendix 6(D) for details of organic organisations and accreditation bodies.

22 COSMOS. Trust in organic and natural cosmetics, https://cosmos-standard.org/for-consumers/ (accessed 7 March 2019).

23 Brotto L and Pettenella D. (eds) (2018) *Forest Management Auditing: Certification of Forest Products and Services*, London: Routledge.

24 Wenban-Smith M, Bowyer J, Fernholz K, et al. (2006) *Combining Organic and FSC Certification of Non-timber Forest Products: Reducing Costs, Increasing Options*, Minneapolis: Dovetail Partners.

25 Guidelines are published, such as Department for Environment, Food and Rural Affairs (DEFRA). (2009) *Protecting our Water, Soil and Air: A Code of Good Agricultural Practice for Farmers, Growers and Land Managers*, Norwich: The Stationery Office.

26 World Health Organization (WHO). (2003) *WHO Guidelines on Good Agricultural and Collection Practices (GACP) for Medicinal Plants*, Geneva: WHO.

27 Committee on Herbal Medicinal Products (HMPC). (2006) Guideline on good agricultural and collection practice (GACP) for starting materials of herbal origin, European Medicines Agency. Available at www.ema.europa.eu/en/documents/scientific-guideline/guideline-good-agricultural-collection-practice-gacp-starting-materials-herbal-origin_en.pdf (accessed 30 June 2019); Schröder M and Cocksedge W. (2004) *Good Practices for Plant Identification for the Herbal Industry; For the Saskatchewan Herb and Spice Association/National Herb and Spice Coalition*, Canada: Centre for Non-timber Resources, Royal Roads University.

28 American Herbal Products Association in cooperation with the American Herbal Pharmacopoeia (2006) *Good Agricultural and Collection Practice for Herbal Raw Materials*, Silver Spring, MD: American Herbal Products Association.

29 Kathe W. (2011) The new FairWild standard – a tool to ensure sustainable wild-collection of plants. *Medicinal Plant Conservation* 14: 14-17.

30 Whitten (1997) pp235-236 has estimated that herb growing on a 0.4 hectare site, fully costed, would require capital investment of AU$11,000 or more.

31 Charities can help too, for example the Woodland Trust in the UK is offering grants for planting, Plant trees, www.woodlandtrust.org.uk/plant-trees/ (accessed 30 March 2019).

32 For example, ARC 2020 briefing note on agroecology, available at www.arc2020.eu/agroecology/briefing-note-agroecology/ (accessed 24 July 2019).

33 In the UK an Organic Herb Growers Co-op formed in December 2018 intending to promote networking between growers and producers, www.organicherbgrowers.uk.

Looking Ahead, pp. 117–121

1 Doyle CJ and Waterhouse T. (2008) Social and economic implications of agroforestry for rural economic development in temperate regions. In: Batish DR, Kohli RK, Shibu J, et al. (eds) *Ecological Basis of Agroforestry*, Boca Raton: CRC Press, pp303-318.

2 In the UK, a network of Permaculture Association LAND centres acts to provide practical demonstrations of permaculture possibilities. See www.permaculture.org.uk/land-centres (accessed 30 June 2019).

3 Urquhart J, Courtney P and Slee B. (2010) Private ownership and public good provision in English woodlands. *Small-scale Forestry* 9: 1-20.

4 See the Sustainable Herbs Program website at http://sustainableherbsproject.com/about (accessed 29 July 2019).

5 Yearsley C. (2017) New United Savers Plant Center seeks to conserve medicinal plants of Appalachia. *HerbalGram* 116: 45-49.

6 Burgess PJ and Rosati A. (2018) Advances in European agroforestry: Results from the AGFORWARD project. *Agroforestry Systems* 92: 801-810.

7 A Permaculture International Research Network has been formed; see https://pirn.permaculture.org.uk (accessed 30 June 2019).

8 Brinckmann JA, Luo W, Xu Q, et al. (2018) Sustainable harvest, people and pandas: Assessing a decade of managed wild harvest and trade in Schisandra sphenanthera. *J Ethnopharmacol* 224: 522-534.

9 James NDG. (1981) *A History of English Forestry*, Oxford: Basil Blackwell, p268.

10 Digby M and Edwardson TE. (1976) *The Organisation of Forestry Co-operatives*, Oxford: Plunkett Foundation for Co-operative Studies.

Part 2, Directory, pp. 122-231

1 Kędzierski B, Kukula-Koch W, Widelski J, et al. (2016) Impact of harvest time of *Aesculus hippocastanum* seeds on the composition, anti-oxidant capacity and total phenolic content. *Ind Crops Prod* 86: 68-72.

2 Henkel (1909) p38.

3 Committee on Herbal Medicinal Products (HMPC). (2009) *Community Herbal Monograph on Aesculus hippocastanum L., semen*, London: European Medicines Agency.

4 Pittler MH and Ernst E. (2012) Horse chestnut seed extract for chronic venous insufficiency. *Cochrane Database Syst Rev* 11: CD003230.

5 World Health Organization (WHO). (2004) *WHO Monographs on Selected Medicinal Plants*. Vol.2, Geneva: WHO.

6 Wilkinson J and Brown A. (1999) Horse chestnut – *Aesculus hippocastanum*: Potential applications in cosmetic skin-care products. *Int J Cosmet Sci* 21: 437-447.

7 Busia K. (2016) *Fundamentals of Herbal Medicine*, vol 2, Xlibris, p124.

8 WHO (2004) vol 2.

9 Engels G and Brinckmann J. (2014) Black chokeberry: *Aronia melanocarpa*: Family: Rosaceae. *HerbalGram* 101: 1-5.

10 Kokotkiewicz A, Jaremicz Z and Luczkiewicz M. (2010) Aronia plants: A review of traditional use, biological activities, and perspectives for modern medicine. *J Med Food* 13: 255-269.

11 Chrubasik C, Li G and Chrubasik S. (2010) The clinical effectiveness of chokeberry: A systematic review. *Phytother Res* 24: 1107-1114.

12 Banjari I, Misir A, Šavikin K, et al. (2017) Antidiabetic effects of *Aronia melanocarpa* and its other therapeutic properties. *Front Nutr* 4: 53; Borowska S and Brzóska MM. (2016) Chokeberries (*Aronia melanocarpa*) and their products as a possible means for the prevention and treatment of noncommunicable diseases and unfavorable health effects due to exposure to xenobiotics. *Comp Revi Food Sci Food Saf* 15: 6.

13 Jurikova T, Mlcek J, Skrovankova S, et al. (2017) Fruits of black chokeberry *Aronia melanocarpa* in the prevention of chronic diseases. *Molecules* 22: E944.

14 Gralec M, Wawer I and Zawada K. (2010) *Aronia melanocarpa* berries: Phenolics composition and anti-oxidant properties changes during fruit development and ripening. *Emir J Food Agric* 31: 214-221.

15 See the Appendix 6(B) section on conservation and climate issues for details of species at risk.

16 Tabeshpour J, Imenshahidi M and Hosseinzadeh H. (2017) A review of the effects of *Berberis vulgaris* and its major component, berberine, in metabolic syndrome. *Iran J Basic Med Sci* 20: 557–568.

17 Harding AR. (1936) *Ginseng and Other Medicinal Plants: A Book of Valuable Information for Growers as well as Collectors of Medicinal Roots, Barks, Leaves, etc.*, Columbus, OH: AR Harding.

18 Misík V, Bezáková L, Máleková L, et al. (1995) Lipoxygenase inhibition and anti-oxidant properties of protoberberine and aporphine alkaloids isolated from *Mahonia aquifolium*. *Planta Med* 61: 372-373.

19 Müller K, Ziereis K and Gawlik I. (1995) The antipsoriatic *Mahonia aquifolium* and its active constituents; II. Antiproliferative activity against cell growth of human keratinocytes. *Planta Med* 61: 74-75.

20 Tegos G, Stermitz F, Lomovskaya O, et al. (2002) Multidrug pump inhibitors uncover remarkable activity of plant antimicrobials. *Antimicrob Agents Chemother* 46: 3133-3141.

21 BHMA Scientific Committee (1983) pp40-41.

22 Hynynen J, Niemistö P, Viherä-Aarnio A, et al. (2010) Silviculture of birch (*Betula pendula* Roth and *Betula pubescens* Ehrh.) in northern Europe. *Forestry* 83: 103-119.

23 Baumgartner A, Sampol-Lopez M, Cemeli E, et al. (2012) Genotoxicity assessment of birch-bark tar – a most versatile prehistoric adhesive. *Advances in Anthropology* 2: 39-49.

24 Sak K, Jürisoo K and Raal A. (2014) Estonian folk traditional experiences on natural anticancer remedies: From past to the future. *Pharm Biol* 52: 855-866.

25 Barker (2001) section 15.

26 Gründemann C, Gruber C, Hertrampf A, et al. (2011) An aqueous birch leaf extract of *Betula pendula* inhibits the growth and cell division of inflammatory lymphocytes. *J Ethnopharmacol* 136: 444-451.

27 Ebeling S, Naumann K, Pollok S, et al. (2014) From a traditional medicinal plant to a rational drug: Understanding the clinically proven wound healing efficacy of birch bark extract. *PLoS One* 9: e86147.

28 Huyke C, Laszczyk M, Scheffler A, et al. (2006) Treatment of actinic keratoses with birch bark extract: A pilot study. *J Dtsch Dermatol Ges* 4: 132-136.

29 Selzer E, Pimentel E, Wacheck V, et al. (2000) Effects of betulinic acid alone and in combination with irradiation in human melanoma cells. *J Invest Dermatol* 114: 935-940.

30 Wardecki T, Werner P, Thomas M, et al. (2016) Influence of birch bark triterpenes on keratinocytes and fibroblasts from diabetic and nondiabetic donors. *J Nat Prod* 79: 1112-1123.

31 Havlik J, Gonzalez de la Huebra R, Hejtmankova K, et al. (2010) Xanthine oxidase inhibitory properties of Czech medicinal plants. *J Ethnopharmacol* 132: 461-465.

32 Baumgartner et al. (2012) p49.

33 Demirci B, Paper DH, Demirci F, et al. (2004) Essential oil of *Betula pendula* Roth. buds. *Evid Based Complement Alternat Med* 1: 301-303.

34 Conedera M, Krebs P, Tinner W, et al. (2004) The cultivation of *Castanea sativa* (Mill.) in Europe, from its origin to its diffusion on a continental scale. *Veg Hist Archaeobot* 13: 161-179.

35 Howkins C. (2003) *Sweet Chestnut: History, Landscape, People*, Addlestone, Surrey: Published by the author.

36 Donno D, Beccaro GL, Mellano MG, et al. (2014) *Castanea* spp. buds as a phytochemical source for herbal preparations: Botanical fingerprint for nutraceutical identification and functional food standardisation. *Sci Food Agric* 94: 2863-2873.

37 Barker (2001) section 19.

38 Carocho M, Barros L, Bento A, et al. (2014) *Castanea sativa* Mill. flowers amongst the most powerful anti-oxidant matrices: A phytochemical approach in decoctions and infusions. *Biomed Res Int* 2014: 232956.

39 Quave CL, Lyles JT, Kavanaugh JS, et al. (2015) *Castanea sativa* (European chestnut) leaf extracts rich in ursene and oleanene derivatives block staphylococcus aureus virulence and pathogenesis without detectable resistance. *PLoS One* 10: e0136486.

40 Chiarini A, Micucci M, Malaguti M, et al. (2013) Sweet chestnut (*Castanea sativa* Mill.) bark extract: Cardiovascular activity and myocyte protection against oxidative damage. *Oxid Med Cell Longev* 2013: 71790.

41 Delwiche C, Zinke P and Johnson C. (1965) Nitrogen fixation by Ceanothus. *Plant Physiol* 40: 1045–1047.

42 Cech R. (2016) *Making Plant Medicine*, Williams, OR: Horizon Herbs, p210.

43 Li XC, Cai L and Wu CD. (1997) Antimicrobial compounds from *Ceanothus americanus* against oral pathogens. *Phytochemistry* 46: 97-102.

44 Salazar-Aranda R, Pérez-López L, López-Arroyo J, et al. (2011) Antimicrobial and anti-oxidant activities of plants from Northeast of Mexico. *Evid Based Complement Alternat Med* 2011: 536139.

45 Carpenter W, Ostmark E and Sheehan T. (1991) Recommendations for germinating fringetree *Chionanthus virginicus* L. seed. *Proc Fla State Hort Soc* 104: 337-340.

46 Conway (2001) p157.

47 Roux F. (1913) Note on the use of *Chionanthus virginiana* in diseases of the liver. *Ind Med Gaz* 48: 394-395.

48 Penman KG, Bone K and Lehmann RP. (2008) Fringe tree (*Chionanthus virginicus* L.) stem bark offers a sustainable alternative to root bark. *Australian Journal of Medical Herbalism* 20: 107-111.

49 Gülçin I, Elias R, Gepdiremen A, et al. (2006) Anti-oxidant activity of lignans from fringe tree (*Chionanthus virginicus* L.). *Eur Food Res Technol* 223: 759.

50 Boyer L, Baghdikian B, Bun SS, et al. (2011) *Chionanthus virginicus* L.: Phytochemical analysis and quality control of herbal drug and herbal preparations. *Nat Prod Commun* 6: 753-758.

51 Sparks TH and Martin T. (1999) Yields of hawthorn *Crataegus monogyna* berries under different hedgerow management. *Agric Ecosyst Environ* 72: 107-110.

52 WHO (2004) vol 2.

53 Barker (2001) section 138.

54 Committee on Herbal Medicinal Products (HMPC). (2016) *Final European Union Herbal Monograph on Crataegus spp., Folium Cum Flore*, London: European Medicines Agency.

55 WHO (2004) vol 2.

56 Hanus M, Lafon J and Mathieu M. (2004) Double-blind, randomised, placebo-controlled study to evaluate the efficacy and safety of a fixed combination containing two plant extracts (*Crataegus oxyacantha* and *Eschscholtzia californica*) and magnesium in mild-to-moderate anxiety disorders. *Curr Med Res Opin* 20: 63-71.

57 Blumenthal M and Foster S. (2000) *Herbal Medicine: Expanded Commission E Monographs: Herb Monographs, Based on those Created by a Special Expert Committee of the German Federal Institute for Drugs and Medical Devices*, Austin, Tex.: American Botanical Council.

58 Tassell MC, Kingston R, Gilroy D, et al. (2010) Hawthorn (*Crataegus* spp.) in the treatment of cardiovascular disease. *Pharmacogn Rev* 4: 32-41.

59 Benabderrahmane W, Lores M, Benaissa O, et al. (2019) Polyphenolic content and bioactivities of *Crataegus oxyacantha* L. (Rosaceae). *Nat Prod Res* Epub 5 March 2019. DOI: 10.1080/14786419.2019.1582044; Busia (2016) vol 2, p142.

60 Barros L, Carvalho AM and Ferreira IC. (2011) Comparing the composition and bioactivity of *Crataegus monogyna* flowers and fruits used in folk medicine. *Phytochem Anal* 22: 181-188.

61 Blumenthal and Foster (2000).

62 Daniele C, Mazzanti G, Pittler MH, et al. (2006) Adverse-event profile of *Crataegus* spp.: A systematic review. *Drug Saf* 29: 523-535.

63 De la Bédoyère C. (2004) *The Handbook of Native Trees and Shrubs: How to Plant and Maintain a Natural Woodland*, London: New Holland, p59.

64 Barker (2001) section 145.

65 González N, Ribeiro D, Fernandes E, et al. (2013) Potential use of *Cytisus scoparius* extracts in topical applications for skin protection against oxidative damage. *J Photochem Photobiol* B 125: 83-89.

66 Abreu AC, Coqueiro A, Sultan AR, et al. (2017) Looking to nature for a new concept in antimicrobial treatments: Isoflavonoids from *Cytisus striatus* as antibiotic adjuvants against MRSA. *Sci Rep* 7: 3777.

67 Larit F, Elokely KM, Chaurasiya ND, et al. (2018) Inhibition of human monoamine oxidase A and B by flavonoids isolated from two Algerian medicinal plants. *Phytomedicine* 40: 27-36.

68 Busia (2016) vol 2, p164.

69 Hamidpour R, Hamidpour S, Hamidpour M, et al. (2016) Russian olive (*Elaeagnus angustifolia* L.): From a variety of traditional medicinal applications to its novel roles as active anti-oxidant, anti-inflammatory, anti-mutagenic and analgesic agent. *J Tradit Complement Med* 16: 24-29.

70 Crawford M. (2015) *Trees for Gardens, Orchards and Permaculture*, East Meon, UK: Permanent Publications, p182.

71 Sadowska B, Budzyńska A, Stochmal A, et al. (2017) Novel properties of *Hippophae rhamnoides* L. twig and leaf extracts – anti-virulence action and synergy with antifungals studied in vitro on *Candida* spp. model. *Microb Pathog* 107: 372-379.

72 Olas B. (2016) Sea buckthorn as a source of important bioactive compounds in cardiovascular diseases. *Food Chem Toxicol* 97: 199-204; Upadhyay NK, Kumar MS and Gupta A. (2010) Anti-oxidant, cytoprotective and antibacterial effects of Sea buckthorn (*Hippophae rhamnoides* L.) leaves. *Food Chem Toxicol* 48: 3443-3448.

73 Ito H, Asmussen S, Traber DL, et al. (2014) Healing efficacy of sea buckthorn (Hippophae rhamnoides L.) seed oil in an ovine burn wound model. *Burns* 40: 511-519.

74 Olas B, Skalski B and Ulanowska K. (2018) The anticancer activity of sea buckthorn [*Elaeagnus rhamnoides* (L.) A. Nelson]. *Front Pharmacol* 9: 232.

75 Barker (2001) section 195.

76 Schaeffer A, Kehr M, Gianetti B, et al. (2016) A randomized, controlled, double-blind, multi-center trial to evaluate the efficacy and safety of a liquid containing ivy leaves dry extract (EA 575®)

vs. placebo in the treatment of adults with acute cough. *Pharmazie* 71: 504-509.

77 Li TS. (2001) Siberian ginseng. *HortTechnology* 11: 79-85.

78 Li (2001).

79 Foster S and Chongxi Y. (1992) *Herbal Emissaries: Bringing Chinese Herbs to the West: A Guide to Gardening, Herbal Wisdom, and Well-being*, Rochester, VT: Healing Arts Press, p78.

80 Huang L, Zhao H, Huang B, et al. (2011) *Acanthopanax senticosus*: Review of botany, chemistry and pharmacology. *Pharmazie* 66: 83-97.

81 Committee on Herbal Medicinal Products (HMPC). (2014) *Community Herbal Monograph on Eleutherococcus senticosus (Rupr. et Maxim.) Maxim., radix*, London, UK: European Medicines Agency.

82 Yance D. (2013) *Adaptogens in Medical Herbalism: Elite Herbs and Natural Compounds for Mastering Stress, Aging, and Chronic Disease*, Rochester, VT: Healing Arts Press; also see Li T, Ferns K, Yan ZQ, et al. (2016) *Acanthopanax senticosus*: Photochemistry and anticancer potential. *Am J Chin Med* 44: 1543-1558.

83 Barth A, Hovhannisyan A, Jamalyan K, et al. (2015) Antitussive effect of a fixed combination of *Justicia adhatoda, Echinacea purpurea* and *Eleutherococcus senticosus* extracts in patients with acute upper respiratory tract infection: A comparative, randomized, double-blind, placebo-controlled study. *Phytomedicine* 22: 1195-1200.

84 Adamczyk K, Olech M, Abramek J, et al. (2019) *Eleutherococcus* species cultivated in Europe: A new source of compounds with antiacetylcholinesterase, antihyaluronidase, anti-DPPH, and cytotoxic activities. *Oxid Med Cell Longev* 2019: 8673521.

85 Busia (2016) vol 2, p208.

86 Ferraz Filho AC, Scolforo JBS and Mola-Yudego B. (2014) The coppice-with-standards silvicultural system as applied to Eucalyptus plantations – a review. *Journal of Forestry Research* 25: 237-248.

87 Leslie A, Mencuccini M and Perks MP. (2011) Eucalyptus in the British Isles. *Quarterly Journal of Forestry* 105: 43-53.

88 Committee on Herbal Medicinal Products (HMPC). (2013) *Community Herbal Monograph on Eucalyptus globulus Labill., folium*, London, UK: European Medicines Agency.

89 Sadlon AE and Lamson DW. (2010) Immune-modifying and antimicrobial effects of eucalyptus oil and simple inhalation devices. *Altern Med Rev* 15: 33-47.

90 Shahi SK, Shukla AC, Bajaj AK, et al. (2000) Broad spectrum herbal therapy against superficial fungal infections. *Skin Pharmacol Appl Skin Physiol* 13: 60-64.

91 WHO (2004) vol 2.

92 Miguel MG, Gago C, Antunes MD, et al. (2018) Antibacterial, antioxidant, and antiproliferative activities of *Corymbia citriodora* and the essential oils of eight Eucalyptus species. *Medicines (Basel)* 5: 61.

93 Williams C. (2011) *Medicinal Plants in Australia. Volume 2: Gums, Resins, Tannin and Essential Oils*, Kenthurst, Australia: Rosenberg Publishing, pp168-169.

94 Ciesla (2002) *Non-wood Forest Products from Temperate Broad-leaved Trees*, Rome: Food and Agriculture Organisation of the United Nations, p30.

95 Transparency Market Research. Global eucalyptus oil market: Snapshot, www.transparencymarketresearch.com/eucalyptus-oil-market.html (2018, accessed 30 April 2019).

96 WHO (2004) vol 2.

97 Ghanbari A, Le Gresley A, Naughton D, et al. (2019) Biological activities of *Ficus carica* latex for potential therapeutics in human papillomavirus (HPV) related cervical cancers. *Sci Rep* 9: 1013; Conforti F, Menichini G, Zanfini L, et al. (2012) Evaluation of phototoxic potential of aerial components of the fig tree against human melanoma. *Cell Prolif* 45: 279-285.

98 Mawa S, Husain K and Jantan I. (2013) *Ficus carica* L. (Moraceae): Phytochemistry, traditional uses and biological activities. *Evid Based Complement Alternat Med* 2013: 974256.

99 Mopuri R, Ganjayi M, Meriga B, et al. (2018) The effects of *Ficus carica* on the activity of enzymes related to metabolic syndrome. *J Food Drug Anal* 26: 201-210.

100 Badgujar SB, Patel VV, Bandivdekar AH, et al. (2014) Traditional uses, phytochemistry and pharmacology of *Ficus carica*: A review. *Pharm Biol* 52: 1487-1503.

101 Barker (2001) section 25.

102 Barolo M, Mostacero N and López S. *Ficus carica* L. (Moraceae): An ancient source of food and health. *Food Chem* 164: 119-127.

103 For further detail of cultivation and propagation see Schafer P. (2012) *The Chinese Medicinal Herb Farm: A Cultivator's Guide to Small-scale Organic Herb Production*, White River Junction, VT: Chelsea Green, p177.

104 Wang Z, Xia Q, Liu X, et al. (2018) Phytochemistry, pharmacology, quality control and future research of *Forsythia suspensa* (Thunb.) Vahl: A review. *J Ethnopharmacol* 210: 318-339.

105 Michalak B, Filipek A, Chomicki P, et al. (2018) Lignans from *Forsythia × intermedia* leaves and flowers attenuate the pro-inflammatory function of leukocytes and their interaction with endothelial cells. *Front Pharmacol* 9: 401.

106 Bao J, Ding RB, Liang Y, et al. (2017) Differences in chemical component and anticancer activity of green and ripe *Forsythiae fructus*. *Am J Chin Med* 45: 1513-1536.

107 See Appendix 6(B) where there is information about conservation and climate issues and the UPS Species At-Risk List.

108 Davidson J. (1942) *The Cascara Tree in British Columbia*, Victoria, British Columbia: Ministry of Agriculture.

109 De Kort H, Mergeay J, Jacquemyn H, et al. (2016) Transatlantic invasion routes and adaptive potential in North American populations of the invasive glossy buckthorn, *Frangula alnus*. *Ann Bot* 118: 1089-1099.

110 Juxton J. (1740?) *Anglica pilula benedicta: Or, the Blessed English Pill, Being an Extract of the Blessed Thistle, and Buckthorn-berries*, London, fol. 4.

111 Edlin HL. (1949) *Woodland Crafts in Britain: An Account of the Traditional uses of Trees and Timbers in the British Countryside*, 1973 edition, Newton Abbott: David and Charles.

112 Committee on Herbal Medicinal Products (HMPC). (2006) *Community Herbal Monograph on Rhamnus Frangula L., Cortex*, London: European Medicines Agency.

113 WHO (2004) vol 2.

114 Țebrencu CE, Crețu RM, Mitroi GR, et al. (2015) Phytochemical evaluation and HPTLC investigation of bark and extracts of *Rhamnus frangula* Linn. *Phytochem Rev* 14: 613–621.

115 Bacha AB, Jemel I, Moubayed NMS, et al. (2017) Purification and characterization of a newly serine protease inhibitor from *Rhamnus frangula* with potential for use as therapeutic drug. 3 *Biotech* 7: 148.

116 Sadowska B, Paszkiewicz M, Podsędek A, et al. (2014) *Vaccinium myrtillus* leaves and *Frangula alnus* bark derived extracts as potential antistaphylococcal agents. *Acta Biochim Pol* 61: 163-169.

117 Xiong HR, Luo J, Hou W, et al. (2011) The effect of emodin, an anthraquinone derivative extracted from the roots of *Rheum tanguticum*, against herpes simplex virus in vitro and in vivo. *J Ethnopharmacol* 133: 718-723.

118 Pickhardt M, Gazova Z, von Bergen M, et al. (2005) Anthraquinones inhibit tau aggregation and dissolve Alzheimer's paired helical filaments in vitro and in cells. *J Biol Chem* 280: 3628-3635.

119 Boussahel S, Speciale A, Dahamna S, et al. (2015) Flavonoid profile, anti-oxidant and cytotoxic activity of different extracts from Algerian Rhamnus alaternus L. bark. *Pharmacogn Mag* 11: S102-109.

120 Bradley P. (ed.) (1992) *British Herbal Compendium: Volume 1.* Bournemouth: British Herbal Medicine Association, p99.

121 Barker (2001) section 183.

122 Vandal J, Abou-Zaid MM, Ferroni G, et al. (2015) Antimicrobial activity of natural products from the flora of Northern Ontario, Canada. *Pharm Biol* 53: 800-806.

123 Evelyn (1670) p40.

124 Barker (2001) section 258.

125 Sarfraz I, Rasul A, Jabeen F, et al. (2017) *Fraxinus*: A plant with versatile pharmacological and biological activities. *Evid Based Complement Alternat Med* 2017: 4269868.

126 European Medicines Agency. (2012) Assessment report on *Fraxinus excelsior* L. or *Fraxinus angustifola* Vahl, *folium*. Available at: www.ema.europa.eu/en/documents/herbal-report/final-assessment-report-fraxinus-excelsior-l-fraxinus-angustifolia-vahl-folium_en.pdf (accessed 6 May 2019).

127 Kostova I and Iossifova T. (2007) Chemical components of *Fraxinus* species: Review article. *Fitoterapia* 78: 85-106.

128 Zulet M, Navas-Carretero S, Lara y Sánchez D, et al. (2014) A *Fraxinus excelsior* L. seeds/fruits extract benefits glucose homeostasis and adiposity related markers in elderly overweight/obese subjects: A longitudinal, randomized, crossover, double-blind, placebo-controlled nutritional intervention study. *Phytomedicine* 21: 1162-1169.

129 Klein-Galczinsky C. (1999) Pharmacological and clinical effectiveness of a fixed phytogenic combination trembling poplar (*Populus tremula*), true goldenrod (*Solidago virgaurea*) and ash (*Fraxinus excelsior*) in mild to moderate rheumatic complaints. [Article in German]. *Wien Med Wochenschr* 149: 248-253.

130 Hillier J and Lancaster R. (eds) (2014) *The Hillier Manual of Trees and Shrubs*. Eighth ed. London: Royal Horticultural Society, p489.

131 Laurain D. (2003) Cultivation of *Ginkgo biloba* on a large scale. In: VanBeek TA (ed) *Ginkgo biloba*, Boca Raton: CRC Press, pp68-88.

132 Committee on Herbal Medicinal Products (HMPC). (2015) *European Union Herbal Monograph on Ginkgo biloba L., folium*, London: European Medicines Agency.

133 Wu Y, Li S, Cui W, et al. (2007) *Ginkgo biloba* extract improves coronary blood flow in patients with coronary artery disease: Role of endothelium-dependent vasodilation. *Planta Med* 73: 624-628.

134 Woelk H, Arnoldt K, Kieser M, et al. (2007) *Ginkgo biloba* special extract Egb 761 in generalized anxiety disorder and adjustment disorder with anxious mood: A randomized, double-blind placebo-controlled trial. *J Psychiatr Res* 41: 472-480.

135 Brondino N, De Silvestri A, Re S, et al. (2013) A systematic review and meta-analysis of *Ginkgo biloba* in neuropsychiatric disorders: From ancient tradition to modern-day medicine. *Evid Based Complement Alternat Med* 2013: 915691; Hashiguchi M, Ohta Y, Shimizu M, et al. (2015) Meta-analysis of the efficacy and safety of *Ginkgo biloba* extract for the treatment of dementia. *J Pharm Health Care Sci* 1: 14.

136 Ramassamy C, Longpré F and Christen Y. (2007) *Ginkgo biloba* extract (EGb 761) in Alzheimer's disease: Is there any evidence? *Curr Alzheimer Res* 4: 253-262.

137 Busia (2016) vol 2, p147.

138 Greenfield J and Davis JM. (eds) (2004) *Medicinal Herb Production Guide: Ginkgo (Ginkgo biloba L.)*, North Carolina: Consortium on Natural Medicines and Public Health.

139 Crawford M. (2015) p87.

140 Booker A, Frommenwiler D, Reich E, et al. (2016) Adulteration and poor quality of *Ginkgo biloba* supplements. *J Herb Med* 6: 79-87; Gafner S. (2016) Ginkgo extract adulteration in the global market: A brief review. *HerbalGram* 109: 58-59.

141 Williamson et al. (2009) p207.

142 Crawford M. (2016) Witch hazel: *Hamamelis virginiana*. *Agroforestry News* 24: 36-38.

143 Lloyd JU and Lloyd JT. (1935) History of *Hamamelis* (witch hazel) extract and distillate. *J Am Pharm Assoc* 24: 220.

144 Henkel (1909) p28.

145 Committee on Herbal Medicinal Products (HMPC). (2009) *Community Herbal Monograph on Hamamelis Virginiana L., Folium*, London, UK: European Medicines Agency.

146 WHO (2004) vol 2.

147 Hughes-Formella BJ, Bohnsack K, Rippke F, et al. (1998) Anti-inflammatory effect of *Hamamelis* lotion in a UVB erythema test. *Dermatology* 196: 316-322.

148 Theisen L, Erdelmeier C, Spoden G, et al. (2014) Tannins from *Hamamelis virginiana* bark extract: Characterization and improvement of the antiviral efficacy against influenza A virus and human papillomavirus. *PLoS One* 9: e88062.

149 Sánchez-Tena S, Fernández-Cachón ML, Carreras A, et al. (2012) Hamamelitannin from witch hazel (*Hamamelis virginiana*) displays specific cytotoxic activity against colon cancer cells. *J Nat Prod* 75: 26-33.

150 Busia (2016) vol 2, p466.

151 Lane C. (2005) *Witch Hazels*, Portland and Cambridge: Timber Press, p31.

152 Paudel P, Satyal P, Dosoky NS, et al. (2013) *Juglans regia* and *J. nigra*, two trees important in traditional medicine: A comparison of leaf essential oil compositions and biological activities. *Nat Prod Commun* 8: 1481-1486.

153 Henkel (1909) p15.

154 Barker (2001) section 12; see also the blog post by the Balkan Ecology Project, 'Plants that can be grown around walnuts and hickories – juglone tolerant plants', https://balkanecologyproject. blogspot.com/2015/09/plants-that-can-be-grown-around-walnuts. html (2015, accessed 7 May 2019).

155 Evelyn (1670) p56.

156 Committee on Herbal Medicinal Products (HMPC). (2013) *Community Herbal Monograph on Juglans Regia L., Folium*, London, UK: European Medicines Agency.

157 Zakavi F, Hagh LG, Daraeighadikolaei A, et al. (2013) Antibacterial effect of *Juglans regia* bark against oral pathologic bacteria. *Int J Dent* 2013: 854765.

158 Hosseini S, Jamshidi L, Mehrzadi S, et al. (2014) Effects of *Juglans regia* L. leaf extract on hyperglycemia and lipid profiles in type two diabetic patients: A randomized double-blind, placebo-controlled clinical trial. *J Ethnopharmacol* 152: 451-456.

159 Rabiei K, Ebrahimzadeh MA, Saeedi M, et al. (2018) Effects of a hydroalcoholic extract of *Juglans regia* (walnut) leaves on blood glucose and major cardiovascular risk factors in type 2 diabetic patients: A double-blind, placebo-controlled clinical trial. *BMC Complement Altern Med* 18: 206.

160 Hwang HJ, Liu Y, Kim HS, et al. (2019) Daily walnut intake improves metabolic syndrome status and increases circulating adiponectin levels: Randomized controlled crossover trial. *Nutr Res Pract* 13: 105-114.

161 Catanzaro E, Greco G, Potenza L, et al. (2018) Natural products to fight cancer: A focus on *Juglans regia*. *Toxins (Basel)* 10: E469.

162 Cosmulescu S. and Ion T. (2011) Seasonal variation of total phenols in leaves of walnut (*Juglans regia* L.). *J Med Plants Res* 5: 4938-4942.

163 De la Bédoyère (2004) p69.

164 Broome A. (2003) *Growing Juniper: Propagation and Establishment Practices*, Edinburgh: Forestry Commission.

165 Bais S, Gill NS, Rana N, et al. (2014) A phytopharmacological review on a medicinal plant: *Juniperus communis*. *Int Sch Res Notices* 2014: 634723; Committee on Herbal Medicinal Products (HMPC). (2009) *Community Herbal Monograph on Juniperus Communis L., Pseudo-fructus*, London: European Medicines Agency.

166 Carpenter CD, O'Neill T, Picot N, et al. (2012) Anti-mycobacterial natural products from the Canadian medicinal plant *Juniperus communis*. *J Ethnopharmacol* 143: 695-700.

167 Pepeljnjak S, Kosalec I, Kalodera Z, et al. (2005) Antimicrobial activity of juniper berry essential oil (*Juniperus communis* L., Cupressaceae). *Acta Pharm* 55: 417-422.

168 Maurya AK, Devi R, Kumar A, et al. (2018) Chemical composition, cytotoxic and antibacterial activities of essential oils of cultivated clones of *Juniperus communis* and wild *Juniperus* species. *Chem Biodivers* 15: e1800183.

169 Ved A, Gupta A and Rawat AK. (2017) Anti-oxidant and hepatoprotective potential of phenol-rich fraction of *Juniperus communis* Linn. Leaves. *Pharmacogn Mag* 13: 108-113.

170 Tsai W-C, Tsai N-M, Chang K-F, et al. (2018) *Juniperus communis* extract exerts antitumor effects in human glioblastomas through blood-brain barrier. *Cell Physiol Biochem* 49: 2443-2462.

171 Carroll JF, Tabanca N, Kramer M, et al. (2011) Essential oils of *Cupressus funebris*, *Juniperus communis*, and *J. chinensis* (Cupressaceae) as repellents against ticks (Acari: Ixodidae) and mosquitoes (Diptera: Culicidae) and as toxicants against mosquitoes. *J Vector Ecol* 36: 258-268.

172 Och M, Och A, Cieśla Ł, et al. (2015) Study of cytotoxic activity, podophyllotoxin, and deoxypodophyllotoxin content in selected *Juniperus* species cultivated in Poland. *Pharm Biol* 53: 831-837.

173 Barker (2001) section 72.

174 Dall'Acqua S, Cervellati R, Speroni E, et al. (2009) Phytochemical composition and anti-oxidant activity of *Laurus nobilis* L. leaf infusion. *J Med Food* 12: 869-876.

175 Fidan H, Stefanova G, Kostova I, et al. (2019) Chemical composition and antimicrobial activity of *Laurus nobilis* L. essential oils from Bulgaria. *Molecules* 24: E804.

176 Lee EH, Shin JH, Kim SS, et al. (2019) *Laurus nobilis* leaf extract controls inflammation by suppressing NLRP3 inflammasome activation. *J Cell Physiol* 234: 6854-6864.

177 Basak SS and Candan F. (2013) Effect of *Laurus nobilis* L. essential oil and its main components on α-glucosidase and reactive oxygen Species scavenging activity. *Iran J Pharm Res* 12: 367-379.

178 Fidan H, Stefanova G, Kostova I, et al. (2019) Chemical composition and antimicrobial activity of *Laurus nobilis* L. essential oils from Bulgaria. *Molecules* 24: E804.

179 Crawford M. (2015) p27.

180 Johnson RL. (1964) Coppice regeneration of sweetgum. *J For* 62: 34-35.

181 Krochmal A and Krochmal C. (1984) *A Field Guide to Medicinal Plants*, New York: Times Books.

182 Grieve (1980) provides a description of the process used in producing storax from *Liquidambar orientalis* (p775).

183 Zhang M, Ma Y, Chai L, et al. (2019) Storax protected oxygen-glucose deprivation/reoxygenation induced primary astrocyte injury by inhibiting NF-κB activation in vitro. *Front Pharmacol* 9: 1527.

184 Hutchens A. (1991) *Indian Herbalogy of North America*, Boston: Shambhala, p276.

185 Felter HW and Lloyd JU. (1898) *King's American Dispensatory*, 18th edition, 2 vols, Cincinatti: Ohio Valley Co.

186 Lingbeck J, O'Bryan C, Martin E, et al. (2015) Sweetgum: An ancient source of beneficial compounds with modern benefits. *Pharmacogn Rev* 9: 1-11.

187 Eid HH, Labib RM, AbdelHamid NS, et al. (2015) Hepatoprotective and anti-oxidant polyphenols from a standardized methanolic extract of the leaves of *Liquidambar styraciflua* L. *Bulletin of Faculty of Pharmacy, Cairo University* 53: 117-127.

188 Wyllie S and Brophy J. (1989) The leaf oil of *Liquidambar styraciflua*. *Planta Med* 55: 316-317.

189 Foster S. (2017) Forest gems: Exploring medicinal trees in American forests. *HerbalGram* 116: 50-71.

190 Conway (2001) p212.

191 Lee Y, Lee Y, Lee C, et al. (2011) Therapeutic applications of compounds in the Magnolia family. *Pharmacol Ther* 130: 157-176.

192 Hipps YG, Hacker YE, Hoffmann DL, et al. (2009) Self-reported quality of life in complementary and alternative medicine treatment of chronic rhinosinusitis among African Americans: A preliminary, open-label pilot study. *J Altern Complement Med* 15: 67-77.

193 Luo H, Wu H, Yu X, et al. (2019) A review of the phytochemistry and pharmacological activities of *Magnoliae officinalis* cortex. *J Ethnopharmacol* 236: 412-442.

194 Poivre M and Duez P. (2017) Biological activity and toxicity of the Chinese herb *Magnolia officinalis* Rehder & E. Wilson (Houpo) and its constituents. *J Zhejiang Univ Sci* B 18: 194-214.

195 Shen Y, Li CG, Zhou SF, et al. (2008) Chemistry and bioactivity of Flos Magnoliae, a Chinese herb for rhinitis and sinusitis. *Curr Med Chem* 15: 1616-1627.

196 Park CH, Park SY, Lee SY, et al. (2018) Analysis of metabolites in white flowers of *Magnolia denudata* Desr. and violet flowers of *Magnolia liliiflora* Desr. *Molecules* 23: E1558.

197 Zai-Kang T, Yan-Ru Z and Jin-Ping S. (2002) Variation, heredity and selection of effective ingredients in *Magnolia officinalis* of different provenances. *J For Res (Harbin)* 13: 7-11.

198 Barker (2001) section 24.

199 Lim SH and Choi C. (2019) Pharmacological properties of *Morus nigra* L. (black mulberry) as a promising nutraceutical resource. *Nutrients* 11: 437; Yang MY, Huang CN, Chan KC, et al. (2011) Mulberry leaf polyphenols possess antiatherogenesis effect via inhibiting LDL oxidation and foam cell formation. *J Agric Food Chem* 59: 1985-1995.

200 Rodrigues EL, Marcelino G, Silva GT, et al. (2019) Nutraceutical and medicinal potential of the *Morus* species in metabolic dysfunctions. *Int J Mol Sci* 20: E301.

201 Hwang S, Li H, Lim S, et al. (2016) Evaluation of a standardized extract from *Morus alba* against α-glucosidase inhibitory effect and postprandial antihyperglycemic in patients with impaired glucose tolerance: A randomized double-blind clinical trial. *Evid Based Complement Altern Med* 2016: 8983232.

202 Sisay M and Gashaw T. (2017) Ethnobotanical, ethnopharmacological, and phytochemical studies of *Myrtus communis* Linn: A popular herb in Unani system of medicine. *J Evid Based Complementary Altern Med* 22: 1035–1043.

203 Hennia A, Miguel MG and Nemmiche S. (2018) Anti-oxidant activity of *Myrtus communis* L. and *Myrtus nivellei* Batt. & Trab. extracts: A brief review. *Medicines (Basel)* 5: 89.

204 Alipour G, Dashti S and Hosseinzadeh H. (2014) Review of pharmacological effects of *Myrtus communis* L. and its active constituents. *Phytother Res* 28: 1125-1136.

205 Mansouri S, Foroumadi A, Ghaneie T, et al. (2008) Antibacterial activity of the crude extracts and fractionated constituents of *Myrtus communis*. *Pharm Biol* 39: 399-401.

206 Zohalinezhad ME, Hosseini-Asl MK, Akrami R, et al. (2016) *Myrtus communis* L. freeze-dried aqueous extract versus omeprazole in gastrointestinal reflux disease: A double-blind randomized controlled clinical trial. *J Evid Based Complementary Altern Med* 21: 23-29.

207 Masoudi M, Miraj S and Rafieian-Kopaei M. (2016) Comparison of the effects of *Myrtus communis* L, *Berberis vulgaris* and metronidazole vaginal gel alone for the treatment of bacterial vaginosis. *J Clin Diagn Res* 10: QC04–QC07.

208 Fern K. (2000) *Plants for a Future: Edible and Useful Plants for a Healthier World*, East Meon, Hampshire: Permanent Publications, p36.

209 Barker (2001) section 520.

210 Kačániová M, Vukovič N, Horská E, et al. (2014) Antibacterial activity against Clostridium genus and antiradical activity of the essential oils from different origin. *J Environ Sci Health* B 49: 505-512.

211 Hoai NT, Duc HV, Thao DT, et al. (2015) Selectivity of *Pinus sylvestris* extract and essential oil to estrogen-insensitive breast cancer cells *Pinus sylvestris* against cancer cells. *Pharmacogn Mag* 11: S290-S295.

212 Amalinei RL, Trifan A, Cioanca O, et al. (2014) Polyphenol-rich extract from *Pinus sylvestris* L. bark–chemical and antitumor studies. *Rev Med Chir Soc Med Nat Iasi* 118: 551-557.

213 American Botanical Council (2019) *Proprietary Botanical Ingredient Scientific and Clinical Monograph for Pycnogenol (French Maritime Pine Bark Extract) Pinus pinaster Aiton subsp. atlantica* [Fam. Pinaceae]: 2019 update, American Botanic Council, Austin, TX.

214 Rohdewald PJ. (2018) Review on sustained relief of osteoarthritis symptoms with a proprietary extract from pine bark, Pycnogenol. *J Med Food* 21: 1-4.

215 Hatfield G. (2004) *Encyclopedia of Folk Medicine: Old World and New World Traditions*, Santa Barbara, CA: ABC-CLIO, p71.

216 Barker (2001) section 141.

217 Egea T, Signorinia MA, Bruschi P, et al. (2015) Spirits and liqueurs in European traditional medicine: Their history and ethnobotany in Tuscany and Bologna (Italy). *J Ethnopharmacol* 175: 241-255.

218 Sak K, Jürisoo K and Raal A. (2014) Estonian folk traditional experiences on natural anticancer remedies: From past to the future. *Pharm Biol* 52: 855-866.

219 Donno D, Mellano MG, De Biaggi M, et al. (2018) New findings in *Prunus padus* L. fruits as a source of natural compounds: Characterization of metabolite profiles and preliminary evaluation of anti-oxidant activity. *Molecules* 23: E725.

220 Bastos C, Barros L, Dueñas M, et al. (2015) Chemical characterisation and bioactive properties of *Prunus avium* L.: The widely studied fruits and the unexplored stems. *Food Chem* 173: 1045-1053.

221 Luna-Vázquez F, Ibarra-Alvarado C, Rojas-Molina A, et al. (2013) Nutraceutical value of black cherry *Prunus serotina* Ehrh. fruits: Anti-oxidant and antihypertensive properties. *Molecules* 18: 14597-14612.

222 Zou J and Cates R. (1995) Foliage constituents of Douglas fir (*Pseudotsuga menziesii* (Mirb.) Franco (Pinaceae)): Their seasonal variation and potential role in Douglas fir resistance and silviculture management. *J Chem Ecol* 21: 387-402.

223 Anderson MK. (2003) Plant guide: Douglas fir: *Pseudotsuga menziesii*. United States Department of Agriculture and Natural Resources Conservation Service. Available at: https://plants.usda.gov/plantguide/pdf/cs_psme.pdf (accessed 16 August 2018).

224 Gunther E. (1973) *Ethnobotany of Western Washington: The Knowledge and Use of Indigenous Plants by Native Americans*, Seattle: University of Washington Press.

225 Kucharska M, Szymańska JA, Wesołowski W, et al. (2018) [Comparison of chemical composition of selected essential oils used in respiratory diseases]. *Med Pr* 69: 167-178.

226 de Christo Scherer MM, Marques FM, Figueira MM, et al. (2019) Wound healing activity of terpinolene and α-phellandrene by attenuating inflammation and oxidative stress in vitro. *J Tissue Viability* 28: 94-99.

227 Garcia G, Garcia A, Gibernau M, et al. (2017) Chemical compositions of essential oils of five introduced conifers in Corsica. *Nat Prod Res* 31: 1697-1703.

228 Phillips M. (2012) *The Holistic Orchard: Tree Fruits and Berries the Biological Way*, White River Junction, VT: Chelsea Green Publishing, pp320-323.

229 Ferlemi A and Lamari F. (2016) Berry leaves: An alternative source of bioactive natural products of nutritional and medicinal value. *Antioxidants (Basel)* 5: E17.

230 Committee on Herbal Medicinal Products (HMPC). (2017) *European Union Herbal Monograph on Ribes Nigrum L., Folium*, London: European Medicines Agency.

231 Ieri F, Innocenti M, Possieri L, et al. (2015) Phenolic composition of 'bud extracts' of *Ribes nigrum* L., *Rosa canina* L. and *Tilia tomentosa* M. *J Pharm Biomed Anal* 115: 1-9.

232 Haasbach E, Hartmayer C, Hettler A, et al. (2014) Antiviral activity of Ladania067, an extract from wild black currant leaves against influenza A virus in vitro and in vivo. *Front Microbiol* 5: 171.

233 Diaconeasa Z, Leopold L, Rugină D, et al. (2015) Antiproliferative and anti-oxidant properties of anthocyanin rich extracts from blueberry and blackcurrant juice. *Int J Mol Sci* 16: 2352-2365; Gopalan A, Reuben S, Ahmed S, et al. (2012) The health benefits of blackcurrants. *Food Funct* 3: 795-809; Li D, Wang P, Luo Y, et al. (2017) Health benefits of anthocyanins and molecular mechanisms: Update from recent decade. *Crit Rev Food Sci Nutr* 57: 1729-1741.

234 Yoshida K, Ohguro I and Ohguro H. (2013) Black currant anthocyanins normalized abnormal levels of serum concentrations of endothelin-1 in patients with glaucoma. *J Ocul Pharmacol Ther* 29: 480-487.

235 Barker (2001) section 113.

236 Donno D, Mellano M, Cerutti A, et al. (2016) Biomolecules and natural medicine preparations: Analysis of new sources of bioactive compounds from *Ribes* and *Rubus* spp. buds. *Pharmaceuticals (Basel)* 9: E7.

237 Borges G, Degeneve A, Mullen W, et al. (2010) Identification of flavonoid and phenolic anti-oxidants in black currants, blueberries, raspberries, red currants, and cranberries. *J Agric Food Chem* 58: 3901-3909.

238 Liu P, Kallio H and Yang B. (2014) Flavonol glycosides and other phenolic compounds in buds and leaves of different varieties of black currant (*Ribes nigrum* L.) and changes during growing season. *Food Chem* 160: 180-189.

239 Kumar N, Bhandari P, Singh B, et al. (2009) Anti-oxidant activity and ultra-performance LC-electrospray ionization-quadrupole time-of-flight mass spectrometry for phenolics-based fingerprinting of Rose species: *Rosa damascena, Rosa bourboniana* and *Rosa brunonii*. *Food Chem Toxicol* 47: 361-367.

240 Barker (2001) section 119.

241 Živković J, Stojković D, Petrović J, et al. (2015) *Rosa canina* L.–new possibilities for an old medicinal herb. *Food Funct* 6: 3687-3692.

242 Winther K, Apel K and Thamsborg G. (2005) A powder made from seeds and shells of a rose-hip subspecies (*Rosa canina*) reduces symptoms of knee and hip osteoarthritis: A randomized, double-blind, placebo-controlled clinical trial. *Scand J Rheumatol* 34: 302-308.

243 Phetcharat L, Wongsuphasawat K and Winther K. (2015) The effectiveness of a standardized rose hip powder, containing seeds and shells of *Rosa canina*, on cell longevity, skin wrinkles, moisture, and elasticity. *Clin Interv Aging* 10: 1849-1856.

244 Seifi M, Abbasalizadeh S, Mohammad-Alizadeh-Charandabi S, et al. (2018) The effect of Rosa (L. *Rosa canina*) on the incidence of urinary tract infection in the puerperium: A randomized placebo-controlled trial. *Phytother Res* 32: 76-83.

245 Niazi M, Hashempur M, Taghizadeh M, et al. (2017) Efficacy of topical Rose (*Rosa damascena* Mill.) oil for migraine headache: A randomized double-blinded placebo-controlled cross-over trial. *Complement Ther Med* 34: 35-41.

246 Maruyama N, Tansho-Nagakawa S, Miyazaki C, et al. (2017) Inhibition of neutrophil adhesion and antimicrobial activity by diluted hydrosol prepared from *Rosa damascena*. *Biol Pharm Bull* 40: 161-168.

247 Engels G and Brinckmann J. (2016) Dog rose hip: *Rosa canina*: Family: Rosaceae. *HerbalGram* 111: 8-19.

248 Lakusić D, Ristić M, Slavkovska V, et al. (2013) Seasonal variations in the composition of the essential oils of rosemary (*Rosmarinus officinalis*, Lamiaceae). *Nat Prod Commun* 8: 131-134.

249 Farkhondeh T, Samarghandian S and Pourbagher-Shahri AM. (2019) Hypolipidemic effects of *Rosmarinus officinalis* L. *J Cell Physiol*. Epub ahead of print 29 January 2019. DOI: 10.1002/jcp.28221.

250 Habtemariam S. (2016) The therapeutic potential of rosemary (*Rosmarinus officinalis*) diterpenes for Alzheimer's disease. *Evid Based Complement Alternat Med* 2016: 2680409.

251 Busia (2016) vol 2, p494.

252 Snell H, Richter C and Berzins R. (1998) *Transcripts from the Third Annual Richters Commercial Herb Growing Conference*, October 24, 1998, Ontario, Canada: Richters, p108.

253 Oszmiański J, Wojdyło A, Nowicka P, et al. (2015) Determination of phenolic compounds and anti-oxidant activity in leaves from wild *Rubus* L. species. *Molecules* 20: 4951-4966.

254 Phillips (2012) pp286-296.

255 Busia (2016) vol 2, p586.

256 Committee on Herbal Medicinal Products (HMPC). (2014) *Community Herbal Monograph on Rubus Idaeus L., Folium*, London, UK: European Medicines Agency.

257 Holst L, Haavik S and Nordeng H. (2009) Raspberry leaf – should it be recommended to pregnant women? *Complement Ther Clin Pract* 15: 204-208.

258 Tito A, Bimonte M, Carola A, et al. (2015) An oil-soluble extract of *Rubus idaeus* cells enhances hydration and water homeostasis in skin cells. *Int J Cosmet Sci* 37: 588-594.

259 Krauze-Baranowska M, Głód D, Kula M, et al. (2014) Chemical composition and biological activity of *Rubus idaeus* shoots – a traditional herbal remedy of Eastern Europe. *BMC Complement Altern Med* 14: 480.

260 Skrovankova S, Sumczynski D, Mlcek J, et al. (2015) Bioactive compounds and anti-oxidant activity in different types of berries. *Int J Mol Sci* 16: 24673-24706.

261 Noleto-Dias C, Ward JL, Bellisai A, et al. (2018) Salicin-7-sulfate: A new salicinoid from willow and implications for herbal medicine. *Fitoterapia* 127: 166-172.

262 Upton R. (ed.) (1999) *Willow Bark, Salix* spp. *Analytical, Quality Control and Therapeutic Monograph*, Santa Cruz: America Herbal Pharmacopoeia, p6.

263 Bradley (1992) p224.

264 Committee on Herbal Medicinal Products (HMPC). (2017) *European Union Herbal Monograph on Salix [Various Species Including S. purpurea L., S. daphnoides L., S. fragilis L.] Cortex*, London: European Medicines Agency.

265 Shara M and Stohs SJ. (2015) Efficacy and safety of white willow bark (*Salix alba*) extracts. *Phytother Res* 29: 1112-1116.

266 Bonaterra GA, Heinrich EU, Kelber O WD, et al. (2010) Anti-inflammatory effects of the willow bark extract STW 33-I (Proaktiv(*)) in LPS-activated human monocytes and differentiated macrophages. *Phytomedicine* 17: 1106-1113.

267 Schmid B, Lüdtke R, Selbmann HK, et al. (2001) Efficacy and tolerability of a standardised willow bark extract in patients with arthritis: Randomized placebo-controlled, double blind clinical trial. *Phytother Res* 15: 344-350.

268 Vlachojannis J, Cameron M and Chrubasik S. (2009) A systematic review on the effectiveness of willow bark for musculoskeletal pain. *Phytother Res* 23: 897-900.

269 Radvar M, Moeintaghavi A, Tafaghodi M, et al. (2016) Clinical efficacy of an herbal mouth wash composed of *Salix alba, Malva sylvestris* and *Althaea officinalis* in chronic periodontitis patients. *J Herb Med* 6: 24-27.

270 Qureshi MA, Khatoon F, Rizvi MA, et al. (2015) Ethyl acetate *Salix alba* leaves extract-loaded chitosan-based hydrogel film for wound dressing applications. *J Biomater Sci Polym Ed* 26: 1452-1464.

271 Busia (2016) vol 2, p425.

272 Williamson et al. (2009), p399.

273 Veberic R, Jakopic J, Stampar F, et al. (2009) European elderberry (*Sambucus nigra* L.) rich in sugars, organic acids, anthocyanins and selected polyphenols. *Food Chem* 114: 511-515.

274 Porter R and Bode R. (2017) A review of the antiviral properties of Black Elder (*Sambucus nigra* L.) products. *Phytother Res* 31: 533-554.

275 Committee on Herbal Medicinal Products (HMPC). (2018) *European Union Herbal Monograph on Sambucus Nigra L., Flos*, London: European Medicines Agency.

276 Hawkins J, Baker C, Cherry L, et al. (2019) Black elderberry (*Sambucus nigra*) supplementation effectively treats upper respiratory symptoms: A meta-analysis of randomized, controlled clinical trials. *Complement Ther Med* 42: 361-365.

277 Tiralongo E, Wee S and Lea R. (2016) Elderberry supplementation reduces cold duration and symptoms in air-travellers: A randomized, double-blind placebo-controlled clinical trial. *Nutrients* 8: 182.

278 Busia (2016) vol 2, p219.

279 Han X and Parker TL. (2017) Arborvitae (*Thuja plicata*) essential oil significantly inhibited critical inflammation- and tissue remodeling-related proteins and genes in human dermal fibroblasts. *Biochim Open* 20: 56-60.

280 Duke JA. (1983) Handbook of energy crops, unpublished text from https://hort.purdue.edu/newcrop/duke_energy/Thuja_occidentalis.html (accessed 26 August 2018).

281 Naser B, Bodinet C, Tegtmeier M, et al. (2005) *Thuja occidentalis* (*Arbor vitae*): A review of its pharmaceutical, pharmacological and clinical properties. *Evid Based Complement Alternat Med* 2: 69-78; Henneicke-von Zepelin H, Nicken P, Naser B, et al. (2019) Non-interventional observational study broadens positive benefit-risk assessment of an immunomodulating herbal remedy in the common cold. *Curr Med Res Opin*. 35: 1711-1719.

282 Pudełek M, Catapano J, Kochanowski P, et al. (2019) Therapeutic potential of monoterpene α-thujone, the main compound of *Thuja occidentalis* L. essential oil, against malignant glioblastoma multiforme cells in vitro. *Fitoterapia* 134: 172-181.

283 Mills and Bone (2005) pp600-601.

284 Pranskuniene Z, Dauliute R, Pranskunas A, et al. (2018) Ethnopharmaceutical knowledge in Samogitia region of Lithuania: Where old traditions overlap with modern medicine. *J Ethnobiol Ethnomed* 14: 70.

285 Barker (2001) section 186.

286 Negri G, Santi D and Tabach R. (2013) Flavonol glycosides found in hydroethanolic extracts from *Tilia cordata*, a species utilized as anxiolytics. *Revista Brasileira de Plantas Medicinais* 15: 217-224.

287 Czerwińska ME, Dudek MK, Pawłowska KA, et al. (2018) The influence of procyanidins isolated from small-leaved lime flowers (*Tilia cordata* Mill.) on human neutrophils. *Fitoterapia* 127: 115-122.

288 Wissam Z, Nour AA, Bushra J, et al. (2017) Extracting and studying the anti-oxidant capacity of polyphenols in dry linden leaves (Tilia cordata). *J Pharmacogn Phytochem* 6: 258-262; Cárdenas-Rodríguez N, González-Trujano ME, Aguirre-Hernández E, et al. (2014) Anticonvulsant and anti-oxidant effects of *Tilia americana* var. *mexicana* and flavonoids constituents in the pentylenetetrazole-induced seizures. *Oxid Med Cell Longev* 2014: 329172.

289 Busia (2016) vol 2, p601.

290 Riva A, Togni S, Franceschi F, et al. (2017) The effect of a natural, standardized bilberry extract (Mirtoselect®) in dry eye: A randomized, double blinded, placebo-controlled trial. *Eur Rev Med Pharmacol Sci* 21: 2518-2525.

291 Sadowska B, Paszkiewicz M, Podsędek A, et al. (2014) *Vaccinium myrtillus* leaves and *Frangula alnus* bark derived extracts as potential antistaphylococcal agents. *Acta Biochim Pol* 61: 163-169.

292 Chu W, Cheung S, Lau R, et al. (2011) Bilberry (*Vaccinium myrtillus* L.). In: Benzie IFF and Wachtel-Galor S (eds) *Herbal Medicine: Biomolecular and Clinical Aspects*. 2nd ed., Boca Raton, Fl: CRC Press/Taylor and Francis, ch4.

293 Huttunen S, Toivanen M, Arkko S, et al. (2011) Inhibition activity of wild berry juice fractions against *Streptococcus pneumoniae* binding to human bronchial cells. *Phytother Res* 25: 122-127.

294 Brasanac-Vukanovic S, Mutic J, Stankovic DM, et al. (2018) Wild bilberry (*Vaccinium myrtillus* L., Ericaceae) from Montenegro as a source of anti-oxidants for use in the production of nutraceuticals. *Molecules* 23: E1864.

295 Arevström L, Bergh C, Landberg R, et al. (2019) Freeze-dried bilberry (*Vaccinium myrtillus*) dietary supplement improves walking distance and lipids after myocardial infarction: An open-label randomized clinical trial. *Nutr Res* 62: 13-22.

296 Crespo M and Visioli F. (2017) A brief review of blue- and bilberries' potential to curb cardio-metabolic perturbations: Focus on diabetes. *Curr Pharm Des* 23: 983-988.

297 Gafner S. (2016) *Botanical Adulterants Bulletin on Bilberry (Vaccinium Myrtillus) Extracts*, Austin, Texas: American Botanical Council.

298 Gardana C, Ciappellano S, Marinoni L, et al. (2014) Bilberry adulteration: Identification and chemical profiling of anthocyanins by different analytical methods. *J Agric Food Chem* 62: 10998-11004.

299 Barker (2001) sections 376-378.

300 Bruton-Seal and Seal (2008) pp62-63.

301 Lans C, Taylor-Swanson L and Westfall R. (2018) Herbal fertility treatments used in North America from colonial times to 1900, and their potential for improving the success rate of assisted reproductive technology. *Reprod Biomed Soc Online* 5: 60-81.

302 Nicholson JA, Darby TD and Jarboe CH. (1972) Viopudial, a hypotensive and smooth muscle antispasmodic from *Viburnum opulus*. *Proc Soc Exp Biol Med* 140: 457-461.

303 Altun ML, Citoğlu GS, Yilmaz BS, et al. (2008) Anti-oxidant properties of *Viburnum opulus* and *Viburnum lantana* growing in Turkey. *Int J Food Sci Nutr* 59: 175-180; Erdogan-Orhan I, Altun ML, Sever-Yilmaz B, et al. (2011) Anti-acetylcholinesterase and anti-oxidant assets of the major components (salicin, amentoflavone, and chlorogenic acid) and the extracts of *Viburnum opulus* and *Viburnum lantana* and their total phenol and flavonoid contents. *J Med Food* 14: 434-440.

304 Cometa MF, Parisi L, Palmery M, et al. (2009) In vitro relaxant and spasmolytic effects of constituents from *Viburnum prunifolium* and HPLC quantification of the bioactive isolated iridoids. *J Ethnopharmacol* 123: 201-207.

305 Rop O, Reznicek V, Valsikova M, et al. (2010) Anti-oxidant properties of European cranberry bush fruit (*Viburnum opulus* var. edule). *Molecules* 15: 4467-4477.

306 Kollmann J and Grubb PJ. (2002) *Viburnum lantana* L. and *Viburnum opulus* L. (*V. lobatum* Lam., *Opulus vulgaris* Borkh.). *J Ecol* 90: 1044-1070.

307 Mills and Bone (2005) p148.

308 Gill B, Mehra R, Navgeet, et al. (2018) *Vitex negundo* and its medicinal value. *Mol Biol Rep* 45: 2925-2934.

309 Committee on Herbal Medicinal Products (HMPC). (2018) *European Union Herbal Monograph on Vitex Agnus-Castus L., Fructus: Final*, London, UK: European Medicines Agency.

310 Keikha N, Shafaghat M, Mousavia SM, et al. (2018) Antifungal effects of ethanolic and aqueous extracts of *Vitex agnus-castus* against vaginal isolates of *Candida albicans*. *Curr Med Mycol* 4: 1-5.

311 van Die MD, Burger HG, Teede HJ, et al. (2013) *Vitex agnus-castus* extracts for female reproductive disorders: A systematic review of clinical trials. *Planta Med* 79: 562-575.

312 Verkaik S, Kamperman AM, van Westrhenen R, et al. (2017) The treatment of premenstrual syndrome with preparations of *Vitex agnus castus*: A systematic review and meta-analysis. *Am J Obstet Gynecol* 217: 150-166.

313 Wuttke W, Jarry H, Christoffel V, et al. (2003) Chaste tree (*Vitex agnus-castus*) – pharmacology and clinical indications. *Phytomedicine* 10: 348-357; Busia (2016) vol 2, p608.

314 Xiang L, Liu Y, Xie C, et al. (2016) The chemical and genetic characteristics of Szechuan pepper (*Zanthoxylum bungeanum* and *Z. armatum*) cultivars and their suitable habitat. *Front Plant Sci* 7: 467.

315 Busia (2016) vol 2, p437.

316 Bafi-Yeboa N, JT Arnason, J Baker, et al. (2005) Antifungal constituents of Northern prickly ash, *Zanthoxylum americanum* Mill. *Phytomedicine* 12: 370-377; Gibbons S, Leimkugel J, Oluwatuyi M, et al. (2003) Activity of *Zanthoxylum clava-herculis* extracts against multi-drug resistant methicillin-resistant *Staphylococcus aureus* (MDR-MRSA). *Phytother Res* 17: 274-275.

317 Zhang M, Wang J, Zhu L, et al. (2017) *Zanthoxylum bungeanum* Maxim. (Rutaceae): A systematic review of its traditional uses, botany, phytochemistry, pharmacology, pharmacokinetics, and toxicology. *Int J Mol Sci* 18: E2172.

Selected Bibliography

Here are some starting points for further reading on selected topics, and see also the notes to chapters giving research articles in journals and further publications.

Agroforestry and permaculture

Crawford M. (2015) *Trees for Gardens, Orchards and Permaculture*, East Meon, UK: Permanent Publications.

European Innovation Partnership Agricultural Productivity and Sustainability (EIP-AGRI) Focus Group. (2017) *Agroforestry: Introducing Woody Vegetation into Specialised Crop and Livestock Systems: Final Report*, Brussels: EIP-AGRI.

Fern K. (2000) *Plants for a Future: Edible and Useful Plants for a Healthier World*, East Meon, Hampshire: Permanent Publications.

Mudge K and Gabriel S. (2014) *Farming the Woods: An Integrated Permaculture Approach to Growing Food and Medicinals in Temperate Forests*, White River Junction, VT: Chelsea Green Publishing.

Phillips M. (2017) *Mycorrhizal Planet: How Symbiotic Fungi Work with Roots to Support Plant Health and Build Soil Fertility*, White River Junction, VT: Chelsea Green.

Remiarz T. (2017) *Forest Gardening in Practice: An Illustrated Practical Guide for Homes, Communities and Enterprises*, East Meon, Hampshire: Permanent Publications.

Weiseman W, Halsey D and Ruddock B. (2014) *Integrated Forest Gardening: The Complete Guide to Polycultures and Plant Guilds in Permaculture Systems*, White River Junction, VT: Chelsea Green Publishing.

Environment, biodiversity and climate change

Allen D, Bilz M, Leaman DJ, et al. (2014) *European Red List of Medicinal Plants*, Luxembourg: Publications Office of the European Union.

Department for Environment, Food and Rural Affairs (DEFRA). (2008) *The Invasive Non-native Species Framework Strategy for Great Britain: Protecting our Natural Heritage from Invasive Species*, London: DEFRA.

Food and Agriculture Organisation (FAO). (2018) *The State of the World's Forests, 2018 – Forest Pathways to Sustainable Development*, Rome: FAO.

Nicoll B. (2016) *Agriculture and Forestry Climate Change Report Card Technical Paper 8. Risks for Woodlands, Forest Management and Forestry Production in the UK from Climate Change*, Roslin: Forest Research.

Tree I. (2018) *Wilding: The Return of Nature to a British Farm*, London: Picador.

Willis KJ. (2017) *State of the World's Plants 2017*, Kew: Royal Botanic Gardens.

Field guides and native plants

Barker J. (2001) *The Medicinal Flora of Britain and Northwestern Europe: A Field Guide Including Plants Commonly Cultivated in the Region*, West Wickham: Winter Press.

Foster S and Chongxi Y. (1992) *Herbal Emissaries: Bringing Chinese Herbs to the West: A Guide to Gardening, Herbal Wisdom, and Well-being*, Rochester, VT: Healing Arts Press.

Hall JE, Kirby KJ and Whitbread AM. (2004) *National Vegetation Classification: Field Guide to Woodland*, Peterborough: Joint Nature Conservation Committee.

Hawes Z. (2010) *Wild Drugs: A Forager's Guide to Healing Plants*, London: Gaia.

Kloos S. (2017) *Pacific Northwest Medicinal Plants: Identify, Harvest, and Use 120 Wild Herbs for Health and Wellness*, Portland, OR: Timber Press.

Moore M. (1979) *Medicinal Plants of the Mountain West*, Santa Fe: Museum of New Mexico Press.

Rose F. (2006) *The Wild Flower Key: How to Identify Wild Plants, Trees and Shrubs In Britain and Ireland*, Revised ed., London: Frederick Warne.

Stace C. (2019) *New Flora of the British Isles*, 4th edition, Middlewood Green, Suffolk: C&M Floristics.

Herb growing and harvesting

American Herbal Products Association in cooperation with the American Herbal Pharmacopoeia. (2006) *Good Agricultural and Collection Practice for Herbal Raw Materials*, Silver Spring, MD: American Herbal Products Association.

Carpenter J and Carpenter M. (2015) *The Organic Medicinal Herb Farmer: The Ultimate Guide to Producing High-Quality Herbs on a Market Scale*, White River Junction, VT: Chelsea Green.

Davis J and Scott Persons W. (2016) *Growing and Marketing Ginseng, Goldenseal and other Woodland Medicinals*, Gabriola Island, Canada: New Society Publishers.

Harding AR. (1936) *Ginseng and other Medicinal Plants: A Book of Valuable Information for Growers as well as Collectors of Medicinal Roots, Barks, Leaves, etc.*, Columbus, OH: AR Harding.

Schafer P. (2012) *The Chinese Medicinal Herb Farm: A Cultivator's Guide to Small-Scale Organic Herb Production*, White River Junction, VT: Chelsea Green.

Sturdivant L and Blakley T. (1999) *Medicinal Herbs in the Garden, Field and Marketplace*, Friday Harbour, WA: San Juan Naturals.

Whitten G. (1997) *Herbal Harvest: Commercial Organic Production of Quality Dried Herbs*, Hawthorn, Victoria, Australia: Bloomings Books.

Herbal pharmacology and therapeutics

Barnes J, Anderson LA and Phillipson JD. (2007) *Herbal Medicines: A Guide for Healthcare Professionals*, London: Pharmaceutical Press.

Blumenthal M and Foster S. (2000) *Herbal Medicine: Expanded Commission E Monographs: Herb Monographs, Based on those Created by a Special Expert Committee of the German Federal Institute for Drugs and Medical Devices*, Austin, Tex.: American Botanical Council.

Busia K. (2016) *Fundamentals of Herbal Medicine*, vols 1 and 2, Xlibris.

Conway P. (2001) *Tree Medicine: A Comprehensive Guide to the Healing Power of over 170 Trees*, London: Piatkus.

Gardner Z and McGuffin M. (eds) (2013) *American Herbal Products Association's Botanical Safety Handbook*, 2nd ed, Boca Raton: CRC Press.

Mills S and Bone K. (2013) *Principles and Practice of Phytotherapy*, Edinburgh: Churchill Livingstone.

Williamson E, Driver S and Baxter K. (2009) *Stockley's Herbal Medicines Interactions*, London: Pharmaceutical Press.

World Health Organization (WHO). (2004) *WHO Monographs on Selected Medicinal Plants. Vols 1-4*, Geneva: WHO.

Herbal remedy making

Bruton-Seal J and Seal M. (2008) *Hedgerow Medicine: Harvest and Make Your Own Herbal Remedies*, Ludlow: Merlin Unwin Books.

Cech R. (2016) *Making Plant Medicine*, Williams, OR: Horizon Herbs.

Green J and Green A. (2000) *The Herbal Medicine-maker's Handbook: A Home Manual*, Freedom, CA: Crossing Press.

Hafferty S. (2018) *The Creative Kitchen: Seasonal Plant-based Recipes for Meals, Drinks, Crafts, Body and Home Care*, East Meon, Hampshire: Permanent Publications.

Hedley C and Shaw N. (1996) *Herbal Remedies: A Practical Beginner's Guide to Making Effective Remedies in the Kitchen*, Avonmouth: Parragon.

History and folklore

Allen DE and Hatfield G. (2004) *Medicinal Plants in Folk Tradition: An Ethnobotany of Britain & Ireland*, Portland, OR: Timber Press.

Francia S and Stobart A. (2014) *Critical Approaches to the History of Western Herbal Medicine: From Classical Antiquity to the Early Modern Period*, London: Bloomsbury.

Grieve M. (1980) *A Modern Herbal: The Medicinal, Culinary, Cosmetic and Economic Properties, Cultivation and Folklore of Herbs, Grasses, Fungi, Shrubs and Trees with all their Modern Scientific Uses*, 1931 edition, London: Penguin.

Hooke D. (2013) *Trees in Anglo-Saxon England: Literature, Lore and Landscape*, Woodbridge: Boydell.

Hutchens A. (1991) *Indian Herbalogy of North America*, Boston: Shambhala.

James NDG. (1981) *A History of English Forestry*, Oxford: Basil Blackwell.

Moerman DE. (2009) *Native American Medicinal Plants: An Ethnobotanical Dictionary*, Portland, OR: Timber Press.

Pollington S. (2008) *Leechcraft: Early English Charms Plant Lore and Healing*, Hockwold-cum-Wilton: Anglo-Saxon Books.

Rackham O. (1990) *Trees and Woodlands in the British Landscape*, London: Phoenix Gunat Publishers.

Tobyn G, Denham A and Whitelegg M. (2010) *The Western Herbal Tradition: 2000 years of Medicinal Plant Knowledge*, Edinburgh: Churchill Livingstone/ Elsevier.

Williamson T, Barnes G and Pillatt T. (2017) *Trees in England: Management and Disease since 1600*, Hatfield: University of Hertfordshire Press.

Medicinal plant trade worldwide

Bodeker G, Ong CK, Grundy C, et al. (eds) (2005) *WHO Global Atlas of Traditional, Complementary and Alternative Medicine*, Kobe, Japan: WHO Centre for Health and Development.

Committee on Herbal Medicinal Products (HMPC). (2006) *Guideline on Good Agricultural and Collection Practice (GACP) for Starting Materials of Herbal Origin*, London: European Medicines Agency.

Foster S and Duke JA. (1990) *A Field Guide to Eastern and Central North American Medicinal Plants*, Boston: Houghton Mifflin Co.

Jenkins M, Timoshyna A and Cornthwaite M. (2018) *Wild at Home: Exploring the Global Harvest, Trade and Use of Wild Plant Ingredients*, Cambridge: Traffic International.

Milliken W and Bridgewater S. (2001) *Flora Celtica: Sustainable Development of Scottish Plants*, Edinburgh: Edinburgh Development Consultants/Royal Botanic Garden/Scottish Executive Central Research Unit.

Sturdivant L and Blakley T. (1999) *Medicinal Herbs in the Garden, Field and Marketplace*, Friday Harbour, WA: San Juan Naturals.

Vines G and Behrens J. (2004) *Herbal Harvests with a Future: Towards Sustainable Sources for Medicinal Plants*, Salisbury: Plantlife International.

World Health Organization (WHO). (2013) *WHO Traditional Medicine Strategy: 2014-2023*, Hong Kong: WHO.

Propagation and seeds

Dirr MA and Heuser CW. (2006) *The Reference Manual of Woody Plant Propagation: From Seed to Tissue Culture*, Second ed, Portland, OR: Timber Press.

Gosling P. (2007) *Raising Trees and Shrubs from Seed*, Edinburgh: Forestry Commission.

Gough R and Moore-Gough C. (2011) *The Complete Guide to Saving Seeds: 322 Vegetables, Herbs, Flowers, Fruits, Trees, and Shrubs*, North Adams, MA: Storey Publishing.

Kock H. (2008) *Growing Trees from Seed: A Practical Guide to Growing Native Trees, Vines and Shrubs*, New York: Firefly Books.

McDonald MF and Copeland LO. (2012) *Seed Production: Principles and Practices*, Dordrecht: Springer Science and Business Media.

McVicar J. (2001) *Seeds: The Ultimate Guide to Growing Successfully from Seed*, London: Kyle Cathie Ltd in association with the Royal Horticultural Society.

Thompson P. (1992) *Creative Propagation: A Grower's Guide*, London: BT Batsford.

Tree physiology and silviculture

De la Bédoyère C. (2004) *The Handbook of Native Trees and Shrubs: How to Plant and Maintain a Natural Woodland*, London: New Holland.

Dirr MA. (1997) *Dirr's Hardy Trees and Shrubs: An Illustrated Encyclopedia*, Portland, OR: Timber Press.

Hillier J and Lancaster R. (eds) (2014) *The Hillier Manual of Trees and Shrubs*, Eighth ed. London: Royal Horticultural Society.

Hirons AD and Thomas PA. (2018) *Applied Tree Biology*, Hoboken, NJ: John Wiley.

Thomas P. (2000) *Trees: Their Natural History*, Cambridge: Cambridge University Press.

Tudge C. (2005) *The Secret Life of Trees: How They Live and Why They Matter*, London: Penguin.

van den Berk Nurseries (2015) *Van den Berk on Trees*, Sint-Oedenrode, the Netherlands: Boomkwekerij. Gebr. Bremmer.

Watson B. (2006) *Trees: Their Use, Management, Cultivation and Biology*, Marlborough, Wilts: Crowood Press.

Acknowledgements

Photographs have been taken at a number of locations in addition to Holt Wood, and I very much appreciate the people and organisations who made this possible: Harriet Bell (Dartington Estate), Helen and Stuart Kearney (Elder Farm), Duncan Ross (Poyntzfield Nursery), Simon Miles (The Forest Garden), Mark Prior (Forestry Commission), Clem Sandison (Alexandra Park Food Forest), Jim Twine (Organic Herb Trading), Bryony Middleton (Sharpham Trust), Claire Hatterseley (Weleda UK). My grateful thanks go to Julie Bruton-Seal, Tedje van Asseldonk and Karen With for additional images. I thank Eugen Ulmer Publications, Germany, for permission to reproduce the European climate zone chart, and the United States Department of Agriculture for the USA climate zone chart.

Sincere thanks are due to so many people who have contributed advice, encouragement, suggestions and support over the years in one way or another. I would like to acknowledge Larry Allain, Ile Ashcroft, Wenderlynn and Iain Bagnall, Jill Baines, Harriet Bell, Alice Bettany, Gail Bradley, Nita Brass, Mike Brook, Julie Bruton-Seal, Paul Burgess, Emma Byrnes, Laura Carpenter, Paul Cawsey, Sandra Chalton, Paul Cleave, Peter Conway, Martin Crawford, Ben Davis, Lisette de Roche, Frank Deimert, Alison Denham, Mary Dixon, Diana East, Chris Etheridge, Susan Farrell, Ken Fern, Chris Flower, Steven Foster, Catriona Gibson, Daniel Halsey, Joanne Harold, Melissa Harvey, Claire Hattersley, Katrina Hevezi, Emma Hockridge, Dawn Ireland, Dave Jacke, Peter Jones, Jon Kean, Helen Kearney, Chris Lane, Linda Lever, Erica Levy, Liz Lillicrap, Ben Lyons, Simon McEwan, Bryony Middleton, Simon Miles, Martin Nesbitt, Shelley O'Berg, Vicki Pitman, Sebastian Pole, Colin Porter, Mark Prior, Michael Roloff, Mark Rumbell, Sagara, Clem Sandison, Angela Segraves, Carole Shaw, Ros Shetler-Jones, Jo Smith, Christina Stapley, Adrian Steele, Paul Strauss, Rosie Trehane, Liz Turner, Jim Twine, Daniel Tyrkiel, Roy Upton, Tedje van Asseldonk, Klaudia van Gool, Marij van Helmond, Carol Vincent-Smythe, Sigrun Wagner, Louise Wall, Frances Watkins, Sally Westaway, Sarah Weston, Karen With, Frances Wright (RIP), Mujeeb Zia, Pietro Zuccheti. I am especially grateful to Johan van den Berk of van den Berk Nurseries in the Netherlands, for help with identification of climate zones. I would like to single out Ken Fern for particular appreciation since the Plants For a Future database has provided a huge resource for all growers including myself. Thanks are due to the staff at Permanent Publications who have been so helpful (and incredibly patient) throughout the production process. Above all, my thanks are due to Kay Piercy, partner and cofounder of Holt Wood, for her constant support.

Image credits

All photographs for this book are by Kay Piercy (kay@studio4art.co.uk) apart from the following contributors:

The author (UPS medicine Trail, Goldenseal, Poisonous hemlock, Planting witch hazel, Greenhouse, Seed pots, Comfrey roots, Agroforestry Trust website, Harvesting stems, Drying rack, Fruit leather, Visitors at Dartington, Lemon balm, Herb beds at Organic Herb Trading, Herb growers sign, Horse chestnut seeds, Ceanothus, Dried forsythia, Ginkgo leaves, Walnut leaves, Sweet bay dried leaves, Scots pine flower, Elder tree in flower, Arbor vitae trees, Bilberries in woodland)

Larry Allain (Ceanothus in flower)

Julie Bruton-Seal (Bilberry leaves and fruit, Sea buckthorn fruit)

Eugen Ulmer Publications (European hardiness zones chart)

United States Department of Agriculture (USA climate zones chart)

Tedje van Asseldonk (Mintal still)

Karen With (Norwegian hytte)

About the author

Anne Stobart is an experienced consultant medical herbalist, herb grower and Honorary Research Fellow at the University of Exeter, UK. She is co-founder of Holt Wood Herbs, transforming a conifer plantation into a medicinal forest garden. Anne is a Bloomsbury author and has worked extensively in education including leading a professional herbal medicine programme at Middlesex University in London, UK.

Index

antifungal 56, 148, 154, 162, 174, 177, 179, 191, 194, 200, 228, 231, 233, 235, 239
antihypoxic 168, 233
antimicrobial 12-3, 19, 21, 104, 136, 148, 157, 162, 174-5, 177, 179, 182, 188, 191, 194, 200, 205, 209, 212, 216, 223, 233
antipyretic 211, 233
antiscorbutic 205, 209, 233
antiseptic 11, 13, 19, 21-2, 30-1, 90, 95, 97, 100, 102, 125, 133, 152, 154, 177, 193-4, 200, 207, 211, 216, 223, 237-43
antispasmodic 21-2, 30, 40, 81, 138, 142, 154, 157, 179, 182, 185, 197, 207, 220, 224, 226, 233, 237-8, 240-3
antitumour 36, 131, 148, 151, 174, 194, 223
antitussive 136, 197, 233
anti-ulcer 133, 136, 151, 159, 164, 182, 209, 217, 223
antiviral 20, 36, 151, 154, 159, 162, 164, 171, 182, 191, 200-2, 205, 215-7, 231, 235, 240, 242
astringent 11, 19, 22, 25, 30-1, 89, 125-6, 131, 135-6, 138, 143, 157, 159, 164, 169, 171, 174, 179, 182, 188, 191, 197, 201, 203-5, 207-9, 211, 223, 226, 233, 236-43
bitter 30, 40, 88-9, 131, 140, 144, 159, 162-4, 185, 197, 207, 211, 226, 233, 238-41, 243
carminative 30, , 151, 157, 179, 191, 205, 207, 231, 233, 237-8, 240-3
cholagogue 130, 133, 140, 162, 233, 238-41, 243
decongestant 194, 234
demulcent 21, 89, 220, 234, 238, 240-1
emmenagogue 30, 179, 185, 207, 216, 234, 237, 240-3
emollient 21, 234
expectorant 19, 30-1, 136, 138, 154, 182, 197, 200, 207, 215-6, 228, 234, 239-40
febrifuge 125, 164, 234
galactagogue 157, 234, 239, 241
haemostatic 191, 209, 234
hepatoprotective 151, 177, 182, 188, 191, 234
hypertension 15-6, 23-4, 143, 202, 220, 233
hypoglycaemic 151, 188, 223, 234, 239, 241
hypolipidaemic 157, 234
hypotensive 143, , 226, 234, 241-3

immune stimulant 148, 151, 154, 205, 237, 241
laxative 19, 30, 35, 40, 91, 96, 130, 140, 157, 159, 161-4, 174, 188, 200, 205, 215-6, 233-242
lymphatic 30, 137-8, 235, 238
oxytocic 144, 235
purgative 174, 188, 215, 233, 236-7
sedative 31, 142, 197, 219-20, 226, 236-7, 239-43
sialogogue 231, 236
tonic 30-1, 39-40, 88-9, 125, 130, 136, 138, 140, 143, 148-9, 151, 159, 162-4, 168, 172, 177, 191, 194, 197, 205-9, 211, 223, 228, 233, 236-43
vasodilator 143, 168, 220, 226, 236, 243
vermifuge 144, 157, 236
vulnerary 22, 182, 236-40, 242
herbal medicine:
    practitioners v, 12, 21, 25-6, 107, 111, 114-5, 117, 119, 232, 247-8
    trade 5, 8, 105, 114
    training 25, 34, 247-8
herbarium 75
Himalayas, plant introductions 11
history:
    ethnobotany 11
    folklore 10, 215
    Native American 126, 129, 138, 169, 182, 200, 211, 216, 226
    plant introductions 11
    traditional medicine 131, 151, 158-9, 182-3, 197, 227
Holt Wood v, 3, 31-3, 44, 48, 51, 53, 55, 61, 74, 78, 80-1, 83, 85, 108, 118-9, 122, 129, 141, 169, 172, 175, 183, 198, 210, 226, 231
honey 85-6, 90, 92, 94-5, 97, 136, 197, 200
honeysuckle, see *Lonicera periclymenum*
Hong Kong, herb importer 8
hops, see *Humulus lupulus*
horsechestnut, see *Aesculus hippocastanum*
Humulus lupulus 30, 36, 38, 63, 73, 240
Hydrastis canadensis 5, 7, 111
hydrosol 23-4, 97-8, 101-4, 191, 200, 205-6, 234
Hypericum perforatum 7, 19, 31, 59, 68-9, 73, 97, 99, 242
hypertension, see circulatory system complaints
hypoglycaemic, see herbal actions

hypolipidaemic, see herbal actions
hypotensive, see herbal actions

immune stimulant, see herbal actions
India, herb exporter 8
infusion 23-4, 30-1, 78, 85-6, 89-91, 97-8, 126-7, 130, 133, 136, 145, 157, 159, 168, 174, 177, 179, 182, 185, 191, 194, 197, 201-2, 204-5, 207, 209, 212, 215-6, 220, 223, 228, 234, 237-43
ingredients:
    organic 7, 85, 107, 109, 148
    provenance 8
    self-sufficiency 85
insects:
    bees 85, 124, 135, 144, 158, 161-2, 178, 189, 194-5, 201, 203, 206, 208, 210, 219-20
    brimstone butterfly 162
    insecticide 11, 145, 191
Inula helenium 30, 59, 64, 73, 239
Ireland, traditional practice 11
Iris versicolor 238
ivy, ground, see *Glechoma hederacea*

Japan:
    herb importer 8
    plant introductions 11
Juglans regia vi, 24, 29, 172
Juniper, see *Juniperus communis*
Juniperus communis vi, 13, 23, 31, 39, 48, 63, 98-100, 106, 175

Kew Gardens 9
kidney, see urinary system complaints

lack of appetite, see digestive system complaints
lady's mantle, see *Alchemilla xanthochlora*
Lady Park Wood 51
Lamium album 242
Laurus nobilis vii, 13, 24, 30-1, 63, 100, 178
Lavandula angustifolia 41, 59, 73, 104, 106
lavender, see *Lavandula angustifolia*
laxative, see herbal actions
lemon balm, see *Melissa officinalis*
Lentinus edodes 36, 39
Leonurus cardiaca 241
lichen 36
limeflowers, see *Tilia cordata*

understorey 2
United Plant Savers 5-6, 111, 118, 247
urinary system complaints:
    kidney 130, 151, 164, 182, 188, 197,
      217, 243
    urinary infection 23-4, 30-1, 87, 126,
      133, 158-9, 167, 177, 179, 188, 191, 195,
      201-2, 205, 221, 223, 226, 237-43
Urtica dioica 13, 29-30, 73, 241
US Food and Drug Administration 257

Vaccinium myrtillus vii, 23, 29-30, 59, 63,
    221
Vaccinium species 13,19, see also
    Vaccinium myrtillus
vaginal discharge, see reproductive system
    complaints
valerian, see *Valeriana officinalis*
Valeriana officinalis 40, 242
varicose veins, see circulatory system
    complaints
vasodilator, see herbal actions
vegetation:
    classification 29
    indicator 29
    native 27-9
Verbascum thapsus 31, 36, 59, 68, 241
Verbena officinalis 59, 68-9, 242
vermifuge, see herbal actions
vervain, see *Verbena officinalis*
Viburnum opulus vii, 22-3, 29, 31, 42, 44,
    54, 62-3, 73, 81, 96, 224
vinegar 23-4, 85-6, 92, 94-5, 148, 165,
    200, 209, 215
Viola tricolor 59, 239
Vitex agnus castus vii, 23, 62, 227
vulnerary, see herbal actions

walnut, see *Juglans regia*
water:
    movement 2-3, 28-30
    management 15, 27, 33-4
    swales to catch 33
Weleda 9, 148, 217
white deadnettle, see *Lamium album*
wild angelica, see *Angelica sylvestris*
wild carrot, see *Daucus carota*
willow, violet, see *Salix daphnoides*
willow, white, see *Salix alba*
witch hazel , see *Hamamelis virginiana*
wood betony, see *Stachys betonica*

woodland:
    ancient 29
    management 47, 54, 66, 109, 111
    simulation 5
    small 5, 117-8
    see also forest
World Health Organization (WHO):
    guidelines on good agricultural and
    collection practices 257
    traditional medicine 12
wormwood, see *Artemisia absinthum*

yarrow, see *Achillea millefolium*
yew, see *Taxus baccata*

Zanthoxylum americanum vii, 24, 36, 42,
    63, 73, 230

Solutions for Changemakers

Every one of us who picks up a seed packet, upcycles a piece of furniture or invests time and energy in a community project is a changemaker. The minute we start to make small but incremental changes in our lives, we become agents for positive change and the ripples of our influence spread out around us.

Permanent Publications produce a range of books to empower and inspire changemakers the world over, from no dig organic growing, food forests and permaculture design, to natural building, renewable technology and connecting with nature.

If you enjoyed *Forest Gardening in Practice*, why not try these titles related to forest gardening and organic gardening:

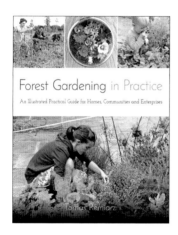

**FOREST GARDENING
IN
PRACTICE**

Tomas Remiarz

£24.95

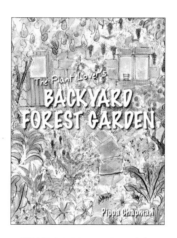

**THE PLANT LOVER'S
BACKYARD FOREST
GARDEN**

Pippa Chapman

£16.00

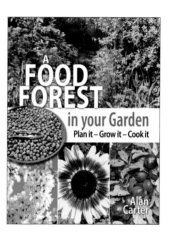

**A FOOD FOREST
IN YOUR
GARDEN**

Alan Carter

£19.95

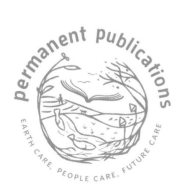

For the full list of our solution-based titles visit
www.permanentpublications.co.uk

Our books are also available via our
American distributor, Chelsea Green at
www.chelseagreen.com/publisher/permanent-publications

Permanent Publications also publishes *Permaculture* magazine

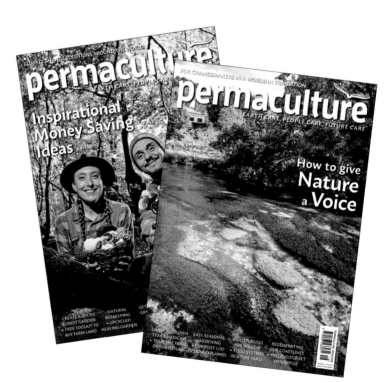